DENTAL PUBLIC HEALTH & RESEARCH

Contemporary Practice for the Dental Hygienist

Third Edition

Christine Nielsen Nathe, RDH, MS
Professor and Graduate Program Director
Division of Dental Hygiene
University of New Mexico
Albuquerque, NM

Pearson

Boston   Columbus   Indianapolis   New York   San Francisco   Upper Saddle River
Amsterdam   Cape Town   Dubai   London   Madrid   Milan   Munich   Paris   Montreal   Toronto
Delhi   Mexico City   Sao Paulo   Sydney   Hong Kong   Seoul   Singapore   Taipei   Tokyo

Library of Congress Cataloging-in-Publication Data

Nathe, Christine Nielsen.
  Dental public health and research : contemporary practice for the dental hygienist / Christine Nielsen Nathe.—3rd ed.
      p. ; cm.
    Rev. ed. of: Dental public health / Christine N. Nathe. 2nd ed. 2005.
    Includes bibliographical references and index.
    ISBN-13: 978-0-13-514205-9
    ISBN-10: 0-13-514205-9
  1. Dental public health.   2. Dental hygiene I. Nathe, Christine Nielsen. Dental public health.   II. Title.
    [DNLM: 1. Dental Care—United States. 2. Dental Hygienists—United States.   3. Delivery of Health Care—United States.   4. Public Health Dentistry—United States. WU 90 N275da 2011]
    RK52.N27 2011
    362.19'760973—dc22

                                              2009037717

Publisher: Julie Levin Alexander
Publisher's Assistant: Regina Bruno
Editor-in-Chief: Mark Cohen
Associate Editor: Melissa Kerian
Assistant Editor: Nicole Ragonese
Director of Marketing: Karen Allman
Executive Marketing Manager: Katrin Beacom
Development Editor: Pamela Lappies, iD8 Publishing Services
Marketing Specialist: Michael Sirinides
Marketing Assistant: Judy Noh
Managing Production Editor: Patrick Walsh
Production Liaison: Christina Zingone
Production Editor: Karen Berry, Laserwords Maine
Senior Media Editor: Amy Peltier
Media Project Manager: Lorena Cerisano
Manufacturing Manager: Ilene Sanford

Manufacturing Buyer: Pat Brown
Art Director: Jayne Conte
Cover Designer: Axell Designs
Manager, Visual Rights and Permissions: Zina Arabia
Manager, Visual Research: Beth Brenzel
Manager, Cover Visual Research and Permissions: Karen Sanatar
Image Permission Coordinator: Vickie Menanteaux
Composition: Laserwords
Printing and Binding: Edwards Brothers Malloy
Cover Printer: Lehigh Phoenix
Cover images: Photograph courtesy of Steve Figar, Equal Health, Australian Health Professionals Overseas Aid Fund Inc. Dental Plaque: Shutterstock.

10 9 8 7 6 5

ISBN-13: 978-0-13-514205-9
ISBN-10: 0-13-514205-9

www.pearsonhighered.com

Dedication

This book is dedicated to my husband, Chris Nathe, and children, Rhen, Marissa, and Chad Nathe, who make every day of my life a joy, and to my parents, John Nielsen and Susan Nielsen, RDH, for their support and example.

In our humanitarian pursuits, we have three encompassing possessions—our time, our talent, and our treasure. Our time, of course, we cannot keep. Only that which we give to others is not lost. We also cannot keep our talent. We must use it or we lose it. Our treasure, at last, is not permanent either. Most of us have lived long enough to know that we really keep only that which we give away.

Author Unknown

Contents

UNIT IV

Practical Strategies for Dental Public Health   299

Appendices

Foreword

When Alfred Civilion Fones followed his dream to create within the dental staff a dental therapist whose focus would be the prevention of dental disease, his intention was not merely to have this person perform in dental offices. He recognized from the start that the most effective way to "spread the word" was to provide direct services, educational and clinical, to groups of people—to the masses. Ideally, those groups would be composed of children who would be taught at an early age the importance of dental health and prevention of dental disease. Where better to interface with children than in grammar schools? And so in time, what was known as the Bridgeport, Connecticut, School Dental Hygiene Corps was established, composed of members of Dr. Fones' classes of 1914, 1915, and 1916. Ergo the first dental hygiene public health program.

I will fast-forward to the early 1950s when thirty-three young women and I were enrolled at the University of Bridgeport's Fones School of Dental Hygiene. As part of our fieldwork rotation, we traveled to long-established dental clinics throughout the city's schools. I remember being extremely fond of that assignment because I liked interacting with the children. But the real thrill of those trips was coming face-to-face with members of those first classes who were still in charge of the various clinics. These women knew Dr. Fones personally. During lunch hours, they had a captive audience and would relate to us how it all began: the first school in the carriage house adjacent to Dr. Fones' and his father's dental building; his perseverance and determination in convincing city fathers, the board of education, and the dental society to allow the early dental hygienists to conduct programs within the schools.

I know how proud and delighted they would be—Dr. Fones and "the pioneers"—to see how dental hygienists have positioned themselves today in various public health settings, and how impressed they would be with Christine Nathe's *Dental Public Health and Research: Contemporary Practice for the Dental Hygienist*. It is a remarkable testimony to the premise that public health dental hygienists have the ability to play a valuable and critical role in the dental health of people everywhere.

Janet Carroll Memoli, RDH, MS
Retired Director, Fones School of Dental Hygiene
Professor Emeritus, University of Bridgeport,
Bridgeport, CT

Preface

The guiding principles that served as the impetus for the first and second editions of *Dental Public Health* remain consistent with an added emphasis on research principles. The twenty-first century mandates a change in the practice and understanding of dental public health concepts. Dental hygiene practitioners who will be practicing in this new century need information on how to effectively position and practice dental hygiene in the dental public health setting.

The third edition expands on public health science from its inception and further explains the essence of dental public health. The chapter on financing dental care is expanded to focus on the current issues concerning that topic and the government's role in this area. Moreover, the chapter regarding advocacy for dental care discusses the importance of collaboration in dental care and building coalitions to help advocate for the oral health of all people. It also includes an introductory discussion on grant writing.

In the second unit, the chapter on cultural competency follows the chapter on target populations. This focus is necessary in a public health setting because it helps future providers define population health and further understand how culture and health relate.

The research unit is greatly expanded to provide detailed information on the study of dental hygiene research. Its focus is a comprehensive discussion of research for the undergraduate dental hygiene student. Areas of expansion include evidence-based research, ethics in research, roles of government and private entities in dental research, oral epidemiology, and the measurement of oral diseases and conditions. Expansion of this unit should help colleges that teach research within the community dental/public health program. Additionally, this unit may be used in conjunction with other materials in stand-alone research courses.

TEACHING AND LEARNING PACKAGE

PEARSON
myhealthprofessionskit™

This Companion Website is a text-specific, interactive, online workbook that provides practice quizzes complete with instant scoring and immediate feedback. It may be used to enrich the students' learning, and comes complete with Internet links and board examination hints. The Website scores the student's results and allows those results to be sent to instructors via e-mail. Select Dental Hygiene, find this book, and then click to log on. To obtain a username and password, please register using the scratch-off access code on the inside front cover of this book.

Instructor's Resource Manual

The Instructor's Resource Manual contains a wealth of material to help faculty plan and manage their course. This manual includes:

- A test bank of more than 550 questions
- Discussion items to provide ideas for classroom discussion
- Laboratory or field experiences with process evaluations for student and faculty member use
- Laboratory exercises

This Instructor's Resource Manual is available for download from myhealthprofessionskit.com and from the Instructor's Resource Center. Instructors should register at the site to obtain a username and password.

Instructor's Resource CD-ROM

The Instructor's Resource CD-ROM (0-13-514207-5) offers many resources in electronic format. It includes the complete 550 question test bank that allows instructors to design customized quizzes and exams. The TestGen wizard guides instructors through the steps in creating a simple test with drag-and-drop or point-and-click transfer. Faculty members can select test questions either manually or randomly and use online spell checking and other tools to quickly polish the test content and presentation. The question formats include multiple choice, fill in the blank, true/false, and essay. Tests can be saved in a variety of formats both locally and on a network, organized in as many as twenty-five variations of a single test, and published in an online format. For more information, please visit www.pearsonhighered .com/testgen.

The Instructor's Resource CD-ROM also includes a PowerPoint lecture package that contains key discussion points for each chapter. This feature provides dynamic, fully designed, integrated lectures that are ready to use and allows instructors to customize the materials to meet their specific course needs.

An electronic version of the Instructor's Resource Manual in both Microsoft Word and PDF formats can be accessed on the Instructor's Resource CD-ROM.

Acknowledgments

The author wishes to acknowledge the contributions of several individuals who have greatly influenced the writing of this book. First, the chapter and section contributions from

Christine French-Beatty, RDH, PhD, Professor, Texas Woman's University, Department of Dental Hygiene, Denton, TX, on the oral epidemiology and biostatistics chapters as well as ideas and suggestions on how to improve the research unit

Claudia Luciak-Donsberger, RDH, PhD, University of Vienna School of Dentistry, Department of Periodontology, Vienna, Austria, on the international dental hygiene chapter

Beth McKinney, RDH, MS, Public Health Dental Hygienist, Montgomery County, Maryland, on research in dental hygiene chapter

Meg Zayan, RDH, MPH, Professor and Dean, Fones School of Dental Hygiene, University of Bridgeport, Bridgeport, Connecticut, on the board review chapter

Irene Connolly, Adjunct Assistant Professor, Old Dominion University, Norfolk, Virginia, on the cultural competency chapter

Shari Peterson, RDH, MEd, Professor and Director, College of Southern Nevada, Las Vegas, Nevada on social advocacy chapter

Elaine Sanchez-Dils, RDH, MA, Assistant Professor, University of New Mexico, Division of Dental Hygiene, Albuquerque, New Mexico on the dental indices section

Important support was provided by Demetra Logothetis, Director and Professor, Division of Dental Hygiene, University of New Mexico. And, of course, editorial support and advice from Mark Cohen, Editor-in-Chief, and Melissa Kerian, Associate Editor, Pearson Health Science. Also, the copyeditor, JaNoel Lowe, and Karen Berry, the production editor at Laserwords Maine. The book would not be possible without support from these individuals.

Reviewers

Sheila Bannister, RDH, BSDH
Assistant Professor, Dental Hygiene
Vermont Technical College
Williston, Vermont

Peggy J. Boyce, RDA, BA
Codirector, Dental Hygiene
Parkland College
Champaign, Illinois

Susan Callahan Barnard, DHSc, RDH
Assistant Professor/Coordinator, Dental Hygiene
Bergen Community College
Paramus, New Jersey

Valerie L. Carter, RDH, BS, MSDH
Associate Professor, Dental Hygiene
St. Petersburg College
Pinellas Park, Florida

Kenneth A. Eaton, BDS, MSc, PhD, MGDS RCS
(Eng), FFGDP (UK), FFPH, FHEA, DHC
Visiting Professor
University College London
Eastman Dental Institute
King's College London, Dental Institute
London, United Kingdom

Jacque Freudenthal, RDH, MHE
Assistant Professor, Dental Hygiene
Idaho State University
Pocatello, Idaho

Beverly H Hardee, RDH, MEd
Instructor/Senior Clinical Coordinator, Dental Hygiene
Cape Fear Community College
Wilmington, North Carolina

Sheranita Hemphill, RDH, MS, MPH
Professor, Dental Hygiene
Sinclair Community College
Dayton, Ohio

Mary E. Jorstad, RDH, MA
Instructor, Dental Hygiene
Lake Land College
Mattoon, Illinois

Aamna Nayyar, DDS
Director, Dental Assisting Program
Santa Fe Community College
Santa Fe, New Mexico

Robert F. Nelson, RDH, MPA
Associate Chairperson/Professor, Dental Hygiene
University of South Dakota
Vermillion, South Dakota

Mary S. Pelletier, RDH, MEd
Assistant Professor, Dental Hygiene
Indian River State College
Fort Pierce, Florida

Connie M. E. Preiser, RDH, MHS
Instructor, Department of Dental Hygiene
Catawba Valley Community College
Hickory, North Carolina

Martha H. Roberson, MSHA, RDH
Associate Professor/Program Head, Dental Hygiene
Virginia Western Community College
Roanoke, Virginia

Judith Romano, MA
Chair, Dental Hygiene
Hudson Valley Community College
Troy, New York

Julie A. Stage, RDH, MPH
Professor, Dental Hygiene
Truckee Meadows Community College
Reno, Nevada

Kim Willey RDH
Instructor, Dental Hygiene
Stark State College
North Canton, Ohio

Sharon C. Stull, CDA, BSDH, MS
Lecturer, Gene Hirschfeld School of Dental Hygiene
Old Dominion University
Norfolk, Virginia

PREVIOUS EDITIONS

Eugenia B. Bearden, Clayton College and State University

Maryellen Beaulieu, University of New England

Lynn Ann Bethel, Mount Ida College

Jacqueline N. Brian, Indiana University–Purdue University Fort Wayne

Janice Brinson, BSDH, MS, Tennessee State University

Diane L. Bourque, Community College of Rhode Island

Sandra George Burns, Ferris State University

Michele M. Edwards, Tallahassee Community College

Kerry Flynn, Palm Beach Community College

Theresa M. Grady, Community College of Philadelphia

Jamar M. Jackson, Hostos Community College

Tara L. Johnson, Idaho State University

Mary E. Jorstad, Lake Land College

Nancy K. Mann, Indiana University–Purdue University Fort Wayne

Patricia Mannie, St. Cloud Technical College

Jill Mason, Oregon Health Sciences University

Marian Williams Patton, Tennessee State University

Barbara Ringle, Cuyahoga Community College

Kari Steinbock, Mt. Hood Community College

Edith Tynan, Northern Virginia Community College

Unit I

Introduction to Dental Public Health

The following excerpt eloquently states the need for educating dental hygienists about the need for dental public health.

> Children live for months with pain that grown-ups would find unendurable. The gradual attrition of accepted pain erodes their energy and aspirations. I have seen children in New York with teeth that look like brownish, broken sticks. I have also seen teenagers who were missing half their teeth. But, to me, most shocking is to see a child with an abscess that has been inflamed for weeks and that he has simply lived with and accepts as part of the routine of life.*

Unfortunately, this statement reflects a problem that exists throughout the world. Dental problems cause pain, infection, disease, and disability and can easily be prevented. Dental hygienists have the skills necessary to help alleviate this problem. This introductory unit focuses on the definition of public health, its historical development as a true public health profession, and evidence-based preventive health modalities that are practiced in public health. This unit also discusses the current status of dental care delivery in the United States and abroad with an emphasis on government structures, financing, and laws affecting dental hygiene care.

---

*Kozol J. *Savage Inequalities: Children in America's Schools*. New York, NY: Crown Publishers; 1991.

Chapter 1

Dental Public Health: An Overview

OBJECTIVES

After studying this chapter, the dental hygiene student should be able to:

- Define public health
- Describe the evolution of public health science and practice
- Define dental public health
- Describe factors affecting dental public health

KEY TERMS

Community dental health
Dental public health
Malpractice
Primary prevention
Public health
Public health goals
Public health services
Secondary prevention
Socioeconomic status (SES)
Tertiary prevention

COMPETENCIES

After studying this chapter and participating in accompanying course activities, the dental hygiene student should be competent to do the following:

- Promote the values of oral and general health and wellness to the public and organizations within and outside of the profession
- Evaluate factors that can be used to promote patient adherence to disease prevention and/or health maintenance strategies
- Evaluate and utilize methods to ensure the health and safety of the patient and the dental hygienists in the delivery of dental hygiene
- Identify career options within the health care industry, education, and research and evaluate the feasibility of pursuing dental hygiene opportunities
- Access professional and social networks to pursue professional goals

Public health is concerned with the health care of all people. It focuses on the health of a population as a whole rather than on the treatment of an individual. The goal of public health is to protect and promote the health of the public across three essential domains: health protection, disease prevention, and health promotion.[1]

Public health has become an essential component of developed societies. Many of the major improvements in the health of populations have resulted from public health measures such as ensuring safe food and water, controlling epidemics, and protecting workers from injury. Most people, however, do not give much thought to the public health system until a crisis occurs or the system fails. Infectious disease outbreaks, the incidence of cancer, and the increasing number of working people unable to afford health care services draw attention to the infrastructure that protects the health of the public.[2]

Public health initially involved caring for a population with a disease, but the focus shifted to controlling the disease itself. It has subsequently evolved to emphasize disease prevention, which enhances quality of life, helps deter illness or outbreaks, and is cost effective. **Primary prevention** is the employment of strategies and agents to forestall the onset of disease, reverse its progress, or arrest its process before treatment becomes necessary. Dental hygiene is a form of primary prevention.

Most people recognize the efficacy of primary levels of prevention, but they are less likely to think of secondary prevention as being effective at preventing disease. **Secondary prevention** employs routine treatment methods to terminate the disease process and/or restore tissues to as nearly normal as possible; can also be called *restorative care.* One example of secondary prevention is the use of fluoride to remineralize tooth surfaces that have been demineralized. Another example is periodontal debridement to reduce periodontal pocketing. **Tertiary prevention** employs strategies to replace lost tissues through rehabilitation. Using dental materials to restore demineralized tooth surfaces to stop an infection and prevent the loss of a tooth due to tooth decay is an example of tertiary prevention.

Dental public health is only one component of public health. An understanding of the foundation of *public health* is important in discussing the topic of dental public health.

PUBLIC HEALTH DEFINED

The World Health Organization (WHO) and others have defined *public health* as the effort to promote physical and mental health and prevent disease, injury, and disability at the population level. It involves a wide range of products, activities, and services aimed at the entire population although it is sometimes delivered to the individual.[3,4] Many postulate that public health is the approach to health care that concerns the health of the community as a whole. The first dentist to be president of the American Public Health Association, John W. Knutson, originally defined public health as:

Public health is people's health. It is concerned with the aggregate health of a group, a community, a state, or a nation. Public health in accordance with this broad definition is not limited to the health of the poor, or to rendering health services or to the nature of the health problems. Nor is it defined by the method of payment for health services or by the type of agency responsible for supplying those services. It is simply a concern for and activity directed toward the improvement and protection of the health of a population group and the aggregate.[5]

In the report *The Future of the Public's Health in the 21st Century,* the Institute of Medicine defined public health as "what we, as a society, do collectively to assure the conditions in which people can be healthy." It identified core functions that were to be conducted by government public health agencies: assessment, policy development, assurance, and serving all functions. [6]

- **Assessment** involves monitoring the health of communities and populations to identify health problems and priorities. It includes activities such as performing public health surveillance, collecting and interpreting data, finding case applications, and evaluating outcomes of programs and policies.
- **Policy development** is the process by which society makes decisions about problems, chooses goals and strategies to address the problems, and allocates resources to reach them. Formulation of public policies usually occurs through collaboration between community, private sector, and government leaders.
- **Assurance** involves making certain that all populations have access to appropriate and cost-effective services to reach agreed-upon public health goals. In addition to treatment services for individuals, assurance activities include health promotion and disease-prevention services.

- **Serving all functions** is the research for new insights and innovative solutions to health problems.[6]

These functions can facilitate public health policy and decision making and further enhance planning public health programs.

Goals and Challenges

The American Public Health Association states that the practice of public health should reduce human suffering, help children to thrive, improve the quality of life, prevent disease, and save money.[7]

Did You Know?

Former US Surgeon General C. Everett Koop once stated that health care matters to all of us some of the time; however, public health matters to all of us all of the time.

Public health goals are goals that guide all public health activities. They dictate services to ensure the promotion of health and prevention of disease and injury (see Boxes 1-1 ■ and 1-2 ■). An example of a public health goal that promotes healthy behaviors is the distribution of mouth guards to student athletes. Screening for dental decay illustrates the monitoring of health status to identify community health problems.

Public health services are those that help attain public health goals. Preventing illness and promoting health through the delivery of efficient and effective public health services lie at the core of society's ability to create an exemplary circle of better health, more productive citizens, and affordable health care.[1] At a time of renewed concern about communicable disease such as avian influenza, tuberculosis, and HIV as well as new anxieties about events such as bioterrorism, people in many countries also face the challenges of lifestyle-related diseases, such as obesity, diabetes, cancer, and

---

BOX 1-1   Public Health Goals

- Prevent epidemics and the spread of disease
- Protect against environmental hazards
- Prevent injuries
- Promote and encourage healthy behaviors
- Respond to disasters and assist communities in recovery
- Assure the quality and accessibility of health services

Source: Fall 1994. Public Health Functions Steering Committee. http://www.health.gov/phfunctions/public.htm

---

BOX 1-2   Public Health Services

- Monitor health status to identify community health problems
- Diagnose and investigate health problems and health hazards in the community
- Inform, educate, and empower people about health issues
- Mobilize community partnerships to identify and solve health problems
- Develop policies and plans that support individual and community health efforts
- Enforce laws and regulations that protect health and ensure safety
- Link people to needed personal health services and assure the provision of health care when otherwise unavailable
- Assure a competent public health and personal health care workforce
- Evaluate effectiveness, accessibility, and quality of personal and population-based health services
- Research for new insights and innovative solutions to health problems

Source: Fall 1994. Public Health Functions Steering Committee. http://www.health.gov/phfunctions/public.htm

cardiovascular disease, which are significantly influenced by diet, physical activity, tobacco use, and alcohol abuse.[1] Public health services aid in educating the public about preventive measures to employ to avoid some diseases.

With health care services placing more and more pressures on budgets as well as a financial burden for individuals and families, the practice of public health has become a cause of great concern for governments and health systems. The World Health Organization (WHO) operates in an increasingly complex and rapidly changing landscape, and the boundaries of public health action extend into other sectors that influence health opportunities and outcomes.[1] WHO responds to these challenges using a six-point agenda to help navigate the health of the public. (See Box 1-3 ■.)

HISTORICAL PERSPECTIVE OF PUBLIC HEALTH

Widespread outbreaks of communicable disease can be traced back to the plague and the black death, which had devastating effects on the population. Public health activities such as quarantines, mass burials, and ship inspections were subsequently developed to prevent such horrendous epidemics.

The first significant recording of public health measures in the United States occurred in South Carolina in 1671 when a water protection measure was enacted to prevent diseases caused by microorganisms in water supplies.[8] In 1798, the United States passed an act that provided for the relief of sick and disabled seamen, which established a federal network of hospitals for the care of merchant seaman, the precursor of the US Public Health Service, which was initiated in 1902.[9] The first supervising surgeon of this network was the predecessor to today's US Surgeon General.

In England in 1777, a Gloucestershire milkmaid told her physician, Dr. Edward Jenner, that she was fortunate to have contracted cowpox because it conferred protection against smallpox. Dr. Jenner, in turn, studied the relationship and established the scientific principle of immunization that eventually resulted in eliminating smallpox.[10]

The identification of a polluted public water well as the source of an 1854 cholera outbreak in London was a major advancement in public health.[11] Dr. John Snow used a logical, epidemiological approach to study the outbreak. At the time, many suspected pollution as the cause of the cholera, but by studying the geographical relation of the sick to a water pump, he was able to help control the outbreak.

BOX 1-3 World Health Organization's Six-Point Agenda

1. **Promoting development** The ethical principle of equity directs health development: Access to life-saving or health-promoting interventions should not be denied for unfair reasons, including those with economic or social roots.

2. **Fostering health security** One of the greatest threats to international health security is from outbreaks of emerging and epidemic-prone diseases.

3. **Strengthening health systems** For health improvement to operate as a poverty-reduction strategy, health services must reach poor and underserved populations.

4. **Harnessing research, information and evidence** Evidence provides the foundation for setting priorities, defining strategies, and measuring results.

5. **Enhancing partnerships** WHO carries out its work with the support and collaboration of many partners, including UN agencies and other international organizations, donors, civil society, and the private sector.

6. **Improving performance** WHO participates in ongoing reforms to improve its efficiency and effectiveness at both the international level and within countries.

Source: http://www.who.int. Accessed June 8, 2009.

Did You Know?

Epidemiology is the study of the amount, distribution, determinant, and control of disease and health conditions among given populations.

The first one-room laboratory for public health was opened in 1887 on Staten Island, New York, and was the forerunner to the National Institutes of Health,[9] which still is the main health care research institution in the United States.

During the first years of the 1900s, Dr. Sara Baker, a physician, led teams of nurses into the crowded neighborhoods of Hell's Kitchen in New York City and taught mothers how to dress, feed, and bathe their babies. Baker established many programs to help the poor in that city keep their infants healthy. After World War I, many states and countries followed her example to lower infant mortality rates.[12]

Did You Know?

Archeologists reported that two molar teeth about 63,400 years old show that the presence of grooves formed by the passage of a pointed object, thought to be a small stick, discovered on the teeth, indicating that Neanderthals may have cleaned their teeth.[13]

The dramatic increase in the average life span during the 1900s is widely credited to public health achievements, such as vaccination programs and control of infectious diseases, effective policies such as motor vehicle and occupational safety, improved family planning, antismoking measures, and programs designed to decrease chronic disease. The US Department of Health and Human Services has incorporated dental public health into many of the more than 300 programs it offers. (See Box 1-4 ■.) One dental public health preventive effort, community water fluoridation, is one of the ten great public health measures adopted during the past century. (See Box 1-5 ■.)

Recent public health efforts include the response to crises such as the September 11, 2001, terrorist attacks and the aftermath of Hurricane Katrina in August 2005. Innovative public health preventive efforts include the increased utilization of dental hygienists in school settings to reduce dental decay and the increase in checkpoints for drunk drivers to help prevent crashes caused by intoxication. See Box 1-6 ■ for historic events involving the US. Public Health Service.

DENTAL PUBLIC HEALTH DEFINED

Dental health is a wide-reaching field of study, but it is grounded in distinct concepts within public health. The American Board of Dental Public Health (ABDPH) defines dental public health as:

the science and art of preventing and controlling dental diseases and promoting dental health through organized community efforts. It is that form of dental practice that serves the community as a patient rather than the individual. It is concerned with the dental health education of the public, with applied dental research, and with the administration of group dental care programs, as well as the prevention and control of dental diseases on a community basis. Implicit in this definition is the requirement that the specialist have broad knowledge and skills in public health administration, research methodology, the prevention and control of oral diseases, and the delivery and financing of oral health care.[14]

Dental public health focuses on oral health care and education of a population with an emphasis on the utilization of dental hygiene sciences. Many agencies of the federal and state governments fund dental care delivery and the dental workforce needed to provide this care. (See Chapter 3.)

Did You Know?

Dental hygiene was initiated as a public health profession.

BOX 1-4 Historical Highlights

The roots of the Dept of Health and Human Services go back to the early days of the nation:

1798: An act for the relief of sick and disabled seamen was passed, establishing a federal network of hospitals for the care of merchant seamen; forerunner of today's US Public Health Service.

1871: The first supervising surgeon (later called Surgeon General) was appointed for the Marine Hospital Service, which had been organized the prior year.

1887: The federal government opened a one-room laboratory on Staten Island for research on disease, thereby planting the seed that was to grow into the National Institutes of Health.

1906: Congress passed the Pure Food and Drugs Act, authorizing the government to monitor the purity of foods and the safety of medicines, now the responsibility of the Food and Drug Administration.

1921: The Bureau of Indian Affairs Health Division, the forerunner to the Indian Health Service, was created.

1946: The Communicable Disease Center, forerunner of the Centers for Disease Control and Prevention, was established.

1955: The Salk polio vaccine was licensed.

1961: The First White House Conference on Aging was held.

1964: The first Surgeon General's Report on Smoking and Health was released.

1965: The Medicare and Medicaid programs making comprehensive health care available to millions of Americans was created. In addition, the Older Americans Act created the nutritional and social programs administered by HHS Administration on Aging, and the Head Start program was created.

1966: The International Smallpox Eradication program led by the US Public Health Service was established; the worldwide eradication of smallpox was accomplished in 1977.

1970: The National Health Service Corps was established.

1990: The Human Genome Project was established, and the Nutrition Labeling and Education Act was passed to authorize nutritional labeling of food.

1993: The Vaccines for Children Program was established, providing free immunizations to all children in low-income families.

1995: The Social Security Administration became an independent agency.

1996: The Health Insurance Portability and Accountability Act (HIPAA) was enacted.

1997: The State Children's Health Insurance Program (SCHIP) that enables states to extend health coverage to more uninsured children was created.

1999: The initiative on combating bioterrorism was launched.

2002: The Office of Public Health Emergency Preparedness was created to coordinate efforts against bioterrorism and other emergency health threats.

Source: Historical Highlights: US Department of Health and Human Services. http://www.hhs.gov/about/hhshist.html. Accessed July 29, 2009.

BOX 1-5 Great Public Health Achievements of the Twentieth Century

- Vaccination
- Motor vehicle safety
- Workplace safety
- Control of infectious diseases
- Decline in deaths from coronary heart disease and stroke
- Safer and healthier food
- Healthier mothers and babies
- Family planning
- Community water fluoridation
- Recognition of tobacco as a hazard

Source: Ten Great Public Health Achievements—United States, 1900–1999. *MMWR Morb Mortal Wkly Rpt.* 1999;48(12):241–243.

BOX 1-6 US Public Health Service Commissioned Corps Timeline

1798: President John Adams signed into law the Act for the Relief of Sick and Disabled Seamen. A year later, Congress extended the act to cover every officer and sailor in the US Navy.

1871: John Maynard Woodworth, the first supervising surgeon, adopted a military model for his medical staff as part of a system reform. He instituted examinations for applicants, put physicians in uniforms, and created a cadre of mobile, career-service physicians who could be assigned to various marine hospitals.

1878: The prevalence of major epidemic diseases such as smallpox, yellow fever, and cholera spurred Congress to enact the National Quarantine Act to prevent the introduction of contagious and infectious diseases into the United States.

1912: Name of the Public Health and Marine Hospital Service was shortened to the Public Health Service. Legislation enacted by Congress broadened its powers by authorizing investigations into human diseases (such as tuberculosis, hookworm, malaria, and leprosy) related to sanitation, water supplies, and sewage disposal.

1930 and 1944: US Public Health Service Corps officers expanded to include engineers, dentists, research scientists, nurses, and other health care specialists (dental hygienists), as well as physicians.

2006: The Commissioned Corps fulfills its mission to protect and promote the nation's public health. With more than 6,000 active-duty officers, it works both nationally and internationally to create a world free of preventable disease, sickness, and suffering.

Source: US Public Health Service. About the US Public Health Service: History. http://www.usphs.gov/aboutus/history.aspx. Accessed August 13, 2008.

Many times dental public health is called **community dental health.** Both terms are correct and share similar meanings. Some consider community health to be a component of public health; others use the terms interchangeably. The major difference between the terms is that *community* focuses on a specific group of people whereas the connotation of *public* is thought to be wider reaching.

The delivery of dental services for individuals and the general population at national and local levels involves a variety of institutions, infrastructures, and activities. Dental public health functions need to be secured and implemented across all areas to ensure the same level of coverage, quality, and performance of services.[2]

Dental public health practice follows steps similar to those taken by a dental hygienist in the private sector, but the focus is primarily on a population, including those who do not seek care, rather than just one patient in the chair. Table 1-1 ■ compares the two types of delivery. Assessment is the core public health function, and the dental public health practitioner collects the necessary information to identify community problems, analogous to an individual dental hygienist diagnosing a patient's condition. Just as a personal dental hygienist develops a treatment plan after the diagnosis, the dental public health practitioner uses the information from the community assessment to develop policies and programs to address the problem(s). Ensuring dental public health is analogous to a dental hygienists' providing care: It involves the delivery of the services to the community.

Many dental hygienists choose to work in dental public health settings. All educational dental hygiene programs present dental public health education to dental hygiene students. The roles of the dental hygienist as related to dental public health are depicted in Table 1-2 ■ and Figure 1-1 ■. Public health is embedded in the educator, researcher, administer/manager, advocate and clinician roles of a dental hygienist.

FACTORS AFFECTING DENTAL PUBLIC HEALTH

Numerous landmark reports suggest that the current dental care system in the United States is not effectively ensuring optimal oral health for all populations.[15–17] Multiple factors exacerbate the challenges to achieving oral health including the current structure of the dental care delivery system; poor distribution of providers; lack of diversity among providers; restrictive regulatory statutes; geographic, educational, and cultural barriers; and cost of care.[15–19]

Table 1-1   A Comparison of Aspects of Dental Private and Public Health Models of Practice

	Dental Hygienist's Role in Private Practice	*Dental Hygienist's Role in Public Health*
Assessment	Conducts initial health assessment by reviewing health and dental history with patient	Conducts a needs assessment of target populations
	Conducts a comprehensive oral examination	Analyzes community needs
Dental hygiene diagnosis	Provides patients' dental hygiene diagnosis	Provides community dental hygiene diagnosis to basically prioritize the needs
Planning	Develops a treatment plan based on the diagnosis, patient interaction, and the priorities and method of payment; utilizes measurable assessment mechanisms	Develops a program based on the analysis of needs assessment data, priorities, and alternatives; community interaction; and resources available for which measurable assessment mechanisms are used
	Selects appropriate health care workers to provide comprehensive care	Selects appropriate labor to implement program
Implementation	Implements self-generated treatment plan effectively, changing it when necessary	Implements self-generated treatment plan effectively, changing it when necessary
Evaluation	Provides treatment via dental, gingival, and periodontal evaluations	Evaluates program via index and community evaluations

Table 1-2   Professional Roles of the Dental Hygienist as Related to Dental Public Health

Role of the Dental Hygienist	*Dental Public Health Responsibilities Embedded Throughout*
Administrator/Manager	Develops and coordinates dental public health programs
Advocate	Provides dental health consultation to various target populations and lobbies to change laws to increase access to care for the underserved population
Clinician	Provides clinical care to the population
Educator	Educates and promotes dental health education and issues to various target populations
Researcher	Conducts research germane to the study of health and disease and utilization of the dental hygienist

Professional Roles of the Dental Hygienist

FIGURE 1-1   Roles of the Dental Hygienist

Source: American Dental Hygienists' Association: Standards for Clinical Dental Hygiene Practice: June 2007. Available at http://www.adha.org/downloads/adha_standards08.pdf. Accessed June 9, 2009.

Access to Care

Although many issues impact dental public health and the care that dental hygienists deliver in the United States today, inadequate access to dental care is undoubtedly one of the most important. The reasons for this widespread problem vary, but one is that in many states, dental hygienists are restricted to providing care only under the supervision of dentists. Moreover, many individuals lack the financial resources or transportation needed to obtain dental care services. The numerous barriers to care in the United States are discussed in more detail in Chapter 10.

Did You Know?

An increasing number of children receive preventive care during school hours from dental hygienists who work in school-based health clinics or as mobile care providers, helping to improve access to care.

Infrastructure

Exacerbating oral health disparities is the ineffective structure of the existing dental care delivery system. The practice of dentistry has remained in the private sector, providing services to a select population. The populations who need dental care the most are often left without access to it.

Many individuals present to the emergency rooms in local hospitals with dental caries that have progressed into major infections. Treatment of these infections costs thousands of dollars in hospital care, medicine, and operating room costs, not to mention the pain and suffering the individuals and families endure. Any level of primary, secondary, or tertiary services could prevent these problems.

Dental care is not as effectively positioned as comprehensive health care, nor is it practiced in a multidisciplinary fashion. Models need to be developed to address the needs of all individuals within society and to incorporate dental health care within comprehensive health care.

Workforce

Nationally, a critical shortage of dentists exists.[20] With fewer dentists nationwide and limited access to preventive care performed by dental hygienists, millions of Americans in rural and urban areas are unable to obtain care. A system is needed to bring oral health care to diverse, underserved populations. Reports suggest that the current dental care delivery system in the United States is not effectively ensuring optimal oral health for all populations.

The Surgeon General's *National Call to Action to Promote Oral Health Care* identifies the need to enhance the oral health workforce in the United States. Many new programs and positions have been developed to address this issue, including the Alaska Dental Health Therapist (ADHT) and the Advanced Dental Hygiene Practitioner (ADHP). The ADHT program created in 2000 addresses the severe dentist shortage in rural areas of Alaska.[21,22] Under ADHT, the therapist provides restorative and urgent care services, including dental

---

DENTAL HYGIENIST SPOTLIGHT:
Dolores Malvitz, RDH, DrPH

The American Dental Hygienists' Association (ADHA) recently established the position of ADHA public health consultant. The function of this position is to consult with members who have questions regarding public health endeavors and to serve as an adviser to the Council on Public Health and ADHA staff on all public health issues. The ADHA chose a true dental hygiene pioneer, Dolores Malvitz, as the first ADHA public health consultant.

After receiving her certificate in dental hygiene and bachelor's degree in English at the University of Michigan and Western Michigan, respectively, Ms. Malvitz went on to earn master's and doctoral degrees in public health from the University of Michigan. She has taught dental hygiene, published numerous articles on studies she led, spoken all over the nation, been active in several professional associations, consulted with various organizations, and recently retired from the Centers for Disease Control and Prevention (CDC). Her exact title at CDC was Surveillance and Research Team Leader, Division of Oral Health, National Center for Chronic Disease Prevention and Health Promotion. She continues to be a role model and mentor to many dental hygienists, and her many accomplishments have truly motivated others in the professions.

Dr. Malvitz has received many awards. Some of the most noteworthy include:

- Special Merit Award of the American Association of Public Health Dentistry

- Distinguished Service Award from the Association of State and Territorial Dental Directors
- Outstanding Alumnus Award, University of Michigan
- Doctor of Humane Letters from the University of Detroit, Mercy (an honorary degree)
- Pfizer/ADHA Excellence in Dental Hygiene Award

Dolores Malvitz, left, received the American Association of Public Health Dentistry's Special Merit Award from Candace Jones, RDH, in 2005.

She continues to be active in dental hygiene and is a true public health practitioner. Even after retirement, she is still promoting the public's health.

I asked her some questions regarding her career.

Can you provide some examples of your consulting this past year?

I attended and provided expertise at meetings of ADHA work groups—for example, Council on Public Health, ADHP Task Force. Also, I reviewed the public health portion of the ADHA Website and suggested specific revisions. I communicated via phone and e-mail with a dental hygiene faculty member assigned to teach community health for the first time; we discussed potential content, learning strategies, and sources of information. I created and oversaw the review of content for the ADHA Website related to the National Research Council report on fluoride. I also provided expert advice to the staff at ADHA and council members on request.

Why did you decide to go into dental hygiene?

Here is the unvarnished truth: Because I was a good student, my high school teachers were pressing me to go to college. I was not enthralled with nursing or teaching, the two careers considered appropriate for young women in that era. My boyfriend's sister-in-law taught in a suburban Detroit school system that employed a dental hygienist, and she suggested exploring this career that required only two years of college yet operated on the school calendar.

How did you get into public health? Did you need additional education?

As I began teaching in a dental hygiene program, it became clear that graduate education would be essential for success in academia. After exploring alternatives, I chose public health for my master's degree. That discipline seemed to offer a wider range of opportunities than the other logical choice, dental hygiene education. Then, my graduate school adviser encouraged me to stay for a doctorate, a decision that proved wise. Knowing more is always better than getting by with incomplete knowledge or skills—and it's critical to have the education that's expected for certain positions.

What type of advice would you give to a practicing hygienist who is thinking of doing something different?

First, the dental hygienist must decide what sorts of things she or he likes—and doesn't like—to do. What are favorite courses from the past? What aspects of the current position provide personal rewards that would be difficult to relinquish? What tasks would be a joy to never perform again?

Then, do some exploring on the Web; start moving outward via links and searches. Find some people who hold the kinds of positions that seem appealing, and ask to spend some time with them. By observing carefully and asking strategic questions, the dental hygienist should be able to decide whether the new role would be satisfying and, given current obligations, whether it's possible to acquire the credentials necessary for credibility in the new role.

Do you have anything else to share or advice to provide?

I emphasize my belief that dental hygiene must ensure an ongoing cadre of well-educated and capable leaders. In education, it is important to be able to work as peers with other health professionals, who often hold masters and doctoral degrees.

Source: Christine Nathe writes the Public Health Column in RDH magazine published by Pennwell Publishing. For more public health spotlights please see RDH magazine online at http://www.rdhmag.com/index.html.

---

restorations and extractions. The main focus of the ADHT is to alleviate infection and restore function.

The American Dental Hygienists' Association developed ADHP to address the shortage of dentists and dentally underserved populations. This program provides diagnostic, preventive, restorative, and therapeutic services directly to the public.[21,23] Although the ADHP's main focus is preventive in nature, he or she is able to provide basic restorative care.

Dental Hygiene

From its inception, dental hygiene has had a strong foundation in managing dental care delivery. The role of the dental hygienist was created to identify and treat dental infections before they became too severe for treatment, to refer patients to the appropriate health care providers, and to prevent dental disease in all populations. Essentially, the dental hygienist is in the unique management position to provide the link to comprehensive oral health care. (See Box 1-7 ■.) Fones wrote in the preface to the 3rd edition (1927) of *Mouth Hygiene*, the first textbook on dental hygiene:

In many states the dentists have chosen to cooperate in an educational movement for mouth hygiene and they have accepted a coworker, the dental hygienist, as the logical means by which dentistry as a profession can discharge her responsibility for improving the mouth health of the masses. It is no longer a theory that the service of the dental hygienist will better the mouth health and general health of all whom she is permitted to serve.... The actual results secured by dental hygienists in private and public service, particularly in public schools, affords incontrovertible proof of the value of this type of preventive dentistry. Those who may still be skeptical are finding it difficult indeed to suggest any other means by which similar good results can be accomplished for large groups of people.[24]

BOX 1-7 Historical Dental Standards in Connecticut

In 1921, Bridgeport's board of education voted to require a definite physical standard for every school child and after conferences with the Connecticut Department of Health, adopted resolutions that included dental standards. The Resolution stated that all school children:

a. provide certification from the dental hygienist that there were no cavities in the permanent dentition

b. demonstrate effectively the use of the toothbrush to remove food debris and to keep the gums in a state of health

c. have teeth and gums in a clean and healthful condition

Source: Fones AC. *Mouth Hygiene.* 3rd ed. Philadelphia, PA: Lea & Febiger; 1927:315.

Did You Know?

The Fones School of Dental Hygiene at the University of Bridgeport in Bridgeport, Connecticut, showcases many of Dr. Fones's original writings, instruments, and equipment.

The introduction of professional dental hygiene care, fluoride, and dental sealants have, more than any other factors, influenced the reduction in oral disease rates. Many feel that the practice of dental hygiene must continue to move into health care systems and models that serve all populations.

Oral Health Disparities

Oral Health in America: A Report of the Surgeon General states that oral health in the United States is rife with profound and consequential disparities within the population. Demographic information shows a correlation between oral health and **socioeconomic status (SES),** which is an individual's comparative social and economic standing within a community. An individual's SES affects the person's access to dental care. Specifically, the lower the individual's SES, the more frequent are untreated dental caries.

The racial and ethnic minority population is already compromised with oral health disparities, and with its projected growth of almost 20% from 2000 to 2050, the disparities will become even greater.[25] In the United States, people who are Hispanic, elderly, and have the lowest SES suffer more periodontal diseases than other populations.[26] Furthermore, about one in three adults living in poverty has untreated dental decay.[26]

Tooth decay remains the single most common chronic disease in children. Untreated dental decay is twice as prevalent in children and adolescents living in poverty as in their peers from families with higher incomes.[26] Children from low-income and ethnic minority households and children with special health care needs are more likely to experience tooth decay and have higher levels of untreated tooth decay compared with children from more economically advantaged households.

Dental Care Needs of the Aging Population

One indication that the increased number of dental hygienists has resulted in dental disease prevention is evident in the aging population. Because of dental hygiene and fluoride treatments, the number of people with teeth lasting a lifetime has increased. Older adults have more preventive and restorative dental care now than ever before and are also much more likely to see dental health as part of their own total health. Also, medical advances have caused longer life expectancies, resulting in the need for dental care for those who are living longer.

Dental hygienists assume a more integral role than ever in the lives of the elderly population. Older people have an increased occurrence of periodontal and other oral disease; consequently, the need for dental hygiene care increases with age.

A number of significant changes occur during aging. Fortunately, most of these normal changes do not cause oral diseases.[27,28] However, oral diseases can be exacerbated by systemic conditions such as xerostomia, caused by medicine taken frequently by older adults. Xerostomia can lead to an increase in root caries, which is frequently seen in the geriatric population. Dental hygiene science has evolved in treating these patients with often debilitating diseases.

Malpractice

Malpractice has also had a direct impact on dental care delivery and quality. **Malpractice** is a dental hygiene professional's negligence by act or omission when the care provided is not within the accepted standards of practice and negatively affects the patient's well-being. The first medical malpractice suit, which was won in 1976, ushered in the advent of patients' rights, allowing patients to sue if the provider does not adequately diagnose and treat periodontal diseases.[29] Malpractice has helped improve dental care by increasing the likelihood that quality assurance mechanisms to aid in validating competent care are in place. Providers are more aware of the way they document office procedures and case notes because of the possibility of malpractice claims.

Although they are employed and supervised by dentists in most states, dental hygienists are liable for all treatment they render or fail to render and consequently should carry malpractice insurance.

Dental Insurance

The introduction of dental insurance has increased the number of patients seeking preventive care in private dental offices. Dental insurance provides comprehensive coverage of dental hygiene services and lends credence to the fact that dental hygiene treatment is cost effective.

> ### Did You Know?
>
> In many states, the dental insurance industry has been collaborating with dental hygienists to provide funding for public health programs that promote preventive dental care to underserved populations.

In many situations, dental insurance has had a positive effect on the quality and quantity of services provided. Because patients routinely seek preventive care that is covered by dental insurance, early restorative care, which is less costly and less invasive, is obtained and less extensive care is needed. Not having dental insurance increases the likelihood that an individual will not obtain dental care.[30]

SUMMARY

Dental hygiene is historically a public health profession. It is vitally important to the public that dental hygienists be educated in the dental public health sciences. The purpose of public health is to promote overall health and prevent diseases and injuries. Public health frequently involves achieving a balance between individual versus population approaches to controlling disease.

Dental public health programs should use organized, interdisciplinary efforts to address the oral health concerns of communities and populations. The activities of dental public health programs can be classified into one of the core functions of public health organizations: assessment, policy development, assurance, and serving all functions. These activities occur at all levels of society.

Factors affecting dental health include access to care, the current infrastructure of dental care delivery including the dental workforce and the practice of dental hygiene, the aging population, malpractice, and the dental insurance industry. The fact that most dental diseases seem to be untreated in specific populations signals the presence of oral health disparities in the United States. Dental hygienists must continue to address factors and strive to promote dental public health.

SELF-STUDY TEST ITEMS

1. What is an example of primary public health prevention?
   a. Disease prevention
   b. Periodontal debridement
   c. Fluoride treatments
   d. Restorative materials

2. Public health is credited with the dramatic increase in the average life span because of which of the following?
   a. Vaccinations
   b. Safety policies
   c. Family planning
   d. All of the above

3. What is an example of secondary public health prevention?
   a. Prevention of disease
   b. Fluoride treatments
   c. Restorations
   d. Patient education

4. What is the main health care research institution in the United States?
   a. Centers for Disease Control and Prevention
   b. Food and Drug Administration
   c. National Institutes of Health
   d. John Hopkins University

5. How has malpractice directly impacted dental care delivery and quality?
   a. Enabled patients to sue
   b. Decreased the number of dental providers because of the fear of malpractice suits
   c. Decreased quality of care
   d. Increased the number of suits against dental providers

REFERENCES

1. World Health Organization Public Health Services. http://www.euro.who.int/publichealth/20070319_4. Accessed May 8, 2008.
2. Tomar S. Public Health Programs. In: Harris NO, Garcia-Godoy F, and Nathe C, ed. *Primary Preventive Dentistry*. 7th ed. Upper Saddle River, NJ: Pearson; 2008.
3. World Health Organization. Preamble to the Constitution. Official Records of the World Health Organization. 1946;(2):100. The Constituton was adopted by the International Health Conference in New York, June 19–July 19, 1946, and was signed July 22, 1946, by the representatives of 61 countries. It became effective April 7, 1948. The definition has not been amended since 1948.
4. Members of the Public Health Functions Steering Committee (July 1995): American Public Health Association, Association of Schools of Public Health, Association of State and Territorial Health Officials, Environmental Council of the States, National Association of County and City Health Officials, National Association of State Alcohol and Drug Abuse Directors, National Association of State Mental Health Program Directors, Public Health Foundation, and US Public Health Service.
5. Knutson JW. What is public health? In: Pelton WJ, Wison JM, eds. *Dentistry in Public Health*. 2nd ed. Philadelphia, PA: W. B. Saunders; 1955.
6. Institute of Medicine. *The Future of the Public's Health in the 21st Century*. Washington, DC: National Academy Press; 2003.
7. American Public Health Association. *Get the Facts: What is Public Health?* www.apha.org. Accessed August 13, 2008.
8. *A Brief History of Environmental Law.* Columbia, SC: South Carolina Dept of Health and Environmental Control, Office of Solid Waster Reduction and Recycling; 2008. OR-0593.
9. US Dept of Health and Human Services. *Historical Highlights and Timelines in Public Health*. www.hhs.gov. Accessed August 13, 2008.
10. American Academy of Family Practitioners. *Practice-Based Research in Family Medicine*. Kansas City. MO: American Academy of Family Practitioners; 1986.
11. Vinten-Johansen P. *Cholera, Chloroform, and the Science of Medicine: A Life of John Snow*. New York, NY: Oxford University Press; 2003.
12. Baker Josephine S. *Fighting for Life*. New York, NY: Arno Press; 1974.
13. Tooth Care: So easy a caveman could do it? *USA Today*. September 12, 2007:5D.
14. American Board of Dental Public Health. *Informational Brochure*. Springfield, IL: American Association of Public Health Dentistry; 2008.
15. US Public Health Service. *Healthy People 2010*. Conf ed. Washington, DC: US Dept of Health and Human Services; 2000.
16. US Dept of Health and Human Services. *Oral Health in America: A Report of the Surgeon General*. Rockville, MD: US Dept of Health and Human Services, National Institute of Dental and Craniofacial Research, National Institutes of Health; 2000.
17. US Dept of Health and Human Services. *A National Call to Action to Promote Oral Health*. Rockville, MD: US Dept of Health and Human Services, Public Health Service, Centers for Disease Control and Prevention, National Institutes of Health, National Institute of Dental and Craniofacial Research; 2003. NIH Publication No. 03-5303.
18. US Dept of Health and Human Services, Health Resources and Services Demonstration, Bureau of Health Professions. *The Professional Practice Environment of Dental Hygienists in the Fifty States and the District of Columbia;* 2001. Contract No. HRSA 230-00-0099. http://bhpr.hrsa.gov/healthworkforce/reports/hygienists/dh1.htm
19. Weaver, RG, Vachovic, RW, Hanlon, LL, Mintz, JS, Chmar, JE. Unleashing the potential; 2006. http://www.adea.org.cepr/documents/unleashing_the_potential.pdf. Accessed April 28, 2008.
20. Bureau of Labor Statistics, US Dept of Labor. *Occupational Outlook Handbook*. 2008-09 ed. http://www.bls.gov/oco/ocos072.htm. Accessed February 7, 2008.

21. McKinnon M, Luke G, Bresch J, Moss M, Valachovic RW. Emerging allied dental workforce models: Considerations for academic dental institutions. *J Dent Educ.* 2007; 71(11):1476–1491.

22. Nash DA, Nagel RJ. A brief history and current status of a dental therapy initiative in the United States. *J Dent Educ.* 2005:69(8):857–859.

23. Competencies for the Advanced Dental Hygiene Practitioner. Chicago, IL: American Dental Hygienists' Association; 2008.

24. Fones AC. *Mouth Hygiene.* 3rd ed Philadelphia, PA: Lea & Febiger; 1927:5.

25. US Census Bureau. US Interim Projections by Age, Sex, Race and Hispanic Origin; Competencies for the Advanced Dental Hygiene Practitioner. http://www.census.gov/ipc/www/usinterimproj/. Accessed June 6, 2006.

26. Beltran-Aguilar ED, Barker LK, Canto MT, Dye BA, Gooch BF, Griffin, SO. Surveillance for dental caries, dental sealants, tooth retention, edentulism and enamel fluorosis—US, 1988–1994 and 1999–2002. *MMWR Morb Mortal Wkly Rpt.* 2005;54(SS-3).

27. Baum BJ, Ship J A. Oral disorders. In: Beck J, ed. *Geriatrics Review Syllabus—A Core Curriculum in Geriatric Medicine.* New York, NY: American Geriatrics Society; 1991:332–336.

28. Beck J D. Epidemiology of dental diseases in the elderly. *Gerodontology.* 1984;3:5–15.

29. Boyce JS. Risk management: An introduction for the dental practice. *Dent Hyg.* 1987;181:504–507.

30. Dental visits among dentate adults with diabetes—United States, 1999 and 2004. *MMWR Morb Mortal Wkly Rpt.* 2005;54(46):1181–1183.

PEARSON
myhealthprofessionskit™

Multimedia Extension Activities

Use this address to access the interactive Companion Website created for this textbook. Simply select "Dental Hygiene" from the choice of disciplines. Find this book and log in using your username and password. To obtain a username and password, please register using the scratch-off access code on the inside front cover of this book.

Chapter 2

The Prevention Movement

OBJECTIVES

After studying this chapter, the dental hygiene student should be able to:

- Describe the history of dental hygiene in relation to dental public health
- Define the historical development and mission of the American Dental Hygienists' Association
- List and describe the current public health preventive modalities practiced today
- Defend the need for preventive modalities in dental public health practice

KEY TERMS

Alternative restorative treatment
Athletic mouth guard
Community water fluoridation
Dental hygiene treatment
Dental sealants
Grass roots
Outreach workers
Tobacco cessation programs
Xylitol

COMPETENCIES

After studying this chapter and participating in accompanying course activities, the dental hygiene student should be competent to do the following:

- Promote the values of oral and general health and wellness to the public and organizations within and outside the profession
- Promote the profession through service activities and affiliations with professional organizations
- Facilitate client access to oral health services by influencing individuals and/or organizations to provide oral health care
- Identify career options within the health care industry, education, and research and evaluate the feasibility of pursuing dental hygiene opportunities
- Access professional and social networks to pursue professional goals

The proliferation of dental hygienists in dental offices and other health care facilities is evidence of the value placed on dental hygiene in the United States. The Bureau of Labor Statistics estimates that the number of employed dental hygienists is expected to increase 30% by the end of 2016, a much higher rate than for the average for other occupations. This increase is due to the increasing demand for dental care and the expanded use of dental hygienists.[1] The insurance industry's comprehensive coverage of dental hygiene services is further proof that the practice of prevention is necessary and logical in health care delivery.

The dental hygiene profession is at the forefront of the prevention and wellness movement that continues to grow. Dental hygiene is the only health care profession based exclusively on *preventive* care. Historically, dental hygiene services have been available in public health forums focused on preventing and controlling disease within the population.[2–6] Thus, the practice of dental hygiene complements the dental public health sciences both from a scientific and practical perspective.

HISTORICAL DEVELOPMENT

Although dental hygiene practice dates further back than its cited inception in 1913, the preventive focus of this new profession was emphasized when Dr. Alfred Civilion Fones coined the term *dental hygienist* in the early 1900s.[6] This change in title from dental nurse to dental hygienist focused on the *preventive* dental sciences. After research results on the preventive benefits of dental hygiene were published, the college discipline of dental hygiene was created.[7]

Even though prevention was being discussed and even practiced in some offices, it was Fones who actually brought dental hygiene into existence. He saw it as a distinct profession and thought it should be positioned within dental public health as opposed to being offered only in private dental practices. In fact, Fones believed that the dental hygienist should provide education and treatment outside the dental office with particular focus on mass pediatric prevention. He emphasized the use of dental hygienists as **outreach workers** "outside" the dental practice to bring patients in need of restorative dental care to private dental practices while providing preventive services outside the dental practice, such as in a school setting.[2–6] (See Table 2-1 ■ for more of Fones's thoughts on the dental hygiene profession.)

Fones educated the first dental hygienist, Irene Newman, for one year before he permitted her to treat patients in his practice. In 1913, he started the Fones School of Dental Hygiene, which continues to educate dental hygienists today within the University of Bridgeport in Connecticut. (See Figures 2-1 ■ and 2-2 ■.) Before he opened his school and began working within the Bridgeport public school system, Fones initiated the dental hygienists' role in dental public health by developing curricula for dental hygienists, but his proposal was rejected. At that time, not all dentists were aware of this new preventive concept and practice. In fact, a dentist on the board of education voted against the plan. Deciding that this action was a blessing in disguise, Fones postponed the opening of his school for a year, during which time he found instructors and chose qualified students.[8]

> **Did You Know?**
>
> Fones secured experienced professors and experts of medicine, basic sciences, public health, and dentistry from Yale University, Harvard University, Columbia University, and the University of Pennsylvania to begin the new college discipline of dental hygiene.[7]

Fones envisioned dental hygienists working collaboratively with other health and social service workers in providing preventive health care to the public. He stated, "Dental hygiene…opens up paths of usefulness, activity and inspiration hitherto undreamed of, allying her with the workers of the world who are helping humanity in masses."[1] After war was declared in 1917, dental hygienists in Bridgeport provided care and education to the military. Additionally, dental hygienists worked to create positions in hospitals and numerous factories in Connecticut.

Fones traveled the country to explain the new profession of dental hygiene to state dental associations, but some dentists were opposed to it.[7,9] Preventive dental science was a new concept, and many dentists had no experience working with a dental hygienist. Consequently, many state dental associations created restrictive laws that prohibited dental hygienists from working in any setting other than a private dental practice with a dentist supervising all treatment.

Table 2-1   Comparison of the Writings of Dr. Alfred Fones, Founder of Dental Hygiene, with Recommendations from the US Surgeon General's Report on Oral Health 2000

US Surgeon General's Report	*Fones'* **Mouth Hygiene,** *textbook of dental hygiene, 1–4 eds., 1916–1934*
Perceptions regarding oral heath and ideas should be changed so that oral health becomes an accepted component of general health.	Since the days of Hippocrates, it has been known that infections of dental origin may be accompanied by serious systemic symptoms. The work of the dental hygienist is most important in the prevention of the systemic infection through the avenue of the mouth.
Accelerate the building of science and advance evidence base and apply science effectively to improve oral health.	It is no longer a theory that the service of the dental hygienist will better the mouth health and general health of all whom she is permitted to serve.
	The research field in preventive dentistry is gradually widening into a study of constitutional causes that are believed to have an influence on the general health, and consequently on dental health.
An effective health infrastructure that meets the oral health needs of all Americans should be built and integrate oral health effectively into general health.	Hundreds of millions of dollars in public and private funds are expended to restore the sick to health, but only a relatively small portion of this amount is spent to maintain the health of well people, even though it is definitely known that the most common physical defects and illnesses are preventable.
	It is not the intention to in any way belittle the efforts being made to aid the sick and needy, nor should such efforts be decreased. The vital point is that we have not commenced to cover the possibilities of true prevention.
Known barriers between people and oral health services should be removed.	The dental hygienist was created from the realization that mouth hygiene was a necessity and that the average dental practitioner could not give sufficient time to it and that the toothbrush alone would never produce it.
	The present need of the dental profession in solving the public health problem of mouth hygiene is an immense corps of women workers, educated and trained as dental hygienists, and therefore competent to enter public schools, dental offices, infirmaries, public clinics, sanitariums, factories, and other private corporations, to care for the mouths of the millions who need this educational service.
Public–private partnerships should be used to improve the oral health of those who still suffer disproportionately from oral disease.	The actual results secured by dental hygienists in private and public services, particularly in public schools, affords incontrovertible proof of the value of the dental hygienists. Those who may still be skeptical are finding it difficult indeed to suggest other means by which similar good results can be accomplished for large groups of people.
	The future of the dental hygienist in public schools work must be determined on a basis of cooperation between the dental profession and the educational authorities.
	The Fones's hygienists who were completing their course in 1917 when war was declared had the unique experience of completing exams and cleanings and supplying each soldier a toothbrush and individual instruction in the care of the mouth.

Source: Nathe C. Dental hygiene's historical roots in modern-day issues. *Contemp Oral Hyg.* 2003;3:24–25.

FIGURE 2-1   Fones School of Dental Hygiene, Bridgeport, Connecticut, Circa Early 1900s

FIGURE 2-2   Fones School of Dental Hygiene Bridgeport, Connecticut, 2008

Ironically, if Fones had introduced the new profession to school teachers, school administrators, hospital administrators, and other professional health care organizations instead of state dental associations, dental hygienists most likely would have been permitted to work in a variety of settings. Dental hygiene was finally accepted in all states with a reduced educational standard for its practice developed in Alabama.[10] Chapter 6 discusses the impending access to care issues that resulted from these restrictive practice acts.

Today, dental practice laws are changing, and at least thirty states now permit the unsupervised practice of dental hygiene in alternative settings, allowing dental hygienists to work more effectively in the public health arena.[11] In fact, some states allow dental hygienists to provide direct services to patients in all settings. Dental hygienists increasingly are bringing dental hygiene services to school children, people who are elderly, and other underserved populations.

EVOLUTION OF ORGANIZED DENTAL HYGIENE

The Connecticut Dental Hygienists' Association was formed with nineteen members on graduation day of the first dental hygiene class in Bridgeport, Connecticut, June 5, 1914. The objective of this newly formed association was "to educate the public in, and to advance the cause of Mouth Hygiene for the mutual improvement of its members, and to assist as far as lie within its power in the prevention of disease."[12] A national association, the American Dental Hygienists' Association (ADHA), was formed in 1923 in Cleveland, Ohio.

> **Did You Know?**
>
> The first president of the Conneticut Dental Hygienists' Association was, fittingly, Irene Newman, the first dental hygienist.

The ADHA's mission has evolved since its inception. Its present mission is:

> to improve the public's total health by working to advance the art and science of dental hygiene by ensuring access to quality oral health care, increasing awareness of the cost-effective benefits of prevention, promoting the highest standards of dental hygiene education, licensure, practice and research and representing and promoting the interests of dental hygienists.[13]

Presently, the ADHA represents more than 125 000 registered dental hygienists and works actively in professional development and governmental affairs. Each of the fifty state dental hygiene associations is a constituent member. All 375 local dental hygiene associations are known as *component organizations.* Constituent organizations

serve the components in their jurisdictions by informing them of national policies and programs and actively working on legislative issues.[7] The components form the first line of involvement, the **grass roots,** or local, efforts to affect change and help guide policy-making decisions. Grass roots members are local dental hygienists who strive for social change to improve their communities' oral health. The components implement community services programs and educational sessions and offer ideas and information about state and national policies. The ADHA has a student membership category and provides student scholarships, networking, mentorship, employment assistance, and continuing education.

> **Did You Know?**
>
> The International Federation of Dental Hygienists is the professional organization that represents dental hygienists from twenty-five countries. It was informally started in 1970 and officially recognized in 1986.

DENTAL HEALTH PREVENTIVE MODALITIES

Dental hygienists provide diagnostic and therapeutic services aimed at attaining and maintaining oral health. The following modalities are practiced to prevent dental diseases.

Dental Hygiene Treatment

Many believe that water fluoridation and the recent introduction of dental sealants have had the biggest impact on public dental health. However, since 1913, dental hygienists have made a tremendous impact through prevention. **Dental hygiene treatment,** sometimes referred to as *dental cleanings* and *oral prophylaxes,* is comprehensive treatment, including assessment, dental hygiene diagnosis, planning, implementation with a focus on periodontal debridement and oral hygiene instruction, and evaluation provided by a registered dental hygienist. Dental hygiene treatment is part of the reason that Americans experience less oral disease. Furthermore, dental hygienists have educated consumers to be more oral health aware. Interestingly, *Healthy People 2010, Oral Health in America: A Report of the Surgeon General* and *A National Call to Action to Promote Oral Health* do not even address the impact dental hygiene has had on preventive dental care in the United States.[14–16]

Since the 1970s, dental hygienists have been employed in clinical positions in the United States, providing preventive, educational, and therapeutic services. However, some private dental offices and many public dental health settings still do not utilize or underutilize dental hygienists. A recent survey conducted by the American Dental Association found that only 68% of dentists employ a part-time or full-time dental hygienist.[17] Nevertheless, the American public indeed places great value on a healthy, beautiful smile, and the United States is often portrayed as a dentally healthy culture with an emphasis on straight, white teeth.

Countries without the benefit of dental hygiene have a higher incidence of dental caries, periodontal diseases, and cancrum oris (noma)—often of a severe nature—than the United States does. In fact, the World Health Organization (WHO) focuses much attention on the treatment of cancrum oris, a serious disease of the mouth and face.[18] Cancrum oris begins with severe gingivitis and is followed by rapidly extending ulceration within the mouth. The infection then spreads through the buccal mucosa, which becomes edematous and necrotic. If septicemia and death do not quickly supervene, a foul smelling purulent discharge precedes massive tissue loss and secondary healing by wound contracture. This often leads to facial disfigurement with limited jaw motion. In the United States, cancrum oris is rarely seen; however, in many developing countries without dental hygienists, it is much too common. (See Figure 2-3 ■.)

FIGURE 2-3   Cancrum Oris

Dental hygiene has not been studied per se as a preventive treatment modality, so no statistics can be cited regarding its benefits to society. The ADHA is currently investigating the cost-effectiveness of dental hygiene, focusing on the use of dental hygienists to treat the underserved.[19] The *role* of the dental hygienist in the oral health care system has been studied, however, and one recent study indicated that dental hygienists were being utilized more in 2000 than they were a decade earlier. The report suggested that dental hygienists have demonstrated their clinical ability to contribute both to quality patient care and improved access to care. Over the past decade, virtually every state has expanded the legal scope of practice of dental hygienists. When taken in conjunction with the findings of expansion initiatives in California and Colorado, which focused on direct care provided by dental hygienists without dentist's supervison, this report suggests that expanding the professional practice environment of dental hygienists improves access to oral health services, use of oral health services, and oral health outcomes.[20]

Community Water Fluoridation

Community water fluoridation is the addition of fluoride to community water supplies. Although fluoride is present naturally in variable amounts in all soils and existing water supplies, it is also present in animal and plant food consumed by people. Community water fluoridation is an excellent method to provide benefits to most people because everyone drinks and cooks with water. Moreover, fluoridated water is used in the processing and bottling of many foods and beverages. Therefore, it is a successful, cost-effective way to decrease dental caries in a population.[21–23] The cost per person is significantly less than the cost of restoring demineralized tooth structure, and fluoride's ability to remineralize demineralized tooth surfaces is of even more value.

Dr. Frederick McKay, a graduate of a Philadelphia dental school who started practicing dentistry in Colorado Springs, Colorado, is partially credited for discovering the effects of fluoridation. He found it accidentally when he was trying to determine why long-term residents of the area had brown enamel opacities and mottling, commonly referred to as *Colorado brown stain*. Dr. McKay knew from his experience in other parts of the country that this was not a normal occurrence. In 1908, with funding from the Colorado Springs Dental Society, he began an investigation that ultimately found that an excess of naturally occurring fluoride in the water supply was causing *dental fluorosis* or chronic fluoride toxicity.[24] However, the same patients exhibited far fewer carious lesions than his other patients, thus revealing the preventive benefit of fluoridated water.[25]

As beneficial as fluoride is to prevention of dental caries, too much of it can be harmful, as McKay found. If systemic fluoride concentration is high enough for a long enough period of time, severe skeletal fluorosis (or chronic fluoride toxicity) can occur as is seen in some parts of the world. Acute fluoride toxicity that can occur after excessive ingestion of fluoride produces nausea and vomiting, which can damage the stomach wall. The condition can be severe enough to be fatal. Emergency treatment includes induced vomiting, protection of the stomach by binding fluoride with orally administered calcium or aluminum preparations (milk), and maintenance of blood calcium levels with intravenous calcium.

Dr. H. Trendley Dean, a US Public Health Service dental officer, and his staff studied fluoride in drinking water and by the late 1930s discovered that fluoride levels of up to 1.0 ppm in drinking water did not cause enamel fluorosis in most people and only mild enamel fluorosis in a small percentage of people.[25]

In the United States, 69.2% of those served by public water systems received fluoridated water in 2006.[26] A *Healthy People 2010* goal calls for 75% of the population on piped-water supplies to be serviced with optimally fluoridated water.[14] Figure 2-4 ■ graphically displays the levels of fluoridation by state.

In areas where it is impossible to fluoridate the water either because the residents have well water or the overwhelming opposition to fluoride, schools can fluoridate the water. School water fluoridation is recommended only when the school has its own source of water and is not connected to a community water system. Each state is responsible for determining whether school water fluoridation is desirable and developing a written agreement between the state and appropriate school officials. Such a program must not be started unless resources are available at the state level to undertake operational and maintenance responsibilities.[27]

Fluoridated water has proved to be an effective means of preventing caries in children with an 8–37% reduction. Although children benefit from the systemic and topical benefits of fluoride, adults benefit only from topical (on the tooth structure) effects. Recent studies show that the topical effect of drinking fluoridated water reduced caries in adults from 20–40%.[22]

Water fluoridation is especially beneficial for communities of low socioeconomic status.[28] These communities have a disproportionate burden of dental caries and

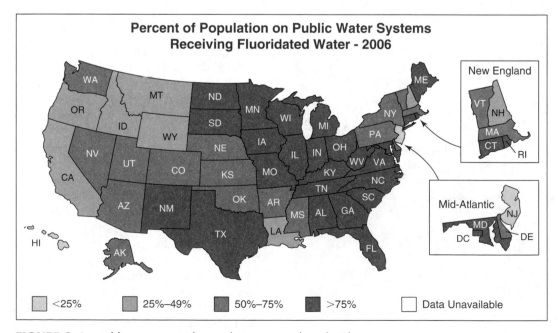

FIGURE 2-4 Public Water Supply Population Using Fluoridated Water
Source: http://www.cdc.gov/nohss.

Table 2-2   Fluoride Levels Recommended by US Public Health Service for Cool and Warm Climates

Annual Average of Maximum Daily Air Temperatures (°F)	Recommended Control Limits of F Concentrations (ppm)		
	Lower	Optimum	Upper
50.0–53.7	1.1	1.2	1.7
53.8–58.3	1.0	1.1	1.6
58.4–63.8	0.9	1.0	1.5
63.9–70.6	0.8	0.9	1.4
70.7–79.2	0.7	0.8	1.3
79.3–90.5	0.6	0.7	1.2

Source: Centers for Disease Control and Prevention. Engineering and administrative recommendations for water fluoridation. *MMWR Morb Mortal Wkly Rpt.* 2001;44(RR-13):1–40.

less access to dental care services and other sources of fluoride than higher income communities do.

See Table 2-2 ■ for the recommended levels of fluoride, depending on climate. In a warmer climate, less fluoride is needed because people drink more water. Because of the increased use of air conditioning in houses and automobiles, however, this theory may be changing.

Dental hygienists should be aware that bottled water often contains no fluoride or fails to identify its fluoride content on the label. See Table 2-3 ■ for bottled water requirements developed in 1995 and still in effect. The FDA has also given permission for bottled water to include enough fluoride to advertise the fluoride claim of reducing dental decay.[29]

Table 2-3   US Food and Drug Administration (FDA) Fluoride Requirements for Water Bottled in the United States

Annual Average of Maximum Daily Air Temperature (°F) of Retail Establishment Selling Bottled Water	Maximum Fluoride Concentration (mg/L) Allowed in Bottled Water	
	No Fluoride Added to Bottled Water	Fluoride Added to Bottled Water
53.7	2.4	1.7
53.8–58.3	2.2	1.5
58.4–63.8	2.0	1.3
63.9–70.6	1.8	1.2
70.7–79.2	1.6	1.0
79.3–90.5	1.4	0.8

Note: FDA regulations require that fluoride be listed on the label only if the bottler adds it during processing, but the bottler is not required to list the fluoride concentration, which might or might not be optimal. FDA does not allow imported bottled water with no added fluoride to contain >1.4 mg fluoride/L or with added fluoride to contain >0.8 mg fluoride/L.

Source: US Dept of Health and Human Services, Food and Drug Administration. Bottled water. 21 Code of Federal Regulations CFR). 1995;60:57124–57130.

BOX 2-1 Some Reasons Cited for Opposition to Water Fluoridation

- Violation of personal freedom
- Cause of disease(s) and/or medical conditions: cancer, AIDS, fatigue, etc.

- Forced medication
- Communist plot
- Abuse of police power

The only valid argument against community water fluoridation is that the addition of fluoride to water prevents personal choice. Refer to Box 2-1■ for some reasons people oppose public water fluoridation.

Did You Know?

Although opponents to community water fluoridation claim that it causes diseases, including cancer and multiple sclerosis, no credible evidence supports such an association.

The US Centers for Disease Control and Prevention recognizes the fluoridation of drinking water as one of ten great public health achievements of the twentieth century. In 2004, the Surgeon General issued a statement promoting the use of community water fluoridation as a cost-effective preventive measure that benefits all individuals without creating oral health disparities.

Defluoridation is the process of removing excess fluoride naturally present in a water supply to prevent dental fluorosis. South Carolina requested the defluoridation of naturally occurring 2.0 ppm fluoride, which would have cost an estimated $12 million. The state found that few of the small communities affected were interested in defluoridating because the degree of fluorosis did not concern them. They did not suffer ill effects, but they had a lower rate of caries.[30]

Fluoride Preventive Modalities

Community water fluoridation works both systemically and topically.[21] Its systemic effects occur as the fluoride becomes incorporated into the structure of the teeth. On the other hand, fluoridated toothpastes, mouth rinses, professional gels, fluoride varnish, and water fluoridation work topically. Laboratory and epidemiological research suggests that fluoride prevents dental caries predominately after eruption of the tooth into the mouth by inhibiting demineralization, enhancing remineralization, and inhibiting bacterial activity in dental plaque.[21]

In addition to community water fluoridation, other systemic fluoride modalities include the use of fluoride supplements. Dietary fluoride supplements are available in the form of tablets, lozenges, or liquids (including fluoride-vitamin preparations) and have been used throughout the world since the 1940s. Most supplements contain sodium fluoride as the active ingredient. Tablets and lozenges are manufactured with 1.0, 0.5, or 0.25 mg fluoride. To maximize its topical effect, tablets and lozenges are intended to be chewed or sucked for one to two minutes before being swallowed. Supplements for infants are available as a liquid and used with a dropper.[21] Although the primary teeth of children aged one to six years would benefit from fluoride's posteruptive action and possibly from the preeruptive benefit to developing permanent teeth, fluoride supplements also could increase the risk for enamel fluorosis at this age.[21]

The benefits of topically applied fluoride are well documented. Fluoride gels and foams professionally applied twice a year reportedly caused an average decrease of 26% in caries in the permanent teeth of children residing in nonfluoridated areas.[21] Fluoride-containing prophy paste is routinely used during dental hygiene treatment and contains 4000–20,000 ppm fluoride, which might restore the concentration of fluoride in the surface layer of enamel removed by polishing, but it this amount is not an adequate substitute for fluoride gel or varnish in treating persons at high risk for dental caries.

Fluoridated toothpastes are thought to decrease the prevalence of dental decay by 25%.[31] Over-the-counter fluoride mouth rinses decrease the prevalence of dental decay by 26%.[32] Patients with xerostomia, high caries rates, orthodontic therapy, or undergoing radiation treatment for cancer can decrease decay by up to 80% when utilizing a fluoride gel in a custom-made tray.[33] Fluoride varnishes applied by the dental hygienist are increasingly being used, although the FDA has approved them only for use as a desensitizing agent.[34] See Table 2-4 ■ for more information on fluoride modalities.

Table 2-4   Quality of Evidence, Strength of Recommendation, and Target Population
of Recommendation for Each Fluoride Modality to Prevent and Control Dental Caries

Modality[a]	Quality of Evidence (Grade)[d]	Strength of Recommendation (Code)[d]	Target Population[ab]
Community water fluoridation	II-1	A	All areas
School water fluoridation	II-3	C	Rural, nonfluoridated areas
Fluoride toothpaste	I	A	All persons
Fluoride mouthrinse	I	A	High risk[c]
Fluoride supplements			
Pregnant women	I	E	None
Children aged <6 years	II-3	C	High risk
Children aged 6–16 years	I	A	High risk
Persons aged >16 years		C	High risk
Fluoride gel	I	A	High risk
Fluoride varnish	I	A	High risk

[a]Modalities are assumed to be used as directed in terms of dosage and age of user.
[b]Quality of evidence for targeting some modalities to persons at high risk is grade III (i.e., representing the opinion of respected authorities) and is based on considerations of cost-effectiveness that were not included in the studies establishing efficacy or effectiveness.
[c]Populations believed to be at increased risk for dental caries are those with low socioeconomic status or low levels of parental education, those who do not seek regular dental care, and those without dental insurance or access to dental services. Individual factors that possibly increase risk include active dental caries; a history of high caries experience in older siblings or caregivers; root surfaces exposed by gingival recession; high levels of infection with cariogenic bacteria; impaired ability to maintain oral hygiene; malformed enamel or dentin; reduced salivary flow because of medications, radiation treatment, or disease; low salivary buffering capacity (ie, decreased ability of saliva to neutralize acids); and the wearing of space maintainers, orthodontic appliances, or dental prostheses. Risk can increase if any of these factors is combined with dietary practices conducive to dental caries (ie, frequent consumption of refined carbohydrates). Risk decreases with adequate exposure to fluoride.
[d]See US Preventive Services Task Force grading and coding systems.
No published studies confirm the effectiveness of fluoride supplements in controlling dental caries among persons aged >16 years.

Source: CDC Recommendations for using fluoride to prevent and control dental caries in the United States. *MMWR Morb Mortal Wkly Rpt.* 2001;50(RR14):1–42.

DENTAL SEALANTS

Dental sealants are plastic resins placed on tooth surfaces to prevent dental decay. Their placement is an effective means of preventing caries in pits and fissures, the areas least affected by fluoride.[35] Dental sealants (sometimes called *pit and fissure sealants*) should be placed as soon as possible after the tooth erupts and can be isolated to prevent moisture contamination. Indications for dental sealants also include a history of caries, xerostomia,

orthodontics, poor oral hygiene, and incipient caries. Some contraindications for sealants include patient behavior that does not permit a dry field and the presence of open occlusal carious lesions.

Sealants are cost-effective means to prevent occlusal, buccal pit, and lingual groove decay. On average, the cost of one surface restoration is more than the cost of a sealant placement.[36] Figure 2-5■ indicates sealant usage of a specific population in the United States.

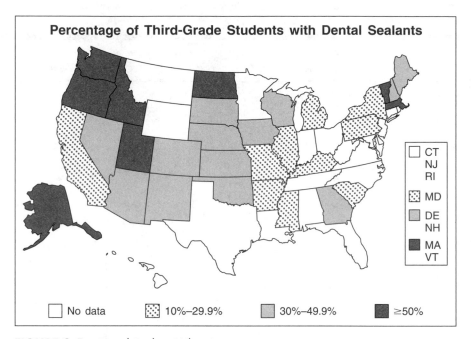

FIGURE 2-5 Dental Sealant Utilization
Source: CDC and the Association of State and Territorial Dental Directors. National Oral Health Surveilance System, 2006. Data from states vary by year of reporting. Available at http://www.cdc.gov/nohss.

Pits and fissures that remain completely sealed are well protected from caries, according to several investigations.[37] Moreover, studies have confirmed that complete retention rates after one year are 85% or better and after five years are at least 50%.[38] Sealants are effective in reducing the occlusal caries incidence in permanent first molars of children with reduction of 76.3% at four years when sealants were reapplied as needed. Caries reduction was 65% at nine years from initial treatment when sealants were not reapplied as needed.[39] Furthermore, sealants were retained on primary molars at a rate of 74–96% at 1.0 year and 71–77% at 2.8 years.[40,41]

Sealants are most effective when administered by a dental hygienist utilizing a dental assistant, a combination that has proved to be an effective force in public health settings. In fact, many communities have dental hygienists who travel to schools placing dental sealants. In some states, dentists are required to supervise their placement by dental hygienists, increasing the cost and subsequently decreasing cost-effectiveness. Moreover, in some states, a dentist must approve tooth surfaces before a dental hygienist places a sealant, a practice that further increases the time spent and decreases cost-effectiveness.

Alternative Restorative Treatment (ART)

When no restorative option is available to a patient, a provider can use a method called **alternative restorative treatment** (ART), formerly known as *atraumatic restorative treatment.* The provider removes carious lesions using hand instruments and restores the resultant cavity and adjoining fissures using a dental sealant, usually glass ionomer material.[42,43] This technique may be modified by the use of rotary instruments.[43]

ART is widely used in developing countries and in rural areas in developed countries. However, it may not be legal in some states for a dental hygienist to apply. The WHO and the International Association for Dental Research have endorsed ART as a means of restoring and preventing dental caries.[43]

Xylitol

Xylitol is a sugar substitute that has shown promising results in reducing dental decay and ear infections. It is found in berries, fruit, vegetables, mushrooms, and birch wood. Xylitol can be delivered in teeth via mints, gums, and lozenges to help reduce dental decay.

Advocates of xylitol use theorize that after chewing it, bacteria do not adsorb well on the surface of the teeth and, as a consequence, the amount of plaque decreases. However, some studies do not support the anticaries benefits.[43–45] In the United States, a dental public health initiative aimed at decreasing dental decay has begun researching the effects of daily xylitol intake.[46]

Nutritional Counseling

In *Mouth Hygiene,* the first textbook for dental hygienists that was published in 1916, the author states that normal nutrition and mouth cleanliness are the two most important factors for preventing dental pathology.[1–4] With this in mind, the dental hygienist must remember to incorporate nutritional counseling into all regimens related to oral health care. In fact, awareness of oral health is a major contributor to good nutrition. The oral cavity is the pathway to the body, and disturbances in the mouth can profoundly affect diet and ultimately nutritional status. Conversely, good nutrition provides the foundation for optimum oral health. Diet plays a major role in the etiology and prevention of dental caries and is an important supporting factor in other oral infections.

The ADHA recommends that dental hygienists maintain a current knowledge of nutrition recommendations and effectively educate and counsel their patients about proper nutrition and oral health.[47] Furthermore, the American Dietetic Association states that collaboration between dietetics and dental professionals is necessary for oral health promotion, disease prevention, intervention, and research.[48] It is important for dental hygienists to work with dietitians in community endeavors to educate and promote the importance of a healthy diet in oral health and, consequently, total health. The dental hygienist should also manage nutritional issues by making referrals to appropriate health care workers.

Oral Cancer Examinations and Tobacco Cessation

Tobacco use in any form is dangerous to a person's health. It is related to tooth staining, periodontal diseases, and oral and pharyngeal cancer. Each year, oral (mouth) and pharyngeal (throat) cancers, which are mainly squamous cell carcinomas, are diagnosed in approximately 30,000 US residents, and approximately 8000 persons die of these diseases.[49,50] Overall, relative five-year survival rates are approximately 54%, and mortality is nearly twice as high among certain minorities, especially African-American men, as among Caucasians.[49,50]

Dental professionals should conduct oral cancer exams annually and provide educational strategies designed to increase public awareness of these diseases. Dental hygienists in many states have the opportunity to provide OralCDX, a brush test method combined with advanced computer analysis to be used when abnormal tissue presents.[51] Another recent technology available for oral cancer screening is Vizilite®, which exposes oral tissues to a light source with a specific wavelength, causing normal healthy tissue and precancerous or cancerous tissues to fluoresce differently. The change in appearance occurs because their cellular composition causes them to reflect light at different rates. Using this handheld device, dental hygienists can visually assess oral tissues for abnormalities.[52] Both of these assessment modalities need more research to determine their overall effectiveness in early diagnosis of oral cancers. The referral to an oral surgeon for any tissue abnormality is paramount.

Dentists and hygienists can provide counseling to patients to stop tobacco use and limit alcohol use, both of which are associated with oral and pharyngeal cancer. In fact, one study suggested that approximately 90% of dentists and dental hygienists ask their patients if they smoke.[53] Unfortunately, many dental professionals stop after they ask the initial question. Programs to help smokers and tobacco chewers quit the habit are plentiful, and many campaigns exist to aid tobacco users. Many dental public health and private dental settings implement **tobacco cessation programs.** These programs encourage patients to quit using tobacco by employing ADHA's Ask, Advice and Refer program. To learn more on this program, go to the ADHA Web site.[54]

Athletic Mouth Guards

An **athletic mouth guard** is a removable oral appliance that protects the hard and soft tissues of the oral cavity and brain during contact sports. Sometimes referred to as *mouth protectors*, mouth guards protect by absorbing energy during an impact, thus decreasing the likelihood of trauma to the oral cavity and brain.[55,56]

Many orofacial injuries can be prevented by wearing athletic mouth guards, yet some individuals participating in athletic activities still do not wear them. The dental hygienist must promote their use by implementing mouth guard programs in school sports and private athletic organizations as well as educating the public on the value of mouth protection during contact sports, and fabricating mouth guards for athletes.

Did You Know?

Young athletes particularly are prone to sports-related orofacial trauma because they are less experienced than professional athletes. This makes the use of athletic mouth guards vitally important to this population.

The three types of mouth guards are the store-bought, boil-n-bite, and the custom-made mouth guards fabricated in the dental office. Dental providers (including dental hygienists in most states) can fabricate them simply by taking an alginate impression of the maxillary dentition, pouring a study model, and melting a thermoplastic material using a vacuum-forming machine. Custom-made mouth guards fit better and are recommended.

Mass Education and Promotion

One of the most important functions of the dental hygienist is to provide dental health education and promote dental health to the public. For these reasons, it is important for the dental hygienist to be well versed as an educator and public speaker. Chapter 8 includes an in-depth look into dental health education and promotion.

Many dental supply companies have developed educational materials for targeted populations. These materials are helpful to the dental hygienist and can be utilized by teachers and other health care workers. Moreover, many popular children's books and videos about dental health issues are also available.

Consumers also receive dental education and promotion through advertising, both in written form and through television. Many times television sitcoms discuss dental issues and even the role of dental hygienists. Sometimes this information is correct; however, these mass messages often give the population inaccurate information. Therefore, it is important for the dental hygienist to provide accurate information to the population.

DENTAL HYGIENIST SPOTLIGHT:
Commander Cathy Hollister, RDH, PhD

The mission of the Public Health Service (PHS) Commissioned Corps is to protect, promote and advance the health and safety of our Nation. Commander Cathy Hollister is a dental hygienist who works as a commissioned officer with the United States Public Health Service. She has been honored with more than ten awards in the Public Health Service and recently received the Navajo Area Director's Award for Health Promotion.

Commander Hollister has published articles on health behavior models and oral health in a variety of periodicals and has presented talks on oral health all over the nation. She has presided as chair of the American Dental Hygienists' Association Council on Public Health and contributed to the ADHA Focus on Advancing the Profession paper. She has been instrumental in enhancing the role of dental hygiene in dental public health in a variety of venues and organizations and is constantly

driven to build coalitions to effectively improve oral health status and the methods used to deliver care.

Commander Hollister has many professional accomplishments. She constantly promotes the skills of dental hygienists by effectively practicing dental hygiene in a variety of roles, subsequently providing quality care to the public.

I asked her several questions regarding her career.

Why did you decide to go into dental hygiene?

I knew I wanted to be in a health-related field. After high school, I volunteered in my dentist's office. I had a chance to observe many dental procedures, and I knew I wanted to work in dental care.

After practicing dental hygiene for a few years, I considered going back to dental school. I thought about it for a long time and decided I really wanted to stay in dental hygiene. I enjoyed the preventive side of dentistry and wanted to help people stay healthy rather than treat disease after it occurred.

How did you get into dental public health? Did you need additional education?

After working in private practices for eight years, I went to work in a community health center. That was my introduction to public health. I conducted a fluoride mouthrinse program in the schools and offered classroom education in many schools. Many of the students in the schools rarely saw a dentist, and the education they received at school was their only opportunity to learn about dental health and take control of their own oral health. I saw this as a real opportunity to improve the oral health of a large group of people, many of whom could not or did not have regular dental visits.

I knew I wanted to work in public health. I also knew I needed more education. At the time, I had an associate's degree in dental hygiene. I entered a certificate completion program to finish my bachelor's degree. Immediately following, I began to work on my master's degree in public health (MSPH). I had some public health education in my dental hygiene programs, but my MSPH gave me an excellent foundation for my present position.

I work in the US Public Health Service and after seven years in PHS, I entered a program to earn a doctorate in health services. I thought this education would help me improve the delivery of oral health services. I did my doctorate at a distance education university that allowed me great flexibility. I was able to study issues in oral health that affected utilization of health services, health education, and health care systems.

What is your current position?

Currently, I am the dental prevention officer with the Indian Health Services Gallup Service Unit, in Gallup, New Mexico. Additionally, I am the director of a dental hygiene clinic I developed and chair of the Medical Ethics Committee at Gallup Indian Medical Center. I also am an adjunct faculty member at the University of New Mexico, Division of Dental Hygiene in Albuquerque.

Please discuss any particularly interesting experiences you have had in your dental public health positions.

I have found it quite interesting to learn about the political side of health care. When I first began working in schools, I found that teachers may want to offer health education or services but could not because of so many demands on classroom time.

Nursing home aides wanted to do oral hygiene for the residents but often did not because of lack of time or because many residents needed dental services and none were available to them.

Public health has caused me to think about more than "How many patients do I have to see in a day?" It also has caused me to look past individual clinical care and look for community partners. I have had the opportunity to work with Head Start; Women, Infants and Children (WIC); diabetes programs; nursing homes; and schools. The most interesting and challenging aspect of working in public health has been finding common ground with nondental groups to increase oral health education, empower individuals to take charge of their own oral health, and increase access to dental services.

What type of advice would you give to a practicing hygienist who is thinking of doing something different?

First, enter a field you have a passion for. Second, make sure it is the right time in your life to make a change. Third, get adequate education or training. On-the-job training may be adequate if the change is very closely related to your current position, but if it is a major change, consider a degree program.

Source: Christine Nathe writes the Public Health Column in RDH magazine published by Pennwell Publishing.
For more public health spotlights please see RDH magazine online at http://www.rdhmag.com/index.html.

SUMMARY

Dental hygiene was the forerunner of the prevention movement now prevalent in public health care. Educating dental hygienists about preventive treatment modalities is vitally important to the public. Those involved in dental hygiene must continue to strive to meet the needs of the public by educating dental hygienists to provide effective preventive public-based care. Since the profession's inception, dental hygienists have worked to increase access to dental hygiene care provided by educated providers throughout the world, decrease barriers to the optimum level of dental hygiene care, and continue to provide care based on the evidence derived from dental hygiene research and practice.

SELF-STUDY TEST ITEMS

1. What is referred to as a constituent member in the ADHA organization?
   a. National organizations
   b. State organizations
   c. Local organizations
   d. Student organizations

2. When is school fluoridation recommended?
   a. When an independent water source is available
   b. For children who have caries
   c. For children who have brown discolored areas on enamel
   d. None of the above

3. Demineralization, enhancement of remineralization, and inhibition of bacterial activity are examples of what?
   a. Water fluoridation
   b. Topical fluoridation
   c. Systemic fluoridation
   d. Fluoride supplements

4. Which type of fluoride increases children's risk of developing dental fluorosis?
   a. Supplements
   b. Systemic
   c. Topical
   d. Both A and B

5. When are sealants most effective?
   a. When applied without etchant
   b. When an assistant is utilized
   c. In the presence of saliva
   d. When material is cured for one minute

REFERENCES

1. Dental Hygienists. *Occupational Outlook Handbook.* 2008-09 ed. http://www.bls.gov/oco/ocos097.htm. Accessed August 14, 2008.
2. Fones AC. *Mouth Hygiene.* Philadelphia, PA: Lea & Febiger; 1916:59–504.
3. Fones AC. *Mouth Hygiene.* 2nd ed. Philadelphia, PA: Lea & Febiger; 1927:307–335.
4. Fones AC. *Mouth Hygiene.* 3rd ed. Philadelphia, PA: Lea & Febiger; 1927:307–335.
5. Fones AC. *Mouth Hygiene.* 4th ed. Philadelphia, PA: Lea & Febiger; 1934:329–359.
6. Fones AC. Origin and history. *J Am Dent Hyg Assoc.* 1929(3): 9–10.
7. Motley W E. *History of the American Dental Hygienists' Association 1923–1982.* Chicago, IL: American Dental Hygienists' Association; 1983.
8. Ottolengui R. The inauguration of a serious effort to establish a system of education for the dental hygienist. *Dent Items of Int.* 1914;36(1):6.
9. Personal Notes. Alfred C. Fones, DDS. Bridgeport, CT. circa 1900s.
10. *Alabama Dental Hygiene Program: 2006–2007 Dentist-Instructor Manual.* Hoover, AL: Board of Dental Examiners of Alabama; 2006.
11. *Direct Access States.* Chicago, IL: American Dental Hygienists' Association; 2008.
12. History of the Connecticut dental hygienists' association. *J Am Dent Hyg Assoc.* 1931;5:26.
13. American Dental Hygienists' Association. 2007–2008 Bylaws Code of Ethics. Chicago, IL: American Dental Hygienists' Association; 2007:3.
14. US Public Health Service. *Healthy People 2010.* Washington, DC: US Dept of Health and Human Services; 2000.
15. US Dept of Health and Human Services. *Oral Health in America: A Report of the Surgeon General.* Rockville, MD: US Dept of Health and Human Services, National Institute of Dental and Craniofacial Research, National Institutes of Health; 2000.
16. US Dept of Health and Human Services. *A National Call to Action to Promote Oral Health.* Rockville, MD: US Dept of Health and Human Services, Public Health Service, Centers for Disease Control and Prevention, National Institutes of Health, National Institute of Dental and Craniofacial Research; 2003. NIH Publication No. 03-5303.
17. American Dental Association. *2003 Survey of Dental Practices.* http://www.ada.org/ada/prod/survey/publications practice.asp
18. Peterson PE. *The World Oral Health Report 2003.* Geneva, Switzerland: World Health Organization; 2003. http://www.who.int/oral_health/media/en/orh_report03_en.pdf. Accessed August 14, 2008.
19. American Dental Hygienists' Association. *National Dental Hygiene Research Agenda.* Chicago, IL: American Dental Hygienists' Association; 2007.
20. The Professional Practice Environment of Dental Hygienists in the Fifty States and the District of Columbia, 2001. National Center for Health Workforce Analysis, Bureau of Health Professions, Health Resources and Services Administration; 2004. Contract No. HRSA 230-00-0099.

21. Recommendations for using fluoride to prevent and control dental caries in the United States. *MMWR Morb Mortal Wkly Rpt.* 2001;50(RR14):1–42.

22. Newbrun E. Effectiveness of water fluoridation. *J Public Health Dent.* 1989;49:279–289.

23. Riley JC, Lennon MA, Ellwood RP. The effect of water fluoridation and social inequalities on dental caries in 5-year-old children. *Int J Epidemiol.* 1999;28:300–305.

24. The relation of mottled enamel to caries. *JADA.* 1928;15:429–437.

25. The Story of Water Fluoridation. Bethesdea, MD: National Institutes of Dental Craniofacial; 2008. http://www.nidcr.nih.gov/OralHealth/Topics/Fluoride/TheStoryofFluoridation.htm. Accessed March 4, 2009.

26. Centers for Disease Control and Prevention. 2006 Water Fluoridation Reporting System (WFRS). http://www.cdc.gov/FLUORIDATION/statistics/2006stats.htm. Accessed April 23, 2008.

27. Engineering and administrative recommendations for water fluoridation, 1995. *MMWR Morb Mortal Wkly Rpt.* 1995;44(RR-13):1–40.

28. Riley JC, Lennon MA, Ellwood RP. The effect of water fluoridation and social inequalities on dental caries in 5-year-old children. *Int J Epidemiol.* 1999;28:300–305.

29. Fluoridated Water Bottle Claims 2008. http://www.cdc.gov/FLUORIDATION/fact_sheets/bottled_water.htm. Accessed August 20, 2008.

30. Newburn E. *Fluorides and Dental Caries.* Springfield, IL: Charles C. Thomas; 1986; National Research Council. *Health Effects of Ingested Fluoride.* Washington, DC: National Academy Press; 1993.

31. Topping G, Assaf A. Strong evidence that daily use of fluoride toothpaste prevents caries. *Acta Odonto Scand.* 2003;61(6):347–355.

32. Marinho VCC, Higgins JPT, Logan S, Sheiham A. Fluoride mouthrinses for preventing dental caries in children and adolescents. *Cochrane Database of Systematic Reviews.* 2003;3(CD002284.DOI:10.1002/14651858.CD002284).

33. Englander HR, Keyes, PH, Gestwicki M. Clinical anticaries effect of repeated topical sodium fluoride applications by mouthpieces. *JADA.* 1967;75:638.

34. Marinho VCC, Higgins JPT, Logan S, Sheiham A. Fluoride varnishes for preventing dental caries in children and adolescents. *Cochrane Database of Systematic Reviews.* 2002;3(CD002279. DOI: 10.1002/14651858.CD002279).

35. Dental sealants in the prevention of tooth decay. *NIH Consens Dev Conf Consens Statement 1983.* 1983;4(11):1–18.

36. Simonsen RJ. Retention and effectiveness of a single application of white sealant after 10 years *JADA.* 1987;115:31–36.

37. Griffin SO, Oong E, Kohn B, Vidakovic B, Gooch, BF, CDC Dental Sealant Systematic Review Work Group, Bader J., Clarkson J, Fontana MR, Meyer DM, Rozier RG, Weintraub JA, Zero DT. The effectiveness of sealants in managing caries lesions. *Dent Res.* 2008;87:169–174.

38. Beltrán-Aguilar ED, Barker LK, Canto MT, Dye BS, Gooch BF, Griffin SO, Hyman J, Jaramillo F, Kingman A, Nowjack-Raymer R, Selwitx RH, Wu T. Surveillance for dental caries, dental sealants, tooth retention, edentulism, and enamel fluorosis—United States, 1988–1994 and 1999–2002. *MMWR Morb Mortal Wkly Rpt.* 2005;54(3):1–44.

39. Bravo M, Montero J, Bravo JJ, Baca P, Llodra JC. Sealant and fluoride varnish in caries: A randomized trial. *J Dent Res.* 2005;84(12):1138–1143.

40. Hotuman E, Rolling I, Poulsen S. Fissure sealants in a group of 3–4 year old children. *Int J Paediatr Dent* 1998;8(1):46–50.

41. Hardison JR, Collier DR, Sprouse LW, Van Cleave ML, Hogan AD. Retention of pit and fissure sealant on the primary molars of 3–4 year old children after 1 year. *JADA* 1987;114(5):613–615.

42. Mjor IA, Gordan VV. A review of atraumatic restorative treatment (ART). *Int Dent J.* 1999;49:127–131.

43. Policy on alternative restorative treatment (ART). *Reference Manual.* 2008;29(7).

44. Stecksén-Blicks C, Holgerson PL, Twetman S. Effect of xylitol and xylitol-fluoride lozenges on approximal caries development in high-caries-risk children. *Int J Paediatri Dent.* 2008;18(3):170–177.

45. Oscarson P, Lif Holgerson P, Sjöström I, Twetman S, Stecksén-Blicks C. Influence of a low xylitol-dose on mutans streptococci colonisation and caries development in preschool children. *Eur Arch Paeditr Dent.* 2006;7(3):142–147.

46. Xylitol Adult Caries Trial (X-ACT) Verified by National Institute of Dental and Craniofacial Research. http://clinicaltrials.gov/ct2/show/NCT00393055?recr= open&cond=%22Dental+Caries%22&rank=7. Accessed June 8, 2009.

47. *American Dental Hygienists' Association: Bylaws.* Chicago, IL: American Dental Hygienists' Association; 2008.

48. Position of the American Dietetic Association: Oral health and nutrition. *J Am Diet Assoc.* 2007;107(8):1418–1428.

49. American Cancer Society. *Cancer Facts & Figures 2001.* Atlanta, GA: American Cancer Society; 2001.

50. Greenlee RT, Hill-Harmon MB, Murray T, Thun M. Cancer statistics, 2001. *CA Cancer J Clin.* 2001;51:15–36.

51. OralCDx BrushTest. http://www.sopreventable.com/brushtest.htm. Accessed April 23, 2008.

52. Ebihara A, Krasieva TB, Liaw LL, Fago S, Messadi D, Osann K, Wilder-Smith P. Detection and diagnosis of oral

cancer by light-induced fluorescence. *Lasers in Surg and Med.* 2003;32:17–24.

53. Tobacco control activities in US dental practices. *JADA.* 1997;18:172.

54. Ask, Advise, Refer Tobacco Cessation Program. American Dental Hygienists' Association. http://www.adha.org/media/facts/tobacco.htm. Accessed April 23, 2008.

55. Nathe CN. Athletic Mouthguards Chapter in Harris, NO, Garcia-Godoy, F, Nathe, CN. *Primary Preventive Dentistry.* 7th ed. Upper Saddle River, NJ: Pearson; 2008, page 388.

56. American Dental Association. Using mouthguards to reduce the incidence and severity of sports-related oral injuries. *J Am Dent Assoc.* 2006;37:1712–1720.

PEARSON

my health professions kit™

Multimedia Extension Activities

Use this address to access the interactive Companion Website created for this textbook. Simply select "Dental Hygiene" from the choice of disciplines. Find this book and log in using your username and password. To obtain a username and password, please register using the scratch-off access code on the inside front cover of this book.

Chapter 3

Dental Care Delivery in the United States

OBJECTIVES

After studying this chapter, the dental hygiene student should be able to:

- Describe the state of dental health in the United States
- Identify the government agencies related to dental hygiene
- Compare the functions of federal, state, and local government in dental care delivery
- Describe dental workforce issues
- Define *need, supply, demand,* and *utilization*

KEY TERMS

Demand
Dental care delivery
Medicaid
Need
Supply
Utilization
Workforce

COMPETENCIES

After studying this chapter and participating in accompanying course activities, the dental hygiene student should be competent to do the following:

- Evaluate the oral health needs of the community and the quality and availability of resources and services
- Facilitate patient access to oral health services by influencing individuals and/or organizations regarding the provision of oral health care
- Identify career options within health care, industry, education, and research and evaluate the feasibility of pursuing dental hygiene opportunities
- Access professional and social networks to pursue professional goals

Dental care delivery refers to the way dental care is provided to the public. In the United States, dental care delivery involves a number of different private and government entities. Although most dental hygienists are employed by private practice dentists, many dental hygiene positions are available with government- or community-based organizations. This chapter describes the infrastructure including the federal and state entities that play a role in dental care as well as concepts germane to the utilization of dental care services and dental workforce models.

Landmark reports suggest that the current dental care system in the United States does not ensure oral health care for all populations.[1–4] Although dental diseases are preventable, the current oral health system has many disparities in prevention. Untreated dental disease is more prevalent in individuals from lower-income households, ethnic minorities, and those with special health care needs.[1–4]

Oral health is an integral part of total health. Research has associated periodontal diseases to heart, lung, and a number of other systemic diseases, diabetes, and premature, low-birth-weight babies.[1] Prevention and early intervention are strategies long recognized across health disciplines as being effective in terms of dollars spent on health care and minimizing or eliminating human pain and suffering. Dental hygiene science, which emphasizes disease prevention and treatment of oral infection, fits perfectly into an interdisciplinary model to provide comprehensive health care to all populations.

DELIVERY OF DENTAL CARE IN THE UNITED STATES

Private dental practices for the most part provide dental care delivery in the United States. Figure 3-1 ■ depicts the agents involved in the delivery of dental care: dentists, dental hygienists, dental assistants, denturists (in some states), dental therapists (in Alaska), expanded function dental personnel, and dental technicians. Most Americans obtain their care from private dental and dental hygiene providers with employer-offered dental insurance as the reimbursement mechanism. The government plays a small role in funding and regulating dental care delivery.

> **Did You Know?**
>
> Denturists are providers who construct and deliver removable oral prosthesis (dentures and partial dentures) directly to the patient.

Many federal and state governmental entities impact dental care delivery. Additionally, states impose practice acts and rules and regulations to govern the practice of dental hygiene, which is discussed in Chapter 6.

FEDERAL STRUCTURE OF DENTAL PUBLIC HEALTH

The executive branch of the federal government has a direct impact on dental care delivery. The Department of Health and Human Services (HHS) is responsible for many entities providing dental care.

Department of Health and Human Services

The HHS is the government's principal agency for protecting the health of all Americans and providing essential human services, especially for those who are least

FIGURE 3-1   Dental Care Delivery in the United States

able to help themselves. The HHS includes more than 300 programs, covering a wide spectrum of activities. (See Box 3-1 ■.) HHS administers more grant dollars than all other federal agencies combined, and its Medicare program provides health care insurance for one in four Americans. HHS works closely with state and local governments, and many HHS-funded services are provided at the local level by state or county agencies or private sector grantees. See Figure 3-2 ■ for the HHS organizational chart. The secretary of the department, who directs the HHS, is appointed by the president of the United States.

US Public Health Service Commissioned Corps

The US Public Health Service (PHS) works to improve and advance the health of our nation's people. It includes several separate entities. The PHS Commissioned Corps, which is directed by the US surgeon general, was established by Congress in 1889. Congress organized it along military lines with titles and pay corresponding to army and navy grades. Officers are currently commissioned in eleven professional categories representing the breadth of health care professionals.

National Institutes of Health

The National Institutes of Health (NIH) headquartered in Bethesda, Maryland, is the government's medical research organization, supporting some 38,000 research projects nationwide in diseases such as cancer, Alzheimer's disease, diabetes, arthritis, cardiovascular diseases, and AIDS. NIH has twenty-seven separate health institutes, including the National Institute of Dental and Craniofacial Research (NIDCR), which focuses on research in the oral health sciences.

Food and Drug Administration

The Food and Drug Administration (FDA) was established in 1906 and headquartered in Rockville, Maryland, ensures the safety of foods and cosmetics as well as the safety and efficacy of pharmaceuticals, biological products, and medical devices. It is responsible for regulating dental materials, dental equipment, and over-the-counter dental care products.

Did You Know?

Products regulated by FDA represent almost 25 cents out of every dollar in consumer spending in the United States.

Centers for Disease Control and Prevention

The Centers for Disease Control and Prevention (CDC) provides a system of health surveillance to prevent the

---

BOX 3-1   Activities of the US Department of Health and Human Services

- Provision of health and social science research
- Prevention of disease including immunization services
- Assurance of food and drug safety
- Provision of Medicare (health insurance for elderly and disabled Americans) and Medicaid (health insurance for specific populations)
- Involvement in health information technology
- Provision of financial assistance and services for low-income families
- Improvement of maternal and infant health

- Support of Head Start (preschool education and services)
- Support of faith-based and community initiatives
- Prevention of child abuse and domestic violence
- Treatment and prevention of substance abuse
- Support of services for older Americans including home-delivered meals
- Provision of comprehensive health services for Native Americans
- Support of medical preparedness for emergencies, including potential terrorism

Source: US Department of Health and Human Services. What We Do; 2008. http://www.hhs.gov/about/whatwedo.html/. Accessed August 7, 2008.

FIGURE 3-2 US Department of Health and Human Services: Organizational Chart

Source: http://www.hhs.gov/about/orgchart.html. Accessed September 2, 2008.

outbreak of diseases and monitor any that do occur. It also maintains national health statistics. Established in 1946 and located in Atlanta, Georgia, it provides immunization services to guard against international disease transmission. The CDC plays a major role in preparing guidelines for the prevention of oral diseases. Its director is also administrator of the Agency for Toxic Substances and Disease Registry.

Indian Health Services

The Indian Health Service (IHS), established in 1955, provides 1.8 million Native Americans, including Alaskan Natives, with medical and dental care. It also assists thirty-four urban Native American health centers. Dental hygienists and dentists can work for the IHS as PHS commissioned officers, civil servants, or independent contractors. In many IHS settings, dental assistants provide some dental hygiene services to the Native American population, including scaling and polishing and some restorative services. In fact, because of the shortage of dentists in Alaska, dental therapists provide restorative services.

Did You Know?

The federal government first offered health services for Indians in the early nineteenth century when US army physicians took steps to curb smallpox and other contagious diseases among tribes living in the vicinity of military posts. By 1880, the first federal hospital was built in Oklahoma making health care available to Indians. By 1913, dentists were visiting reservations and schools to provide dental services.[5]

In addition to the IHS dental services, many individual tribes offer dental services and maintain clinics. Each of the more than 560 federally recognized tribes govern tribal dental clinics and employ dental hygienists, dentists, and dental assistants.

Health Resources and Services Administration

The Health Resources and Services Administration (HRSA) provides health resources for medically underserved populations and works to build the health care **workforce,** the workers whose members deliver health care to the public. It operates a nationwide network of community health centers, migrant health centers, and primary care programs. HRSA also maintains the National Health Service Corps, which provides services to people with AIDS through the Ryan White CARE Act, oversees the organ transplantation system, and works to decrease infant mortality and improve children's health. Dental hygienists may serve with the National Health Service Corps.

Agency for Healthcare Research and Quality

The Agency for Healthcare Research and Quality (AHRQ) supports research on health care systems, health care quality and cost issues, access to health care, and effectiveness of medical treatments. It also provides evidence-based information on health care

outcomes and quality of care. These data include oral health information.

Administration of Aging

The Administration on Aging (AOA) is the principal agency designated to carry out the provisions of the Older Americans Act of 1965 and is responsible for enhancing and supporting the older population's independence. It has been involved in dental education in geriatric dental care.

Administration of Children and Families

The Administration for Children and Families (ACF) is responsible for federal programs that promote the economic and social well-being of families, children, individuals, and communities and is responsible for the Early Head Start and Head Start programs, which provide educational, social, medical, dental, nutritional, and mental health services to pregnant mothers and children up to five years old from low-income families.

Did You Know?

In many states, dental hygienists provide education and preventive treatment to children enrolled in Head Start programs.

Centers for Medicare and Medicaid Services

The Centers for Medicare & Medicaid Services (CMS), formerly known as the Health Care Financing Administration (HCFA), is the federal agency responsible for administering the Medicare, Medicaid, Children's Health Insurance Program (CHIP), Health Insurance Portability and Accountability Act (HIPAA), Clinical Laboratory Improvement Amendments (CLIA), and several other health-related programs. CMS also oversees the federal portion of the Medicaid program and has full responsibility for the Medicare program. Medicare funds cover medical care for people who are elderly and/or disabled. In specific cases, Medicare may provide reimbursement for dental procedures carried out in the hospital on elderly or disabled individuals, but it generally does not fund dental care.

Medicaid is the program that traditionally funds dental care to the indigent population and is administered by states. Medicaid insurance can be paid to dentists and, in some states, dental hygienists in private practice or community clinical settings.

Medicare and Medicaid are the two largest federal health care programs and account for about 80 percent of annual federal health care expenditures. The CMS also runs CHIP, the largest effort by Congress since Medicaid was enacted thirty-two years ago to provide health insurance to vulnerable children throughout the United States. Enacted as part of the Balanced Budget Act of 1997, it addresses the health care needs of 10 million medically uninsured children. CHIP is distinct from Medicaid in that it entitles states, but not individual children, to allotments of federal funds to purchase child health assistance; it pays a 30 percent higher share of program costs than Medicaid, and it gives states more latitude in program design, including eligibility, benefits, cost sharing, and administration. Chapter 5 discusses in detail the financial aspects of Medicaid and CHIPS.

Other Federal Dental Health Programs

Many other federal departments impact dental health, including the Departments of Agriculture, Defense, Education, Justice, Labor, State, Treasury, and Veteran's Affairs. Dental hygienists have the opportunities to work in various federal government positions and settings. (See Table 3-1 ■.) To qualify for a civil service dental hygiene position, a candidate must be a US citizen and undergo a thorough background investigation to receive a security clearance. In some instances, a bachelor's degree may be required.

Food, nutrition counseling, and access to health and dental services are provided to low-income women, infants, and children under the Special Supplemental Nutrition Program for Women, Infants, and Children (WIC). Specifically, its programs collaborate with dental hygiene programs and community dental clinics to offer dental screenings and dental health education. The Food and Nutrition Services of the Department of Agriculture administers WIC at the federal level, providing federal grants to states for their WIC programs. Most

Table 3-1 Federal Dental Hygiene Settings and Positions

Department/Agency	Settings
Agriculture	Women, Infant, Children (WIC)
Defense	Military base
Justice	Federal prison
Health and Human Services	Public Health Service commissioned officer
	Early Head Start and Head Start
	Centers for Disease Control and Prevention
	Researcher/Administrator
	National Institutes of Dental and Craniofacial Research
Peace Corps (Agency)	Dental hygienist in a developing country
State	Civil service position with military, VA hospital, or other governmental agency
Veteran's Affairs	Dental hygienist at a VA hospital

state WIC programs provide vouchers that participants use at authorized food stores.

The Department of Defense oversees the dental care of military dental personnel and their dependents often provided by dentists in the military and enlisted dental technicians. One interesting facet of dental care delivery in the military is that in some military branch dental settings, enlisted dental technicians provide supragingival scalings and coronal polishing, which are termed *prophylaxis* (measures designed to preserve health and prevent the spread of disease) without having graduated from an accredited dental hygiene program or taking the national and regional dental hygiene board examinations. This practice, however, is becoming less common. Dental hygienists may work as civil servants or independent contractors for the Department of Defense, and dental hygienists with bachelor of science degrees may work as military officers. Dependents of military personnel generally receive care through the dental providers participating in the dental insurance program available to them through military benefits.

Did You Know?

Dental hygienists are being hired more frequently to provide dental hygiene care and education in military bases around the United States.

In the United States, inmates have a constitutional right to health care. The Department of Justice is responsible for the Federal Bureau of Prisons and therefore the dental care provided to prisoners. Dentists and dental hygienists may work as US PHS officers, civil servants, or independent contractors. Settings can vary from prison camps for minor offenders to maximum-security prisons. Providing dental hygiene to this population decreases cost by decreasing the need for restorative services.

Many dental hygienists practice in facilities under the Department of Veteran's Affairs (VA), treating veterans with service-connected dental disabilities. Dentists, dental hygienists, assistants, and technicians are usually employed as civil servants. Occasionally, VA dental services treat members who have left military service but did not complete their dental care as well as veterans who live in long-term care facilities at the individual VA

medical centers. Dental hygienists in this setting provide a variety of services, including educating patients and nurses and offering clinical treatment within the dental clinic and at the bedside.

The Bureau of Labor Statistics (BLS), which is organizationally housed within the Department of Labor, is the principal fact-finding agency for the federal government in the broad field of labor, economics, and statistics. It collects, processes, analyzes, and disseminates essential statistical data to the American public, the Congress and federal agencies, state and local governments, business, and labor. The BLS forecasts dental and dental hygiene workforce need and demand for future years.

The Department of Treasury is responsible for the manufacturing and labeling of alcohol and tobacco products. Its work is important in promoting health-related problems that are often acquired by use of these products.

The Department of Education's mission is to ensure equal access to education and to promote educational excellence for all Americans. It provides federal financial aid policies to many dental hygiene students.

The Peace Corps, an independent agency within the executive branch of the federal government, was formally initiated in 1961. The president of the United States appoints the Peace Corps director and deputy director who must be confirmed by the Senate. The Senate Foreign Relations Committee and the House Committee on International Relations have general oversight of Peace Corps activities and programs.

Did You Know?

Dental hygienists can provide dental hygiene treatment and education as Peace Corps volunteers.

STRUCTURE OF STATE DENTAL PUBLIC HEALTH

All states and Washington, D.C., and US territories, have departments that provide health and human services to those in need. The departments may have different names, but all share a similar mission that includes preventing disease and promoting health, ensuring access to health care, and managing public health resources.

State health departments include dental divisions whose directors work as dental consultants within the state. Dental hygienists may be employed as state dental directors in many states. Many of these departments work to implement water fluoridation within communities, school-based prevention programs, school sealant programs, and fluoride mouth rinse programs. Some state health departments are in charge of the CHIPS program as well. The human services division of the state health department usually operates Medicaid programs, which are often operated by a third party, generally an insurance company.

Did You Know?

The American Association of State and Territorial Dental Directors (AASTDD) provides leadership to advocate a governmental oral health presence in each state and territory and to assist in the development of initiatives for prevention and control of oral diseases.

Many states operate community clinics to provide dental care, and some states own and operate community clinics, many of which employ dental hygienists to provide services. Some of these clinics are private, and many are nonprofit but sometimes receive sliding scale reimbursements and Medicaid payments. State dental clinics can be federally qualified heath centers (FQHCs), meaning that they qualify for enhanced reimbursement from Medicaid and other benefits. FQHCs must provide services for an underserved area or population, offer a sliding fee scale, provide comprehensive services, have an ongoing quality assurance program, and have a governing board of directors. Although some of these clinics are in an urban (metropolitan) setting, many operate in rural or other settings where the population is underserved.

State or private organizations operate state prison systems that are separate from the Federal Bureau of Prisons but also provide dental care to inmates.

States may also have tribal dental clinics that usually follow guidelines established within the tribe. In some instances, the IHS provides assistances. Dental hygienists are often employed in these clinics and may provide care in migrant clinics as well.

Many states provide dental care to the elderly and developmentally disabled in institutionalized dental clinic settings. Care to these groups is difficult to obtain in private dental practices because of the difficulty in transportation, low reimbursement rates, treatment specialization needed, and refusal by providers to accept Medicaid insurance.

DENTAL HEALTH CARE WORKFORCE

In the United States, *pluralism* refers to the way of organizing and providing health care services because of the diversity of values, populations, and entities involved.[6] The dental care delivery system is a mixture of organizations, practitioners, financing mechanisms, and innovative approaches to health care.

Those concerned with planning to meet health labor force requirements attach a specific meaning to the concepts of need, demand, utilization, and supply. **Need** can be defined as a normative, professional judgment as to the amount and kind of health care services required to attain or maintain health. The particular or desired frequency of dental care by a population is **demand,** and the amount of dental care services available can be termed **supply. Utilization** is the number of dental care services actually consumed, not just desired, which can be important when speculating on the available supply of personnel to meet the demand and/or need. One example of the difference between need and demand is demonstrated with children's athletic teams. Players on these teams have high rates of oral-facial injuries and concussions, and professional recommendations mandate the use of mouth guards, preferably custom-made ones; however, many young athletes across the country do not wear them. In this case, the need is present—oral health professionals have determined that using mouth guards will maintain health—but the demand by consumers is not because they are not using them as desired. Now, assume that consumers' demand is great, but their communities lack the dental providers to fabricate the mouth guards. This scenario would change the equation by not having the supply to meet the demand and the need.

The federal guidelines forecast the number of dentists needed for a population but do not include the number of dental hygienists necessary. Adequate dental capacity as suggested by the National Health Professional

Shortage Area (HPSA) is designated as one dentist per 2000 population,[7,8] but HHS considers the appropriate dentist-to-population ratio as at least one dentist per 5000. Furthermore, the appropriate dentist-to-population ratio for a special consideration population, such as a state facility or reservation, has been estimated at one dentist per 4000 population.

Dental Workforce Issues

The landmark 2000 Oral Health in America report concluded that the public health workforce was not sufficient to meet the dental needs of the underserved.[1] The reasons for this include barriers to oral health care access, lack of insurance or payment options, tremendous growth of the aging population, limited means of transportation, and insufficient availability of dental providers.[1–4] These issues have resulted in the development of innovative models of delivery and proposed additions to the dental team.

Models of Care

Although the provision of dental hygiene originated in schools, in most states it has not been practiced there. However, school children in an increasing number of states are receiving preventive dental care. In some states, schools also provide restorative care. Sometimes this is accomplished with mobile dental programs, but recently school-based health clinics have begun to hire dental hygienists. Preventive dental care also is being brought into Early Head Start and Head Start programs, WIC programs, and nursing facilities.

Another opportunity to bring prevention to the people is to place dental hygienists in pediatric offices, primary care clinics, and hospitals. Positioning dental hygienists within health care systems allows them to provide the missing link between total health and oral health. This also provides an effective referral mechanism with local dentists. Bringing care *to* populations in need is one solution to the oral health disparities witnessed today.

Dentist Shortage

Although the American Dental Association (ADA) projects an increase in the aggregate number of dentists over the next two decades, the increase will not keep pace with the projected population growth.[9] Additionally, the BLS concluded that the employment of dentists is not expected to keep pace with the escalating demand for their services.[10]

It is logical to assume that in the near future the shortage of dentists will be more pronounced. A large number of aging dentists are projected to retire from practice during the next ten to fifteen years.[11] During the next decade, two dentists will retire for every new graduate.[12] In addition, geographic distribution of dentists remains problematic. In large metropolitan areas, the dentist-to-population ratio was 61 per 100,000 as compared to 29 dentists per 100,000 in rural areas.[13]

Demand for Dental Hygienists

Dental hygiene continues to grow as a profession, and the market continues to dictate the need for dental hygiene providers. Dental hygienists held about 167,000 jobs in 2006, and their employment is expected to increase much faster than the average employment areas.[14]

To meet the increasing demand for dental hygiene, facilities that provide dental care, particularly dentists' offices, will increasingly employ dental hygienists and more per office to perform services that dentists have performed in the past. Older dentists who have been less likely to employ dental hygienists are leaving the profession and will be replaced by recent graduates, who are more likely to employ dental hygienists. In addition, as dentists' workloads increase, they are expected to hire more hygienists to perform preventive dental care, such as cleaning, so that they may devote their own time to more complex procedures.[14]

Denturists

Denturists are trained to provide complete oral examinations and evaluation of patients and to directly provide them removable dentures and fit them properly.[15] They are legally allowed to practice in seven states. Although fairly new to the United States, denturists have the potential to provide care to many older adults.

Dental Therapists

Beginning in 2000, Alaska Native tribal health organizations developed the Alaska Dental Health Therapist Initiative, a new solution to address rural Alaska dental needs.[16] It includes the Alaska dental health aide therapist (DHAT) concept that is an accepted primary model of care in more than fifty countries. The Alaska DHAT student completes a two-year program and focuses on providing restorative care in patients in remote areas under the supervision of a dentist who is responsible for writing standing orders and being the point of contact for the therapists through telehealth.[11] Telehealth is the delivery of health services using telecommunications, such as a non-dentist providing care in an unsupervised setting and communicating any questions to the dentist via the telephone or computer.

At present, DHATs may practice only in the state of Alaska.

Proposed Providers

The *National to Call to Action to Promote Oral Health* identified the need to enhance oral health workforce capacity in the United States. The DHAT program was a response to that call as were the following proposed dental care providers.

Advanced Dental Hygiene Practitioner The American Dental Hygienists' Association developed the position of *advanced dental hygiene practitioner* (ADHP) to improve the underserved public's health.

Specifically, the ADHP as a mid-level provider will provide diagnostic, preventive, therapeutic, and restorative services as well as referrals to dentists and other health care providers in a variety of settings. The focus of care for this provider will still be prevention, but the ADHP will also have the ability to stop infection by restoring demineralized tooth surfaces and prescribing medicine. ADHPs will be educated in master's degree programs.[13]

The concept of a mid-level provider is well accepted in the medical field and integrated into the health care arena. For example, the nursing profession has developed the nurse practitioner position in response to unmet public health needs. Applied to the dental health field, the mid-level practitioner model will allow greater access to care. At present, many states are proposing legislation to approve this provider model.

Community Dental Health Coordinator The American Dental Association has proposed the addition of the community dental health coordinator (CDHC) in response to the *National to Call to Action.*[17] The CDHC would perform many duties, such as oral hygiene instruction and coronal polishing, that dental assistants and dental hygienists do today but must be supervised by a dentist at all times.[11] Table 3-2 ■ compares these proposed new models of dental providers.

Table 3-2 Comparison of New Models of Dental Providers

	Advanced Dental Hygiene Practitioner (ADHP)	Alaska Dental Therapist (DHAT)	Community Dental Health Coordinator (CDHC)
Proposed or currently available	Proposed	Currently practiced in Alaska Indian Health Service Clinics	Proposed
Developing organization	American Dental Hygienists' Association	United States Public Health Service	American Dental Association
Degree	Master's degree	No degree required	No degree required
Physical presence of dentists required for clinical care	No	No	Yes
Clinical focus	Prevention and primary restorative	Restorative	Prevention
State license required	Yes	No	No

DENTAL HYGIENIST SPOTLIGHT:
Beth McKinney, RDH, MS

Beth McKinney is a dental hygienist and case manager with the Montgomery County, Maryland, Public Health Department. She graduated with honors from both the University of Maryland with a Bachelor of Science Degree in Dental Hygiene and from Old Dominion University with a Master's of Science Degree in Dental Hygiene.

Ms. McKinney previously worked as a patient care coordinator with the National Institutes of Health in Bethesda, Maryland. She treated medically compromised and acutely ill patients and provided oral health education for health care providers. She also coordinated hospital care for patients in several research studies and participated in research studies. Ms. McKinney has taught as an adjunct faculty member with dental hygiene programs in the area as well. She has also worked for the US Department of the Navy as a dental hygienist and in the dental insurance industry as a quality assurance coordinator.

Ms. McKinney is a member of Sigma Phi Alpha, the national dental hygiene honor society, and was bestowed the Outstanding Performance Award, Naval Dental Clinic; the Employee Service Award at the National Institutes of Health (NIH); and recently was honored as the recipient of the Sunstar Butler/RDH magazine Award of Distinction, which is presented to dental hygienists of distinction (September 2005 RDH).

Clearly, Ms. McKinney's career in dental public health has been multifaceted. A dental hygienist who has the skills to practice in public health and by advancing his or her education will find opportunities more easily.

I asked Ms. McKinney a few questions.

Why did you decide to go into dental hygiene?

I'm not sure it was a conscious decision. I was a dental assistant for a while out of high school. I wanted to work in the health care profession, but all of my relatives were nurses, and they always complained about their jobs. So I thought dental hygiene might be the way to go.

How did you get into dental public health? Did you need additional education?

Surprisingly, I have to say that I found all of my jobs in public health through ads in the paper. Traditionally, this is not reputed to be the best way to network and make career moves. I got into this right out of school when I took a job doing quality assurance for a dental insurance company. The only days I have ever spent in private practice as a hygienist have been as a temp. I quickly found that I loved the variety and autonomy that come with working in public health.

In order to be successful in public health, I really think a bachelor's degree is necessary. An advanced degree certainly helped me be very competitive for jobs. Familiarity with statistics, research, budgets, and program management are all essential skills for working in the public health sector. Most of that kind of education you get in an advanced program. Having that knowledge made it very easy to adapt to the roles I've been called upon to fill.

What are your current positions?

I currently work for a county health department. I'm responsible for the program that treats children and pregnant women. I deliver care, manage cases, and do statistical reporting. I'm also responsible for clinic management and the supply budgets for three clinics. I teach students on rotation from a nearby dental hygiene program. I'm responsible for OSHA compliance, infection control, and quality assurance audits conducted on all dental programs the county offers. I do some group education, too, when I can fit the requests into my schedule.

Can you discuss any particularly interesting experiences you have had in your dental public health positions?

I have a ton of stories. Once when I was working at NIH, I treated a patient who was there for a bone marrow transplant. He required ten packs of platelets prior to the scaling visit. When I was cleaning up, I picked up the instrument cassette where an explorer was poking out from underneath and punctured my finger. Up at occupational medicine, when responding to the questions about the source, I had to tell them there were eleven sources and they'd have to contact the blood bank. Even so, I still had to get in line behind the guy who had been bitten by a monkey. At NIH, I worked with an oral medicine resident who was researching oral manifestations of McCune-Albright syndrome. One of my jobs while helping him turned out to be spinning urines to look for vitamin D excretion levels. That brought a new meaning to how we're always telling people the mouth is connected to the body.

When I worked for the navy, the clinic had a mobile dental van. It was always fun to get the opportunity to go out to the submarines and see patients. When I worked for the dental insurance company, I used to travel all over the country inspecting dental offices. I saw some interesting things back in the late 1980s. There was the dentist who sterilized his instruments in a toaster oven. There was another who sterilized his instruments in a GE kitchen oven he kept in an operatory.

What type of advice would you give to a practicing hygienist who is thinking of doing something different?

Do it. You won't regret it, and you'll never "burn out." You may need to expand your skills or get additional education. Expect to make less money at first. But also expect a better benefit package. And remember, benefits add about 30 percent to your salary. All in all, public health is much less stressful and much more fun than private practice.

Source: Christine Nathe writes the Public Health Column in RDH magazine published by Pennwell Publishing. For more public health spotlights please see RDH magazine online at http://www.rdhmag.com/index.html.

SUMMARY

Many barriers to dental care delivery exist in the United States. In fact, the current system has proven ineffective in providing care to all segments of the population. Creating dental hygienist positions in existing interdisciplinary public health settings can help alleviate this problem. The governmental structure in relation to dental hygiene care is intricate and offers numerous opportunities for dental hygiene employment. New solutions and innovative approaches to dental care delivery will most definitely occur in the next decade as organizations respond to the current issues.

Note

Much of the information on the federal government was taken directly from the Web sites http://www.hhs.gov, http://www.ed.gov, http://www.va.gov, http://fns1.usda.gov, and http://www.dol.gov.

SELF-STUDY TEST ITEMS

1. What has been recognized as a major unmet need in the United States?
   a. Geriatric awareness
   b. Oral health
   c. Access to health care
   d. All of the above

2. What branch of the federal government has a direct impact on dental care delivery?
   a. Legislative
   b. Executive
   c. Judicial
   d. All of the above

3. Who or what directs the US Public Health Service?
   a. US Surgeon General
   b. Centers for Disease Control and Prevention
   c. John Hopkins University
   d. Dental Public Health Committee

4. Which organization provides a system of health surveillance to monitor and prevent outbreak of diseases and maintain national health statistics?
    a. National Institutes of Health
    b. Centers for Disease Control and Prevention
    c. Food and Drug Administration
    d. Indian Health Service

5. Which organization is responsible for the Head Start program?
    a. Administration on Aging
    b. Centers for Medicare and Medicaid Services
    c. Administration for Children and Families
    d. Indian Health Services

REFERENCES

1. US Department of Health and Human Services. *Oral health in America: A Report of the Surgeon General.* Rockville, MD: Department of Health and Human Services, National Institute of Dental and Craniofacial Research, National Institutes of Health; 2000.
2. US Department of Health and Human Services. *Healthy People 2010: Understanding and Improving Health.* 2nd ed. Washington, DC: US Government Printing Office; 2000.
3. US Department of Health and Human Services. *A National Call to Action to Promote Oral Health.* Rockville, MD: US Department of Health and Human Services, Public Health Service, Centers for Disease Control and Prevention, National Institutes of Health, National Institute of Dental and Craniofacial Research; 2003. NIH Publication No. 03-5303.
4. *Keep America Smiling: Oral Health in America.* 2003. The Oral Health America National Grading Project 2003. Oral Health America.
5. Gundrum C. Dental hygiene in the Indian Health Service with information from Ann Witherspoon. Paper presented at: DEHY 442: Dental Public Health Course, University of New Mexico, October 1, 2008.
6. DeFriese G, Barker B. *Assessing Dental Manpower Requirements.* Cambridge, MA: Ballinger Publishing; 1982.
7. Health Resources and Service Administration Guidelines on Designation of Population Groups with Health Manpower Shortages. Bethesda, MD: US Department of Health and Human Services; 1995.
8. Shortage Designation Branch, Bureau of Health Professions, Health Resources and Services Administration. http://bhpr.hrsa.gov/shortage. Accessed June 8, 2006.
9. Weaver RG, Valachovic RW, Hanlon LL, Mintz JS, Chmar JE. *Unleashing the Potential.* Washington, DC: American Dental Education Association; 2006. http:www.adea.org/cepr/Documents/Unleashing_the_Potential.pdf. Accessed August 5, 2008.
10. Dentists. *Occupational Outlook Handbook.* 2008–2009 ed. http://www.bls.gov/oco/ocos072.htm. Accessed August 22, 2008.
11. McKinnon M, Luke G, Bresch J, Moss M, Valochovic RW. Association Report: Emerging Allied Dental Workforce Models: Consideration for Academic Dental Institutions. *J Dent Ed.* 2007;71(11):1476–1491.
12. Beazoglou T, Bailit H, Jackson-Brown L. Selling your practice at retirement: Are there problems ahead? *J Am Dent Assoc.* 2000;31(12):1693–1698.
13. Competencies for the Advanced Dental Hygiene Practitioner. Chicago: American Dental Hygienists' Association; 2008.
14. Dental Hygienists. *Occupational Outlook Handbook.* 2008–2009 ed. http://www.bls.gov/oco/ocos097.htm. Accessed August 22, 2008.
15. National Denturists Association. What denturists do. http://www.nationaldenturist.com/about%20us.html. Accessed August 22, 2008.
16. Alaska Native Tribal Health Consortium. Dental Health Therapist. http://www.anthc.org/cs/chs/dhs/index.cfm. Accessed August 22, 2008.
17. Fox K. ADA House creates new options for dental team. American Dental Association; 2006. http://www.ada.org/prof/resources/pubs/adanews/adanewsarticle.asp?articleid=2231. Accessed August 22, 2008.

Chapter 4

Dental Hygiene Care Delivery in the Global Community

Claudia Luciak-Donsberger, RDH, PhD

OBJECTIVES

After studying this chapter, the dental hygiene student should be able to:

- Describe the evolution of dental hygiene in countries other than the United States
- Identify global oral health challenges and the positioning of dental hygiene care
- Describe the historical perspective of global dental hygiene
- Describe the global workforce distribution and access to dental hygiene care
- Explain changes in dental hygiene education and work roles
- Explain changes in professional regulation
- Define gender issues related to the dental hygiene profession
- Describe portability of licensure and other professions providing care
- Explain the challenges of global oral health

KEY TERMS

Dental nurses
Dental therapists
Fédération Dentaire Internationale (FDI)
International Federation of Dental Hygienists (IFDH)
World Health Organization (WHO)

COMPETENCIES

After studying this chapter and participating in accompanying course activities, the dental hygiene student should be competent to do the following:

- Promote the profession through service activities and affiliations with professional organizations
- Communicate effectively with individuals and groups from diverse populations both verbally and in writing
- Promote the values of oral and general health and wellness to the public and organizations within and outside the profession

Finding solutions to the unmet oral health needs of global populations is a challenge being addressed by a variety of public health initiatives, most notably the **World Health Organization (WHO),** the directing and coordinating authority for health within the United Nations system, in its commitment to improve oral health as an integral part of general health.[1] Over the past decades in wealthier industrialized regions such as the United States, Canada, Japan, and parts of Europe, effective preventive strategies have contributed to a decreased incidence of dental disease. These strategies included the addition of fluoride to toothpastes, community water systems, milk products, and table salt; community efforts to educate the public about oral health risk factors; the application of dental sealants, the use of noncariogenic sweeteners; and the introduction of the dental hygiene profession as a discipline of prevention.[1] Life expectancy is increasing, and teeth are more likely to be retained.

However, dental health care is also polarized: Disadvantaged and poor populations in wealthier nations are affected and experience a significant burden of untreated dental diseases in economically less-developed countries.[2] According to the WHO's *World Oral Health Report 2003,* "although common dental diseases are preventable, not all community members are informed of or are able to benefit from appropriate oral health-promoting measures."[3] The WHO has identified "profound oral health disparities...[that] may relate to socioeconomic status, race or ethnicity, age, gender or general health status. Underserved population groups are found in both developed and developing countries."[4]

These findings have led to the development of public health strategies guided by the need to identify at-risk groups and individuals and to modify risk behaviors with an established negative effect on oral health, such as poor oral hygiene, sugar intake, tobacco use, and excessive alcohol consumption. However, risk reduction is possible only if oral health systems are oriented to primary health care and prevention.

On a global basis, political, cultural, and socioeconomic factors affect public dental health delivery systems, resulting in significant variations in access to care and in clinical outcomes. These differences can be observed in local oral health policies, costs, health beliefs, and attitudes of dental professionals and the public.[5] In some countries, oral health has a high priority, and structured policies often govern its provision. Budgets made available for community oral health care and educational structures are more extensive and frequently pay for a specialized dental team,

which generally includes dental hygienists. In some countries, oral health appears to have low priority as evidenced by absence of a specialized workforce—dental hygienists in particular—who might provide access to preventive care for a significant part of the population.

Thus, to plan for the provision of oral health care for a given society, it is important to gather reliable evidence-based information on treatment needs, oral health care systems, costs, workforce numbers, and education for the dental team.[4] In some regions of the world, dental hygienists, due to their primary preventive orientation, play an important role in providing access to oral health care. The majority of the world's dental hygienists practice in wealthier societies that have a high demand for prevention, aesthetics, and wellness, as well as the recognition that oral health is an integral part of general health and quality of life.[5] Because of this, most dental hygienists provide care on an individual basis in dental or dental hygiene offices and serve the increasing number of persons who have maintained a functional dentition as a consequence of crown- and bridgework and dental implants.[6] In Norway, dental hygienists already act as primary oral health care providers in the public health system, and for decades Norway has ranked first on the Human Development Index (HDI), which measures and compares worldwide life expectancy, literacy, education, and standard of living, and thus serves as a quality of life indicator.

In lower-income populations with a lack of basic dental care, as in the Dominican Republic and Nepal, some dental hygienists have been involved in public health initiatives and other grassroots projects promoting oral health.[7-9] Even in developed nations, however, the need is ever increasing for dental hygienists to facilitate oral health equity for underserved disadvantaged populations and to respond to the current and future demographic changes of an aging population with natural teeth, some of whom require services in permanent care facilities.

This chapter examines the global distribution of dental hygienists set against national and regional community oral health care needs and demands. It explores work roles and extended professional positions that would enable dental hygienists to make a greater contribution to global public oral health care provision in response to specific regional needs. Finally, the chapter presents examples of the role dental hygienists in oral public health to stimulate other projects of global and local impact.

ACCESS TO INFORMATION ON GLOBAL ORAL HEALTH NEEDS

Action plans for promoting the prevention of oral disease frequently rely on surveys that monitor disease patterns. To ensure outcome-driven oral health programs, the WHO maintains statistics on the prevalence of dental diseases from more than 170 countries in its Global Oral Data Bank. Data on both dental caries and periodontal diseases are accessible.[10,11] WHO methodology has stimulated the gathering of epidemiological data in a large number of countries. These data are combined with information from the WHO Country Profiles Project and are available to administrators for planning and evaluating oral care services.

> **Did You Know?**
>
> Dental caries and periodontal diseases are the most widespread of all human diseases.

Another data bank is maintained by the **Fédération Dentaire Internationale (FDI),** the organization that represents the international community of dentists.[12] In addition to some epidemiological data on nearly 130 countries, the FDI Web site provides detailed information about dentistry and the dental team in participating member countries including demographics and numbers concerning the dental workforce, institutions for dental and dental hygiene education, type of oral health care system, fluoridation levels, existence of a public health policy, and information on free dental coverage for children. However, figures pertaining to the dental hygienists workforce must be viewed with caution, especially for countries where the profession has not been officially introduced or schools are reported but are not accredited. In such cases, dental associations are often not aware of or do not wish to report the actual numbers of internationally educated dental hygienists who provide care in a legal "grey zone" as in Austria, Belgium, France, Germany, and Greece. For instance, France reports no dental hygienists and no chairside dental assistants as part of its workforce.

The Council of European Chief Dental Officers (CECDO) maintains another databank.[13] Key data relate to the oral health workforce, dental education, costs, and oral health indicators including epidemiological data on decayed, missing, and filled teeth (DMFT). CECDO data also include information on the numbers of registered and active dental hygienists in Europe.

The Council of European Dentists (CED) maintains a databank on 30 European countries containing detailed descriptions of national oral health systems, workforce, and public health care demographics.[14]

Since 1987, Dr. Patricia Johnson has monitored patterns and changes pertaining to the dental hygiene profession in membership countries of the **International Federation of Dental Hygienists (IFDH),** the organization representing the international community of dental hygienists.[15] Her international longitudinal study began with thirteen countries, had been extended to twenty-two by 2001 and to twenty-six by 2007. Her latest survey may be accessed through the IFDH Web site.[16,17]

Meaningful international comparisons concerning the equity and quality of oral health care must be based on a precise epidemiologic assessment of treatment needs, demands, and information on how these are being met.[5] For strategic planning, it is imperative that data be evidence based, consistent, reproducible, and comparable. Unfortunately, finding reliable data is still a major challenge in global dental public health.[5]

Epidemiology of Dental Caries

The prevalence of caries tends to be most commonly measured with the DMFT index. Key ages for data collection are twelve years, thrity-five to forty-four years, and sixty-five years and older. A mean DMFT between 0.0 and 1.1 is considered low; one of 6.6 or more is high. Although some populations report that the WHO goals for the year 2000 were achieved or even exceeded, they remain a remote hope for a significant part of the world's population.[18] (See Table 4-1 ■.)

Table 4-1 WHO Goals for "Health for All" by the Year 2000

By the age of	Goal
5–6 years	50% should be caries free
12 years	Fewer than 3 decayed, missing, and filled teeth
18 years	85% should have retained all their teeth
34–44 years	50% reduction in the number of persons with no teeth
65 + years	25% reduction in the number of persons with fewer than 20 teeth

Source: www.who.int/oral_health/action/information/surveillance/en/index.html.

Some question the reliability of these data. Eaton conducted an extensive analysis concerning the validity and comparability of data accessible through internationl data banks.[5] Even though most countries still provide epidemiological evidence in DMFT scores, results showed that existing epidemiological data are inadequate and the studies performed to gather the data are not comparable. No universally accepted criteria appear to be used for the diagnosis of caries, and most international surveys lack interexaminer calibration to ensure consistency.[19] In addition, sampling facilities tend to lack dental chairs, lights, and a supply of compressed air. These factors lead to lower estimates of caries experience.

Did You Know?

Interexaminer calibration means that all examiners have a degree of consistency among themselves when evaluating outcomes during a research study.

The International Caries Detection and Assessment System (ICDAS) is a collaborative initiative with the goal of finding closer agreement between the outcomes of caries epidemiology and caries clinical trials.[20] The system provides consistent criteria based on evidence-based dentistry designed to generate more meaningful and comparable data. ICDAS has been used in pilot studies in a number of countries such as the United States, United Kingdom, Denmark, Columbia, Mexico, and Iceland and has been shown to be valid and practical.

The Significant Caries Index has been proposed to replace the ICDAS because DMFT scores do not account for the skewed distribution of caries prevalence within a given population.[21] This proposed index would bring attention to individuals with the highest caries in each population. As a consequence, public health programs could be targeted to benefit these groups.

Epidemiology of Periodontal Diseases

Data collection on periodontal disease appears to pose an even greater challenge for the scientific community. Over the years, significant differences pertaining to severity and incidence of periodontal diseases have been reported, again due to nonstandardized methods of sampling. To improve methodology, the WHO introduced the Community Periodontal Index of Treatment Needs (CPI, formerly called CPITN) to evaluate periodontal disease in population surveys.[22] (See Box 4-1 ■.)

After the inception of the CPI, a wealth of global data was generated, but no uniform criteria for the assessment of periodontal diseases have yet been established. Furthermore, it has been shown that broad indices such as the CPI produce such severe inconsistencies in the methodologies employed in epidemiological studies that *it is unclear whether this group of diseases represents a growing, stable, or declining problem.*[5] Consequently, it has been concluded that no reliable epidemiological method currently exists for assessing periodontal disease and that data used to assess treatment needs have been of questionable value and are not comparable. The underestimation of periodontitis may not only adversely affect treatment recommendations and public health strategies but also service cost studies, service demand estimation, or workforce planning.[23,24] Currently available information on oral health care systems, costs, and workforce numbers also appears inadequate *for planning the provision of oral health care on a scientific basis.*[5,25] Problems persist in the collection of information with which to calculate the supply of dental hygienists and their ratio to dentists and the population for the same year.[16]

BOX 4-1 Community Periodontal Index (CPI) of Treatment Needs

A specially designed periodontal probe is used for the examination using specifically designated index teeth. The highest score for each sextant is used for treatment recommendations.

0: Healthy: No signs of periodontal disease: Promote self-assessment of oral health, (Oral Hygiene Instruction)

1: Gingival bleeding after gentle probing: OHI
2: Presence of supra- or subgingival calculus: OHI, supra- and subgingival scaling
3: Presence of periodontal pockets of 4–5 mm: OHI, supra- and subgingival scaling
4: Presence periodontal pockets $\geq$ 6 mm: Need for more complex periodontal therapy

Source: WHO Oral Health Country/Area Profile Programme. Community Periodontal Index (CPI). Periodontal country profiles. http://www.whocollab.od.mah.se/expl/orhcpitn97.html Accessed on June 8, 2009.

POTENTIAL ROLES FOR DENTAL HYGIENISTS ACCORDING TO EVIDENCE-BASED DATA COLLECTION

To improve the reliability of epidemiological data for large-scale international populations, interexaminer calibration is essential but cannot be achieved on a global level. Accuracy in diagnostic data collection depends on many factors, such as harmonization of examiners' training, comparable clinical experience, and adequate clinical settings, factors that are nearly impossible to achieve worldwide. For these reasons, the WHO collaborating centers are aspiring to promote good practice, training, and collaboration between teams throughout the world. They recommend the development of a workforce with clinical examination skills and the creation of partnerships between health practitioners and academics in conducting evaluations.[2]

Such collaboration might present an area of application for dental hygiene knowledge. It has been shown that suitably calibrated dental hygienists and periodontists produce more consistent epidemiological data than those relatively unaccustomed to performing periodontal assessments.[26] According to studies in Sweden, dental hygienists exhibit equally high accuracy for the diagnosis of dental caries as dentists.[27] Another area that dental hygienists might participate in is the systematic evaluation of the effectiveness of community oral health care programs. Health care providers and funders must know whether an intervention was effective and evidence based. The WHO has called for higher quality and validity of outcome measures and has developed guidelines for evaluating national and community oral health programs.

Did You Know?

Dental hygienists would be well suited to translate health promotion principles into action at community levels, especially after the acquisition of skills required to engage in collaborative evidence-based project planning and a focus on primary prevention.

Because most dental diseases are preventable, an ever-growing global need for experts in the field of oral health promotion and disease prevention appears to exist. With these potential work roles for dental hygienists, the size and the distribution of the global dental hygiene workforce and its specific roles in different societies should be investigated.

As stated in Chapter 1, dental hygiene was historically developed to address public oral health needs from a preventive orientation. With skills in evidence-based preventive health modalities and in behavior modification, modern dental hygienists are in an excellent position to provide services as principal oral health care professionals at a cost lower than dentists might charge.[28]

In industrialized nations, the concept of the collaboration among the various types of dental personnel to provide care is gaining increasing acceptance. In the last decades, the overall supply of dental hygienists and the hygienist-to-population and hygienist-to-dentist ratios in wealthier countries have increased notably.[16,28] However, when looking beyond the United States, Canada, Japan, South Korea, and a few European countries, the supply of dental hygienists compared to dentists is too small to assess their impact on health outcomes or on the reduction of health care costs.

INTERNATIONAL DENTAL HYGIENE

In a perfect world, the ratio of dental hygienists and dentists to the population would suffice to meet preventive and restorative oral health care needs. However, most countries still report a lack of access to dental hygiene services. Reasons range from insufficient funding for preventive service and educational facilities, limitations inherent in the legal restraints on the profession to a social and cultural lack of awareness of the benefits of preventive care.[16]

Historial Perspective

Soon after Dr. A.C. Fones first introduced the term *dental hygienist*, steps were taken that generally constitute the development of a profession: the foundation of educational institutions and a professional association, access to university education, establishment of a code of ethics, and publication of scientific journals.[29,30]

The international expansion of dental hygiene was inspired by the professionalism and delivery of care in the United States and had early origins in the United Kingdom, Norway, Japan, and Canada to ongoing pioneering work to introduce the profession in countries where it was and still is unknown or politically rejected from the dental community, for example, in Austria, Belgium, France, and Greece. (See Table 4-2 ■.) In most cases, dental hygiene has been "imported" by enthusiastic individuals who have had an opportunity to study or work in the United States and were inspired by this preventive

Table 4-2 Chronology of Dental Hygiene Education and Legal Recognition by Country

Country	Formal Legal Regulation[a]
Norway	1979
Great Britain	1954
Japan	1948
Canada	1947, 1952
Nigeria	1993
South Korea	1973
The Netherlands	1974
Sweden	1991
South Africa	1969
Denmark	1986
Switzerland	1975,[b] 1991[b]
Australia	1972
Finland	1972
Italy	1988
Israel	1978
Iceland	1978
Hong Kong	1970
Poland	1973
Portugal	1988
Saudi Arabia	NA
Spain	1986
Hungary	1995
Latvia	1996
Lithuania	NA
Czech Republic	1996
New Zealand	1993, 1988
Austria	DHs work in legal "grey zone"
Belgium	Not legally recognized[c]
France	Not legally recognized[c]
Germany	DHs work in legal "grey zone"
Greece	Not legally recognized[c]

[a]Practice could have begun earlier; this is when dental hygiene practice was legally defined.
[b]Applies to different cantons.
[c]A few internationally educated dental hygienists work there.
NA = No information available.

approach to oral health. As a consequence, many schools of dental hygiene around the world have based their curriculum on the US style of training, which may explain why overall characteristics of the profession are quite homogeneous in scope of practice.[16]

In 1942, dental hygiene was first introduced in three-month courses to ensure that pilots in the United Kingdom Royal Air Force (RAF) fighter planes during World War II had good dental health and were not troubled by dental pain, which can occur when flying at high altitudes, particularly in unpressurized aircraft. At that time, some RAF dentists had received further training in periodontics in the United States, where they heard about the dental hygiene profession. Their pioneering enthusiasm was instrumental in urging the British government's Department of Health to start dental hygiene education at the Eastman Dental Institute, London, in 1949, after the war had ended.

Did You Know?

A number of schools around the world were influenced by the British example, such as those in Australia, New Zealand, Nigeria, and Hong Kong (all once members of the British Commonwealth).

Global Workforce Distribution and Access to Dental Hygiene Care

Although the ratio of dental hygienists and dentists to the population indicates that they cannot presently meet preventive and restorative oral health care needs, most countries still lack dental hygiene services.

A global analysis indicates that dental hygiene has been introduced in more than thirty countries. However, a closer look at the demographics reveals that access to care mainly exists in wealthier economically developed countries that have an increased life expectancy, an overall decline in caries prevalence, and interest in wellness and esthetics, possibly an improvement in periodontal health (evidence still under investigation) but no significant improvement in the incidence of oral cancer, at least in Europe. Even in these countries, access to dental hygiene varies significantly according to income levels as the Report of the US Surgeon General in 2000 stated.[31] Populations living in remote areas may also lack access to care. This applies to large countries, such as Australia and Canada, where most people are mainly gathered in cities with small numbers scattered in remote rural areas.

However, for most people living in industrialized countries, going to the dentist and seeing a dental hygienist is relatively easy, although costly. Therefore, cost is a major factor in preventing people from accessing dental care. Dental treatment free to patients is usually (if at all) provided only for children. This is the case in Australia, Denmark, Estonia, Finland, Latvia, Lithuania, New Zealand, Norway, Sweden, Switzerland, and the United Kingdom. Free treatment is available in both private and public health settings, and dental hygienists may provide care in both environments. In Norway and Finland, the government funds clinics that provide free treatment to children. National medical insurance covering some dental treatment to adults is available in some countries, such as Australia, Canada and Japan. In other countries, such as in Norway, Portugal, and South Korea, adult patients must pay for treatment. Even in countries with national insurance, coverage varies and is therefore not comparable. Although most such countries include prophylaxis and dental sealants for children, other countries—for instance Austria—do not.

A survey of the dental hygiene workforce in 1998 concluded that Canada, Japan, and the United States had more than fifteen times as many dental hygienists as the former eighteen-member states of the European Economic Area (EEA) although *the combined populations and the total number of dentists working in these three countries are broadly similar* to those in the EEA.[32] Because the countries with the most dental hygienists have the most educational institutions, their workforce naturally will continue to expand the fastest. (See Table 4-3 ■.)

According to estimates, today's European Union (EU), composed of twenty-seven countries, has fewer than 20,000 dental hygienists (no information is available as to whether they are educated in accredited institutions or preceptorship trained) but 330,000 "active dentists" and a population of roughly 485 million people. A comparison of more recent data (2004 to 2007) indicates that the ratios have not improved since 1998. (See Table 4-4 ■.) Japan, Canada, and the United States still have seventeen times more dental hygienists than the expanded European Union. Seven EU countries still report no or few dental hygienists. In some countries, such as Austria and Germany, clinical care is frequently provided by preceptorship-trained dental assistants at a significant loss of quality and safety to the public.[33,34] Access to qualified dental hygiene care is therefore not equitable among EU countries.

With access to dental hygienists in the European Union mainly through private dental offices in industrialized countries, care tends to be preventive, cosmetic, and therapeutic, which favors a team approach to maximize access and profit.[25] Only a few countries, such as Finland, Norway, and Sweden, report the public health sector as the predominant workplace for a dental hygienist.

Did You Know?

In most other parts of the world, the dental hygiene workforce is still underrepresented or nonexistent.

Oral health has experienced no change or even deterioration in many developing or underdeveloped countries. A large workforce is needed to promote oral health and educate the public about fluoride, home care, smoking cessation, and nutrition. The total population in Brazil, China, India, Indonesia, and the Russian Federation is nearly 3 billion. According to estimates cited earlier,[15,16,24] the ratio of dental hygienists and dentists per capita is too small for them to plan and implement programs, provide treatment, or educate hundreds of millions of people about the consequences of increased consumption of sugar and processed foods, and carbonated drinks as well as the positive effects of fluoride toothpaste, and prophylactic care. This explains the vicious cycle of dental caries remaining largely untreated and very little knowledge about preventive measures such as the benefits of fluorides and the effects of cariogenic nutrition on oral health. India, Pakistan, and Thailand train personnel in basic oral health education and oral hygiene instruction. These providers tend to work in public dental health clinics or go out to villages where they demonstrate toothbrushing and encourage individuals to adopt a preventive attitude toward dental diseases. But even they are far too few in number to make a significant impact.

Data compiled by the FDI suggest that the highest number of dental hygienists is found in countries with the highest dentist-to-population ratios and the greatest reduction of dental diseases as in Canada, Sweden, Switzerland, and the United States. (See Table 4-5 ■.) These data suggest that there is no need to fear that dental hygienists will replace dentists but that a larger workforce is needed to treat and maintain the oral health of a growing and aging population that cares for and retains its natural teeth. Dental hygienists and dentists truly work in a collaborative manner.

Table 4-3   Number of Dental Hygiene Educational Institutions, Entry Levels, and Expected Changes

Country	Number of Programs	Study Duration (years)	Diploma	Baccalaureatte Degree	Expected Changes
Australia	2+7 Dual[a]	2, 3	2	7	1 M.A. in Dental Hygiene pending
Canada	43	2–3, 3	41	2	Postgraduate education related areas
Czech Rep.	3	3	3	—	
Denmark	2	2.5, 3.5	1	1[b]	B.A. entry discussed
Fiji	1	2	1	—	B.A. program discussed
Finland	5	3.5	—	All[b]	B.A. entry achieved
Germany	0[c]	—	—	—	B.A. program
Hong Kong	1	2	1	—	—
Hungary	3	2–3	—	1	
Israel	5	2	4		B.A. entry
Italy	20	3	15	5[b]	M.A. in Dental Hygiene pending
Latvia	1	1	1		2-year diploma program
Lithuania	2	3, 4	1	1[b]	—
Netherlands	4	4		All[b]	B.A. entry achieved 1 M.A. in Dental Hygiene
New Zealand	2 Dual[a]	3, 4	—	All	M.A. pending
Norway	3	3	—	All[b]	B.A. entry achieved M.A. and Ph.D. pending
Portugal	2	3	—	All[b]	B.A. entry achieved
R. Ireland	2	2	2		1 B.A. program pending 2008[b]
South Korea	53	3, 4	47	6	—
Slovakia	1	3	Discont.	All[b]	B.A. entry achieved
Slovenia	1	2	1	—	—
South Africa	6	2, 3	5	1	B.A. entry, 3 additional B.A. programs Postgraduate studies in dental hygiene
Sweden	8[d]	2, 3	8		B.A. entry pending M.A. in Dental Hygiene
Switzerland	4	3	4	—	Expanded curriculum
United Kingdom	20	2.5, 3	16 Dual[a]	4[b]	More B.A. programs

[a]Dual education as dental hygienist and dental therapist.
[b]B.A. degree programs adapted to European Credit Transfer System (ECTS).
[c]One three-year Swiss style program was closed in 2006.
[d]All schools in Sweden offer optional third year for B.A. attainment.

Source: Luciak-Donsberger C. Questionnaire presented to delegates of the IFDH and representatives of CECDO, 2007–2008.

Table 4-4 Estimated Ratios of Dental Hygienists to Dentists and to the Population

Country	Population (millions)	Dental Hygienists (number)	Ratio Dental Hygienists:Dentists	Ratio Dental Hygienists:Population
Australia	22.00	900	1:14	1:25,500
Austria	8.00	8	1:350	1:1,000,000
Canada	33.00	18,500	1:1	1:1800
Denmark	5.50	1800	1:3	1:3100
Fiji	0.80	50	1:1	1:16,000
Germany	82.00	150	1:300	1:550,000
Hungary	10.50	900	1:5	1:10,400
Ireland	4.25	300	1:8	1:14,000
Italy	60.00	3000	1:12	1:20,000
Israel	7.20	1030	1:8	1:6700
Japan	127.00	150,000	1:1	1:846
Latvia	2.30	200	1:80	1:11,000
Netherlands	16.50	2000	1:30	1:8000
New Zealand	4.30	250	1:90	1:17,000
Norway	4.50	1200	1:50	1:3700
Portugal	11.00	340	1:15	1:32,000
Slovakia	5.50	300	1:11	1:18,000
South Africa	48.00	2000	1:2.5	1:24,000
South Korea	49.00	31,000	1:0.5	1:1500
Sweden	9.00	3200	1:20	1:2800
Switzerland	7.50	1700	1:2.5	1:4100
United Kingdom	60.00	4500	1:80	1:13,300
United States	300.00	180,000	1:0.9	1:1700

Sources: Luciak-Donsberger C. Questionnaire presented to delegates of the IFDH and representatives of CECDO, 2007–2008; FDI and WHO databanks.

Table 4-5 Regulation of the Dental Hygiene Profession by Country

Country	Regulating Authority
Australia	Dental board
Canada	Self-regulation in 6 provinces (representing 90% of DHs); dental board/council in 4 provinces
Denmark	Board of Health
Finland	Social and Health Ministry
Hungary	Ministries of Health and Education and Culture
	Institute for Basic and Contin. Education of Health Workers
Ireland	Dental Council
Italy	Ministry of Health
Israel	Division of Dental Health of Ministry of Health
Netherlands	Ministry of Health
New Zealand	New Zealand Dental Council
Norway	Health Personnel Act
Portugal	Ministry of Health
South Africa	Health Professions Council of South Africa
South Korea	Ministry of Health and Welfare
Sweden	Board of Social Welfare
Switzerland	Swiss Red Cross
United Kingdom	General dental council
United States	Individual state boards

CURRENT STATUS OF DENTAL HYGIENE EDUCATION

Education serves to socialize and legitimize knowledge, and credentials ensure a standard of care. Currently, dental hygiene education is eclectic. Studies indicate that it varies in prerequisites, duration, and institutional settings. Dental hygiene education in Europe is becoming increasingly academic.[35] (See Table 4-3). Requiring specific education to gain entry into the profession is a response to the increasing complexity in dental hygienists' work roles.

In most countries, dental hygiene education seeks to qualify students in evidence-based clinical care, diagnostic assessment and intervention planning, lifestyle consulting, and risk behavior modification counseling as well as in public health promotion, teaching, research, and program administration. In some countries, dental hygienists are educated to polish amalgam restorations, administer local anesthesia and/or local antibiotic therapy, place and remove temporary restorations and/or orthodontic bands, and even prepare and treat primary caries. These applications require increased responsibility and critical thinking based on research. As the profession is becoming increasingly autonomous, dental hygiene education must transmit technical efficiency with critical evidence-based decision making coupled with the ability to recognize one's own professional limitations in order to judge when it is time to refer to a dentist.[16,33]

Did You Know?

Generally, dental hygiene is studied at institutions of higher education and requires university entry qualifications. Candidates must be over eighteen years of age. Some schools have adopted a two-tier entry level, requiring the candidate either to demonstrate a high standard of matriculation or to have studied and qualified as a dental assistant.

In most countries, entry into the dental hygiene profession is preceeded by graduation from an accredited program and independent testing of clinical ability and theoretical knowledge.[16,33] Dental hygiene study facilities range from private schools to technical colleges and universities that award diplomas as well as associate's, bachelor's, master's, and doctoral degree levels. Duration of study to enter the profession varies from two to four years with an average of three years. Globally, and even within the European Union, a variety of models of dental hygiene education exists.

Two- to three-year diploma programs still exist in many countries, but in Europe the tendency is to replace them with degree programs or, as is the case in Sweden, offer an optional third year of education to attain bachelor's degree levels at all schools. Some countries already require a bachelor's degree for entry into practice, and several more report a planned academic upgrade of the educational process.

The European Union is increasingly adapting degree program curricula to the European credit transfer system (ECTS). The European Ministers of Education introduced this system in Bologna in 1999 to make academic studies more attractive, transparent, and transferable and to promote quality assurance. Under this system, students earn sixty credits per year (forty-two weeks of study) for a total of 1680 hours of study. Bachelor's programs in Denmark, Finland, Italy, the Netherlands, Portugal, the Republic of Ireland, Sweden, and the United Kingdom either already have or are about to introduce this system. The European Dental Hygienists' Federation proposed 198 ECTS units for the study of dental hygiene, which totals 5200 hours.

Postgraduate-level programs such as those for master's or doctoral (PhD) degrees in related health fields are open to all dental hygienists with bachelor's degrees. The Netherlands, Sweden, and the United States offer master's programs in dental hygiene. The United States has the highest number of master's programs (eleven) in dental hygiene. Three more are pending in Australia, Italy, and Norway in responce to the need for evidence-based research in dental hygiene care by providing scientifically oriented educational opportunities.

In some countries, such as Australia and the United Kingdom, students may graduate with a degree in both dental hygiene and dental therapy. However, these dual degree programs have caused some concern about the disappearance of stand-alone dental hygiene education because professionals educated in preventive and restorative care might lose their predominantly preventive orientation.

Germany has chosen so far an eclectic model of dental hygiene education. It is a continuing education model for actively working dental assistants, not comparable to the two-, three-, and four-year full-time diploma or degree courses found in accredited dental hygiene education. The only three-year full-time diploma course in Germany, which followed the Swiss model of education, closed in 2006. However, there is discussion about implementing programs at bachelor's levels at technical colleges.

Although the length of study and entry requirements to the profession vary, all students in countries where the profession is registered complete examinations at the end of their courses to obtain a national qualification. In the larger countries, such as in the United States, Australia, and Canada, state or province examinations (sometimes called *boards*) are also required to practice in that particular region.

Did You Know?

The length of dental hygiene education tends to be extended as curricula are being expanded with an increase in academic orientation.

The movement toward extended education is associated with an increase in the scope of practice and a decrease in regulation. In the Netherlands, for instance, students acquire skills in extended functions, including the restoration of primary caries. This change occurred in response to an aging population coupled with a significant decline in the dentist workforce due to retirement.

PROFESSIONAL REGULATION

Regulation of health occupations under public statute ensures quality and safety of patient care. Although the dental profession still exercises control over the dental hygiene profession, requirements for becoming a dental hygienist in many countries include legislative changes and self-regulation.[36] (See Table 4-5.)

Refer to Table 4-2 whose data indicate that the dates of the onset of dental hygiene education rarely coincide with the profession's legal recognition. This means that, in several countries, dental hygienists were providing patient care, usually under the supervision of dentists, long before their services were legally regulated. In some cases, the legal acceptance of the profession, which organized dentistry often opposed, required years of lobbying by supporters, most of them also dentists. Foreign-educated dental hygienists working in Austria, Belgium, Germany, and France still face this situation; these countries continue to resist developing the profession or employing dental hygienists, especially because preceptorship- (on-the-job) trained dental assistants work for less than educated and licensed dental hygienists, even though the fees charged to the public are often roughly the same.[29]

National differences in legislative practices affecting dental hygiene tend to reflect the impact of the dental profession's organized lobby to retain control of dental hygiene care. Some countries still legally prohibit anyone other than dentists to provide patient care. In those countries, dental hygiene may not be implemented at all. Barriers to change include the fear that this will financially affect too many dentists who might provide dental hygiene care themselves and that they will lose control and status. Frequently, such fears can result from a lack of understanding of exactly what dental hygienists and dental therapists can do. Dental schools that favor a team approach by integrating dental and dental hygiene education may foster mutual understanding and a recognition of task-related boundaries.

However, data show that regulations imposed to tie dental hygiene care to work settings controlled by dentists are gradually beginning to disappear. Increasingly, dental hygienists may practice autonomously, free of any supervision of dentists. In such settings, they may be consulted as primary oral health care providers.

MOVEMENT TOWARD AUTONOMY

International dental hygienist regulation is decreasing, resulting in increased autonomy. (See Table 4-6 ■.) However, the definition of independent practice in one country is not necessarily the same in another. Some countries allow dental hygienists to operate their own practices and provide treatment without the referral of a dentist. Other countries may not allow them to operate their own practices but to work in the public sector without supervision.

Models of Supervision

The shift toward an increase in professional autonomy is reflected in the definition of a dental hygienist found in the Dutch curriculum for dental hygiene education: The dental hygienist is an independent preventive professional within the dental healthcare sector, with his/her own responsibility and specific expertise[7] Discussion of the models of supervision (or lack thereof) summarized in Table 4-6 follows.

Direct Supervision

In countries employing direct supervision, legal requirements state that dentists not only decide and authorize dental hygiene treatment but must be physically on-site during the delivery and, in some cases, may have to be in the room or examine the patient after treatment. Once the predominant model of care, this supervisory method has essentially disappeared or is applied to selected treatments such as the administration of local anesthesia.[8]

General Supervision

Countries such as the Czech Republic and Israel legally stipulate that dentists prescribe and authorize dental hygiene care but need not be physically on-site while treatment is rendered. Generally, care is provided at a facility owned or managed by dentists or at public health clinics managed by them.

Independent Referred Practice

Legislation in some countries permits dental hygienists to practice in their own facilities or in institutions that provide preventive services only if the patient is referred by a dentist. Treatment decisions are thus made in collaboration with dentists. This practice is found in some Canadian provinces, Germany (one practice in Munich), the United Kingdom, and Latvia.

Unsupervised, Autonomous, or Independent Practice

Some countries have enacted legislation that permits dental hygienists to practice without the supervision of a dentist. Dental hygienists autonomously decide treatment plans and render care in their own facilities or in the public sector without the referral of a dentist and refer patients to dental care when they diagnose a problem that is beyond their scope of practice or are uncertain about a diagnostic decision. This practice has been introduced in some Canadian provinces, Denmark, Finland, Italy, the Netherlands, Norway, and Sweden and in all but one of the Swiss cantons. In these cases, the public may choose dental hygienists as primary oral health care providers. South Africa and Fiji so far permit this practice only in the public sector.

Data in Table 4-6 reflect a strong movement toward independent dental hygiene practice. Standardization of autonomy would facilitate dental hygiene services in remote areas, public health care settings, permanent care facilities, and mobile dental units, which are underserved by dentists in all countries surveyed. For instance, dental hygienists in South Africa may not own their own practice (change is pending) but may perform their full scope of services in all public health settings independently of a dentist. They provide care in much needed fissure-sealant and brushing programs, HIV and home-based care projects, correctional services programs, and rural programs. Dental hygiene education increasingly prepares students for independent decision making and the ability to recognize when to refer patients to dentists.

Professional self-regulation and autonomy in providing care may be the key to a gradual change in the profession's image.[16] Independent practice is empowering—not only to operators but also to patients who may freely choose care providers. One-third of all dental hygienists in the Netherlands have their own practice, probably the highest percentage worldwide. Globally,

Table 4-6 Requirements for Supervision of Dental Hygiene Practice per Country

Country	Independ. Practice	Indep. Ref. Practice	Off Site Supervision	On-site Supervision	Expected Changes
Australia	✓[a]	✓[b]	✓		More autonomy
Canada	✓[b]	✓			More autonomy; direct insurance. reimbursement
Czech Republic			✓		Move toward independent practice
Denmark	✓				Expanded functions
Fiji	✓[a]				Missing
Finland	✓				Missing
Germany		✓[c]	✓[d]		Missing
Hungary				✓	—
Iceland		✓			Missing
Israel			✓[e]		More autonomy
Italy	✓				More independent practices
Japan			✓		Missing
Latvia		✓	✓		Missing
Lithuania			✓		Missing
Netherlands	✓				More independent practices
New Zealand			✓[e]		More autonomy
Norway	✓				More independent practices
Portugal			✓		Expanded functions
R. Ireland			✓[e]		Independent practice
R. S. Korea		✓[a]		✓	Missing
R. Slovakia			✓		Independent practice
South Africa	✓[a]				Autonomous practice in private settings
Spain			✓		Greater autonomy
Sweden	✓				More independent practices
Switzerland	✓[e]				More independent practices
UK		✓			Removal of referral

[a]Only in public sector.
[b]One autonomous practice in Munich run by US-educated and Swiss-licensed DH.
[c]Eclectic dental hygienist (DH) education; DH not licensed.
[d]DH treatment plan decided with dentist
[e]Direct supervision during administration of local anaesthesia

Source: Luciak-Donsberger C. Questionnaire presented to delegates of the IFDH and representatives of CECDO, 2007–2008.

relatively few dental hygienists work in this manner. Financial considerations of investing in an office and the responsibilities of office maintenance and administration may be deterrents. As role models increase, however, more and more dental hygienists may recognize the rewards of being in charge of their own business, job sharing, flexible work and vacation times, and choice of how and where to practice. The need for a cooperative arrangement between independent dental hygienists and general dentists and dental specialists is not in question.

In summary, in the Scandinavian countries, dental hygienists increasingly work as independent professionals, academics, and public health experts with significant decision-making responsibilities and may be chosen as primary oral health care providers by the public. In Eastern Europe, Asia, and in the Middle East, dental hygienists frequently work as rigidly controlled and supervised auxiliaries who perform dental assisting functions and are underutilized in clinical care.[37,38]

DENTAL HYGIENIST SPOTLIGHT:
Ron Knevel, RDH

Ron Knevel is a graduate of the University of Amsterdam's School of Dental Hygiene. He has worked full-time as a dental hygienist at the department of periodontology at the Academic Centre for Dentistry (ACTA) and in a general practice. After earning his teacher's degree at the Free University, he became a teacher at the Dental Hygiene Program in Amsterdam. He has become more and more involved in dental hygiene curriculum development and is now planning to begin work on a doctoral degree.

I asked him some questions concerning his work and the status of dental hygiene in the Netherlands.

What is your current position?

When the European Union began funding projects for exchange within it, and Amsterdam Dental Hygiene School started to develop partnerships with others for student exchange, I became an international coordinator and therefore came into contact with many colleagues in other countries. I introduced the concept of the international week, and at international conferences, I discussed the benefits of internationalizing dental hygiene. I believe that student and teacher mobility can lead to more respect and understanding for different cultures and treatment options.

I started a project in Nepal to promote oral health based on sustainability and equity. It focuses on oral health promotion based on the culture of Nepal, not on Western approaches. I am also involved in the curriculum development of the dental hygiene school in Katmandu. This project also involves conducting research to determine the impact of the oral health promotion activities on the oral health of children and oral-related aspects of quality of life. I will probably start a similar project in Sri Lanka.

How does the department of periodontology charge for its services?

Patients pay a small nominal fee for the complete treatment, which almost all patients can afford and whose quality is important. The prevalence of caries is decreasing, but the incidence of periodontal diseases is growing. General oral health promotion focuses on identifying and targeting groups at risk for oral health problems.

Have economic and social changes in the Netherlands influenced the way the university operates?

Yes, in the Netherlands, it is important for departments to generate their own financial resources.

How have the same factors influenced the national health insurance?

Although the demand for dental care is high and there is a shortage of dentists and dental hygienists, the national health insurance and basic dental insurance began covering fewer treatments for economic reasons. Dental care is covered by national insurance for children and young adults up to eighteen years (depending on the parents' financial situation; otherwise, the parents need extra insurance to cover the children). People older than eighteen are required to have extra dental insurance, which can be rather expensive and not affordable for many. This situation eventually led people to avoid dental checkups.

How has the country's approach to dental care changed?

A special advisory group of the government concluded that to improve the availability of dental care,

a new team approach was needed. The team includes dentists, dental specialists, dental hygienists, dental assistants, and dental technicians who work closely together to offer patients integrated dental care. This approach has led to a different type of dental hygiene education. The program (which had been changed from two to three years not long before) was changed to a four-year course of study. Now dental hygienists in the Netherlands must have a bachelor of health degree, and their duties have been extended to include the preparation and restoration of simple (primary) cavities with composite.

The prolonged education was necessary because additional preparation was required. To provide this training, the dental faculty offered some teachers the opportunity to become skilled in restorative techniques and be trained in evidence-based practice.

Source: Christine Nathe writes the Public Health Column in RDH magazine published by Pennwell Publishing. For more public health spotlights please see RDH magazine online at http://www.rdhmag.com/index.html.

Effects of Gender Politics on Dental Hygienists

Worldwide, approximately 98% of all dental hygienists are women. This raises the question of whether this female-dominated profession, perceived as auxiliary to dentistry, has been affected by gender politics.[34] A 2003 report commissioned by the Austrian Federal Ministry of Science, Education, and Culture explored whether a correlation exists between national differences found in the dental hygiene profession and gender-related disparities found in other work-related areas. Results showed that, while the scope of practice tends to be similar around the world, the gender bias in the dental hygiene profession has impaired equal access to education and equal occupational opportunities for dental hygienists within the European Union and beyond.

In northern Europe, higher educational attainment in the field of dental hygiene, increased professional responsibility, and opportunities for self-employment in autonomous practice tend to correlate with increased equality in the workforce at large. In Eastern Europe, lower educational and professional opportunities in dental hygiene correlate with gender disparities found in other work-related areas. In some western European countries, the profession has not been implemented because of the political impact of male-dominated organized dentistry.

Portability of Licensure

Many hygienists would like to be able to travel and work in countries other than their own. Large countries such as Australia, Canada, and the United States require state or provincial and national qualifications. Within the European Union, an equivalency ruling exists, permitting the regulatory body to assess whether training in one EU country is equivalent to another. If the finding is positive, the dental hygienist is permitted to work. Of course, hygienists are permitted to work only in those European countries that recognize them. One disadvantage could be the inability to speak the language of the country in which one wishes to work.

The European Union regulates a profession when it is legally registered in at least two-thirds of the member countries. This goal is almost reached and actively pursued by the European Federation of Dental Hygienists. Such a regulation would lead to free movement of the dental hygiene workforce within the European Union.

Other Dental Professions Providing Care

Dental therapists provide restorative care under the general supervision of dentists. They are mostly found in the

United Kingdom and in former countries of the British Commonwealth, such as Australasia, Canada, and Nigeria. Until recently, their services were restricted to public health facilities and school dental services where they would examine and treat children under the prescription of dentists. Therefore, in New Zealand, they are also referred to as school **dental nurses.** Generally, their services include dental hygiene care, but their main focus is on children's restorative needs. Dental nurses may restore both the primary and permanent dentition of children and extract primary teeth. While they initially worked only at community dental services, dental therapists now may provide services for children and adults in private practice settings.

Orthodontic assistants are trained in Canada and Australia and will soon be in the United Kingdom. They tend to be qualified dental assistants who attend a postgraduate course in orthodontics. They assist orthodontists in technical tasks by making and fitting bands, taking impressions, and fitting arch wires. They also ensure that the patient undergoing treatment maintains a high standard of oral hygiene.

Developing countries have programs for oral health educators who dispense information in a culturally sensitive manner to raise oral health awareness of large poor populations who frequently live in remote areas. Little can be gained by training a highly skilled professional to undertake costly and complex clinical tasks when the population requires simple oral hygiene education and oral health promotion programs.

Some countries require *dental assistants* to graduate from training programs that have high standards, meet specified qualifications, and be registered before being considered a professional member of the dental team. In other countries, however, their skills may not be rated so highly and not be recognized by regulatory authorities. Many receive only preceptorship training with no formal theoretical education to support evidence-based practice. Clearly, the standard of training is inconsistent.

A formally trained and registered professional is more likely to receive public confidence. No regulation or deregulation allows more opportunity for negligent care by nonprofessionals with no recourse to an authority should the need arise. For instance, assistants in Austria operating in a legal "grey zone" perform prophylactic treatments and nonsurgical periodontal therapy, sometimes without any coursework at all, which has been shown to have a detrimental effect on treatment efficacy and patient safety.[33] Countries endeavoring to standardize education are slowly recognizing this risk. Society has the right to expect that educated and qualified professionals will provide its oral health care. In this context, the International Federation of Dental Hygienists, representing the views of its members, objects to calling these grey-zone assistants "dental hygienists." The title is protected in a number of countries and has an international definition, which is (in most cases) tied to the advanced educational requirements described in this chapter.

CHALLENGES TO THE PROFESSION

The WHO Oral Health Report 2003 shows that for some societies, dental diseases (especially caries) have declined while certain at-risk groups carry the bulk of the burden of oral diseases around the globe.[2] It is estimated that in developing countries, nearly 90% of the population is unable to receive standardized caries treatment.[3] There is a dire need to promote oral health on a large-scale basis.

The Role of the WHO in Promoting Global Oral Health Equity

The World Health Organization (WHO) in conjunction with the Fédération Dentaire Internationale (FDI) established the first global oral health goals in 1981 to combat rising levels in dental caries due to an increase in sugar consumption. These goals were formulated to be achieved by some industrialized countries by 2000.[39] (See Table 4-1.) In 2003, the FDI, the WHO, and the International Association for Dental Research (IADR), jointly presented new global oral health goals for 2020. (See Box 4-2 ■.) This document presents two goals, ten objectives, and sixteen targets at which community public health programs may be directed.[40] Objectives are population based and guided by the principles of disease prevention and health promotion. The new goals emphasize an evidence-based approach to practice and a stronger public health orientation with a focus on modifiable oral risk behaviors. The targets are formulated in more general terms without absolute values and are intended to serve as a useful framework for health planners at regional, national, and local levels, taking into account global variations in the epidemiology of oral diseases and socioeconomic realities. One specific target is the decrease periodontal disease.[41]

In 2007, WHO issued the document "Oral Health: Action Plan for Promotion and Integrated Disease Prevention," which includes step-by-step suggestions for framing policies and strategies for oral health.[42] It is hoped that this initiative will unite public health providers in effective strategies to reduce barriers to oral health care.

BOX 4-2 Global Goals for Oral Health 2020

- To promote oral health and to minimise the impact of diseases of oral and craniofacial origin on general health and psychosocial development, giving emphasis to promoting oral health in populations with the greatest burden of such conditions and diseases

- To minimise the impact of oral and craniofacial manifestations of general diseases on individuals and society, and to use these manifestations for early diagnosis, prevention and effective management of systemic diseases.

Note: Adopted by the FDI General Assembly September 18, 2003.

Source: FDI policy. http://www.whocollab.od.mah.se/expl/globgoals20.html. Accessed June 8, 2009.

Impact of Global Dental Hygiene on Oral Health Equity

Generally, it appears that public dental health is not perceived as a priority service in many countries. Dental hygienists can play a major role in influencing health services to place more importance on their dental public health programs. In addition to improving the quality of life and general health, preventing oral diseases translates into long-term cost savings.

Many countries have community and school dental services within the public health sector in which dental hygienists provide a significant part of services. Some hygienists are actively involved in clinical work; others work solely in oral health promotion.

Did You Know?

In Norway, the majority of hygienists work in community dental services.

Dental hygienists worldwide have been involved in oral health promotion for children and in giving oral hygiene instruction to disadvantaged groups in the community. Under the stewardship of the WHO, community programs and health care settings provide opportunities to expand oral disease prevention and health promotion knowledge and practices among the public. To implement global oral health strategies and community programs, the WHO promotes partnerships with national and international nongovernmental organizations through its Collaborating Centres on Oral Health.[43] Dental hygienists in their traditional role as oral health prevention specialists are ideally qualified to become proactive in this collaboration.[44] Dental hygienists have also been effective in achieving another WHO objective, that of promoting healthy lifestyles by incorporating tobacco cessation programs and nutritional counseling into their practices.[4] In a study with periodontal patients, success rates in smoking cessation (up to one year later) following the advice of dental hygienists trained in smoking cessation counseling were better than national quit rates achieved in specialist smoking cessation clinics.[45]

An increased collaboration of the WHO with dental hygienists would not only save financial resources but might relax many barriers and legislative restrictions that currently interfere with the full use of dental hygienists in the delivery of public oral health promotion and care.[44]

Autonomous dental hygiene care has the potential to significantly impact the quality of mobile dental care, a service model in which oral health care facilities are transported to a nonmobile population. With the aging of society, mobile dentistry is gaining importance not only in less developed countries but also as in industrialized nations.[46] Extended function dental hygienists (such as in the Netherlands) could meet many challenges presented by the care for this population through their minimal interventive approach. This includes the assessment of the risk of disease with a focus on early detection and prevention, techniques for remineralization, and the treatment of primary coronary or root caries, erosion, abrasion, demineralization, compensation for salivary dysfunction, and management of high plaque levels.[47]

Many countries have structures in place, but the dental hygiene workforce is too scarce and the scope of practice too restricted to have a significant impact on access to care. (See Table 4-7 ■.)

Table 4-7   Countries with Access to Mobile Dentistry

Argentina	Cyprus	Haiti	Malaysia	Philippines	Thailand
Australia	Germany	India	Mexico	Portugal	United Kingdom
Austria	Dominican Republic	Indonesia	New Zealand	Russia	Uruguay
Brazil	Denmark	Ireland	Netherlands	Singapore	United States
Cambodia	Finland	Iceland	Norway	South Africa	Venezuela
Canada	France	Israel	Panama	Spain	Vietnam
Chile	French Polynesia	Italy	Paraguay	Sweden	
China	Guatemala	Japan	Peru	Switzerland	

Source: Correa da Fonseca, A. *An Analysis of Mobile Dentistry in Austria in Comparison to International Scenarios* [master's thesis]. Krems, Austria; Danube University; 2007. Used with permission.

National Oral Health Policies

Few countries have formal national published oral health policies or strategies provided by the government, but Japan, South Korea, and the United Kingdom do provide them. Denmark, France, Germany, Kenya, New Zealand, Nigeria, Norway, Portugal, Slovenia, and Sweden also have policies in place.[12] They range from statements about entitlement to dental treatment to strategies explaining in detail what the government is striving to achieve. In the past, the Council of European Chief Dental Officers proposed an oral health strategy for Europe.[13]

Mass fluoridation programs were popular at one time. However, research has shown that they have decreased in number due in part to the success that fluoride toothpaste has had on reducing caries. Examples of fluoridated drinking water are found, for instance, in the United States and the Republic of Ireland. However, in the poorest nations, even access to community water resources is generally scarce.

Public Health Initiatives and Campaigns

Most countries have some public dental health services administered by states or provinces within the country. In some countries, such as Germany and the United Kingdom, specifically trained oral health promoters offer the programs. In the United Kingdom, a dental professional (dental hygienist, dental therapist, or dental assistant) often provides the service. Many governments are, however, reducing their financial support for national oral health promotion programs in part because of the absence of evidence-based research providing a rational for the continuation of such government spending.

Many countries increasingly are having significant dental public health campaigns and health promotion days, weeks, or months. (See Table 4-8 ■.) Some of the major campaigns are Japan's 8020 campaign, which focuses on retaining twenty teeth by eighty years of age; South Korea's 10 Principles of Dental Health poster campaign; the Netherlands' extensively documented Bottle It Up, Take a Cup campaign to reduce the incidence of nursing caries; and the United Kingdom's Early Years campaign that reflects principles similar to those of the Netherlands. Refer to Table 4-8 for examples of groups lobbying for oral health.

SUCCESSFUL PUBLIC HEALTH INITIATIVES INVOLVING DENTAL HYGIENISTS

"Sonrisas," an Oral Health Care Project for the Underpriviledged in the Dominican Republic

In 1986 while on vacation in the Dominican Republic, Elina Katsman, a Canadian dental hygienist, noticed the poor oral health condition of the local youth and initiated a project to provide free dental treatment and oral health education to underprivileged children. She started

Table 4-8 Oral Health Lobbying Groups by Country

Country	Lobbying Groups
Germany	Toothfriendly Germany (Aktion Zahn-freundlich e.v.) for sugar-free confectionery and drinks
New Zealand	New Zealand Dental Health Foundation
Switzerland	Toothfriendly Switzerland (Aktion Zahn-freundlich) for sugar-free confectionery and drinks
United Kingdom	Action and Information on Sugars (watchdog on misinformation on sugars through poor labeling and advertising)
	Food Commission (watchdog on food industry including sugar issues)
	Chuck Sweets Off the Checkout
	Toothfriendly UK for sugar-free confectionery and drinks

giving lectures with two local nurses whom she trained in the principles of oral hygiene and related primary health care. Through relentless lobbying, she was able to gain support and funding for dental clinics to provide much needed care. Today, the Sonrisas project runs eight dental clinics and five mobile units that serve remote areas and have benefited more than 1.7 million people. This project was honored with the 2007 Sunstar World Dental hygienists' award.[8]

Oral Health Care on the Phelophepa Train in South Africa

The Phelophepa (meaning "good clean health") Train is a project to provide health care to rural South Africans. It began in 1903 as an eye clinic with three coaches. Today, the train has thirteen coaches traveling through rural areas to deliver comprehensive, affordable, accessible health care to remote rural areas in which people have limited access to care. The train reaches more than 130,000 people each year. The dental coach has six dental chairs for providing hygiene care, restorations, and extractions and a special x-ray unit. Prescreenings are performed outside the coach.[48]

Dysphagia Management for the Elderly in Japan

A three-year dental hygiene curriculum in Japan introduced a dysphagia management course in a residential care facility for elderly people.[49] Dental hygiene care was performed on a patient who was bedridden after suffering from a stroke. Oral health personnel had difficulty providing daily oral hygiene routines because the patient suffered from severe muscle tension around the oral cavity. After monthly treatments for five months, results showed a relaxation of oral muscles and a decrease in plaque accumulation and gingival inflammation. Through the positive results of this intervention, students gained first-hand knowledge of the importance of professional oral care to organic and functional oral health improvements for elderly people.

National Periodontal Screening in Austria

When the Austrian national health insurance updated its periodic health examination in 2005, a US-educated dental hygienist was approached to design a periodontal screening program to be administered by general physicians as part of this examination. Austria, where the dental hygiene profession has not been introduced, has a high incidence of untreated periodontitis because prevention and treatment are excluded from national social insurance coverage. Goals of this periodontal screening are to raise public awareness of prevention and treatment, refer persons at risk to periodontal care, include treatment coverage in the national insurance coverage, and make evident the need for qualified care provided by dental hygienists. This project may be viewed as an initiative to integrate oral health into primary health functions, a step the WHO recommends.[50]

FUTURE OF DENTAL HYGIENE WORLDWIDE

Dental hygiene is an expanding profession. Changes in demographics, epidemiology of oral diseases, and longevity call for cost-effective, flexible health care that is best provided by a team approach. In health care, knowledge utilization commonly manifests through evidence-based decision making in practice as well as in public health initiatives.[51] Many examples have shown that autonomous dental hygienists with expanded functions and higher educational attainment are better able to provide quality, cost-effective clinical care and to initiate and manage scientifically based public oral health initiatives. Such dental hygienists may contribute to a wider practical application of scientific knowledge, which has been shown to improve oral health and general health.

The change toward an increasingly academic orientation in dental hygiene education enables a growing number of graduates to engage in research and interpret research results and apply new scientific achievements to benefit the public. Researchers in dental hygiene are needed to gather evidence-based data about the effectiveness of clinical dental hygiene care, behavior modification strategies, and public initiatives. They are needed to collaborate in epidemiological research with relevant organizations in the collection of reliable data. In their traditional role as oral health prevention specialists, dental hygienists may also play a more significant role in workforce partnerships with other health practitioners and academics in conducting evaluations of national and community oral health programs. However, a 2007 survey of all members of the House of Delegates of the IFDH revealed that dental hygienists so far have not participated in such initiatives in any significant way.

In addition to their clinical skills, dental hygienists have an established role as oral health promoters and educators. The new WHO goals emphasize an evidence-based approach to practice and a stronger public health orientation with a focus on modifiable oral risk behaviours. A policy statement of the Proceedings of the 2003 European Workshop on Oral Care and General Health acknowledges that as *clinicians, dental hygienists have the advantage of meeting patients on a regular basis.* This allows dental hygienists to play a key role in changing behavior patterns, thus improving both oral health and quality of life for the patient.[52] Dental hygienists may apply their excellent motivational skills to modify risk behaviors by providing smoking and alcohol cessation counseling and promoting healthy nutrition.

With expanded skills, the dental hygiene workforce may be utilized in a more flexible and accessible way—from private practice to mobile oral health care. The aging population in industrialized regions presents new challenges. Many in this population have heavily restored dentitions and implants that require extensive flexible maintenance care for the rest of their lives.[5] In some countries, dental hygienists are beginning to respond to the need to work in such facilities. Barriers preventing educated members of the dental

team to provide autonomous cost-effective preventive and minimal interventive restorative care must be removed.[46]

In addition, some countries, in an effort to detect oral cancer, dental hygienists have been allowed to administer minimally invasive brush biopsies combined with an advanced computer analysis of nuclear DNA contents, taken from suspicious oral lesions. This process may lead to early referral and to a better prognosis for a cure.

> **Did You Know?**
>
> Dental hygienists have been effective in lobbying for oral health campaigns and programs and are acting as local and national policy advisers in health promotion.

In developing countries, autonomous dental hygienists with extended functions may not only initiate preventive oral health programs but also begin to tend to the primary, minimal interventive restorative needs of millions of untreated children and adults.

Concerns have been voiced about dental hygienists being replaced by preceptorship-trained assistants. However, a closer look at the information presented in this chapter reveals a steady growth of the dental hygiene workforce, a tendency toward higher academic educational attainment and extended functions as well as increased autonomy and self-regulation. Evidence supports the increased employment and extended roles for dental hygienists after appropriate training. When viewing this development in the context of an increased need for care due to demographic changes coupled with a decline in the dentist workforce, the future of the dental hygiene profession appears to be secure.

KEY INTERNATIONAL ORGANIZATIONS

In addition to the World Health Organization, a number of other organizations seek to promote dental health worldwide.

Fédération Dentaire Internationale (FDI)

One of the oldest international health organizations, the FDI was founded in 1900 in Paris. It has member associations in about 120 countries and has established standing commissions and programs on a number of dental-related issues including oral health. FDI began official relations with the World Health Organization (WHO) in 1948 and collaborates with the WHO on the planning and development of global goals for oral health.

International Association for Dental Research (IADR)

The mission of the International Association for Dental Research (IADR) is to advance research and increase knowledge for the improvement of oral health worldwide. It consists of divisions and sections that establish and support programs to promote oral health research and IADR activities. IADR collaborates with other international dental associations, industries, health agencies, and scientific and educational professional organizations.

Council of European Chief Dental Officers (CECDO)

The Council of European Chief Dental Officers (CECDO) promotes dental public health and ethics and exchanges views on dental matters throughout EU and European Economic Area member countries with the goal to harmonize dental professions and access to care within Europe.[13]

Council of European Dentists (CED)

The Council of European Dentists (CED) represents the interests of more than thirty dental associations across Europe. It maintains a databank on thirty European countries with detailed descriptions of national oral health systems, workforce, and public health care demographics.[14] Its Web page contains information on public health strategies of the European Union.

European Federation of Periodontology (EFP)

The main goal of the European Federation of Periodontology (EFP), which first met officially in 1994, is "the promotion of periodontal health in Europe."[53] The EFP strongly believes that some minimum standards in all fields of dental education should be provided and enforced and has published recommendations concerning undergraduate and specialist education in periodontology. Its Web site also includes EFP guidelines for the dental hygiene profession.[54]

International Federation of Dental Hygienists (IFDH)

The International Federation of Dental Hygienists (IFDH) was officially formed in 1986 in Oslo, Norway. It is an international nonprofit organization uniting dental hygiene associations from around the world in their common cause of promoting access to quality preventive oral services and to raise public awareness about the prevention of dental disease.[17] The IFDH is a growing organization with twenty-six countries current members.

IFDH has forged strong links with international organizations that have similar outlooks on oral health promotion such as the FDI, EFP, and WHO (Oral Health Unit). Resources on its Web site include information about work requirements for each member country.

Did You Know?

IFDH publishes the quarterly periodical *International Journal of Dental Hygiene* that contains peer-reviewed scientific articles and international issues involving dental hygiene.

European Dental Hygienists' Federation (EDHF)

The European Dental Hygienists' Federation (EDHF) was founded in 1999 by Spain, Italy, Portugal, Austria, Germany, the Netherlands, and Switzerland and has since expanded.[55] Its focus is on the recognition of the dental hygiene profession and the harmonization of dental hygiene education within Europe. The work of this organization is essential in light of directives from the European Union pertaining to free movement of EU workers and the right of its citizens to equitable access to health care, education, and work opportunities.

SUMMARY

This chapter has provided an overview of the ways in which dental hygienists are involved in dental public health on a global basis. Many countries lack basic facilities for sophisticated oral health promotion programs and are not able to utilize a dental hygienist in the traditional role developed in the United States. Therefore, dental hygienists should remain flexible in their approach to delivering oral hygiene.

Oral health issues are not recognized as health problems in many countries; consequently, periodontal diseases and oral hygiene are neglected and programs addressing them do not exist or are underfunded.

Oral health should embrace other health issues in order to make a case for priority funding in national health programs such as tobacco cessation, nutrition, and diet in efforts to prevent disease.

This is an exciting time for dental hygienists, and the profession will continue to grow in importance and status within the dental team. It is possible to significantly reduce oral disease on a global basis if dental public health systems include dental hygienists.

SELF-STUDY TEST ITEMS

1. Which European country has a history of establishing the dental hygiene profession?
   a. England
   b. Italy
   c. Germany
   d. Portugal

2. Which of the following is a reason for the lack of access to dental hygiene services worldwide?
   a. Insufficient funding
   b. Lack of social and cultural awareness
   c. Legal restraints
   d. All of above

3. How many countries in the European Union report no or virtually no hygienists?
   a. 3
   b. 7
   c. 10
   d. 17

4. In industrialized nations, where do dental hygienists mainly practice?
   a. Public health clinics
   b. Educational institutions
   c. Government positions
   d. Private dental clinics

5. What organization is a nonprofit group that unites dental hygiene associations from around the world in their common cause of promoting access to qualify preventative oral services and to raise public awareness of the prevention of dental disease?
   a. American Dental Hygiene Association
   b. European Dental Hygienists' Federation
   c. International Federation of Dental Hygienists
   d. European Federation of Periodontology

REFERENCES

1. Petersen PE. The world oral health report 2003: Continuous improvement of oral health in the 21st century—The approach of the WHO Global Oral Health Programme. *Comm Dent Oral Epidemiol.* 2003;31(suppl 1):3–24.
2. Petersen PE, Kwan S. Evaluation of community-based oral health promotion and oral disease prevention—WHO recommendations for improved evidence in public health practice. *Community Dent Health.* 2004;21(suppl 4): 319–329.
3. Robert Y, Sheiham A. The burden of restorative dental treatment for children in Third World countries. *Int Dent J.* 2002;52(1):1–9.
4. World Health Organization. Strategies and Approaches in Oral Disease Prevention and Health Promotion. http://www.who.int/oral_health/strategies/cont/en/index.html. Accessed November 12, 2007.
5. Eaton, KA. *Factors Affecting Community Oral Health Care Needs and Provision* [dissertation]. London, UK: University of London; 2002.
6. Öhrn, K. The role of oral sequelae in health-related quality of life of cancer patients. *Support Care Cancer.* 2002;10(8):656–658.
7. Pine CM, Pitts NB, Steele JG, Nunn JN, Treasure E. Dental restorations in adults in the UK in 1998 and implications for the future. *Br Dent J.* 2001;190(1):4–8.
8. Katsman E. Report on the activities carried out by "Sonrisas" to promote oral health: The experience of a Canadian dental hygienist in the Dominican Republic. *Int J Dent Hyg.* 2007;5(3):139–144.
9. Knevel RJM, Neupane S, Shressta B, de Mey L. Buddhi Bangara Project—a 3–5 year collaborative program combining support, education, and research. *Int J Dent Hyg.* In press.
10. World Health Organization. Global Oral Health Database. http://www.who.int/oral_health/databases/global/en/index.html. Accessed November 12, 2007.
11. World Health Organization. Periodontal Country Profiles. http://www.dent.niigata-u.ac.jp/prevent/perio/contents.html. Accessed November 12, 2007.

12. Fédération Dentaire Internationale. Dental Schools. http://www.fdiworldental.org/resources/6_0schools.html. Accessed November 12, 2007.

13. Council of European Chief Dental Officers. CECDO database. http://www.cecdo.org/pages/database%20intro.html. Accessed November 12, 2007.

14. Council of European Dentists. About the CED. http://www.eudental.eu/. Accessed November 12, 2007.

15. Johnson PM. Dental hygiene practice: International profile and future directions. *Int Dent J.* 1992;42:451–459.

16. Johnson PM. International profiles of dental hygiene 1987 to 2001: A 19-nation comparative study. *Int Dent J.* 2003;53:299–313.

17. International Federation of Dental Hygienists. Home page. About the IFDH. www.ifdh.org. Accessed November 12, 2007.

18. Hobdell M, Petersen PE, Clarkson J, Johnson N. Global goals for oral health 2020. *Int Dent J.* 2003;53:28.

19. Bader JD, Shugars D. Need for change in standards of caries diagnosis—Epidemiology and health services research perspective. *J Dent Educ.* 1993;57:415–421.

20. Ismail AI, Sohn W, Tellez M, Amaya A, Sen A, Hasson H, Pitts NB. The International Caries Detection and Assessment System (ICDAS): An integrated system for measuring dental caries. *Community Dent Oral Epidemiol.* 2007;35(3):170–178.

21. Bratthall D. Introducing the Significant Caries Index together with a proposal for a new global oral health goal for 12 year-olds. *Int Dent J.* 2000;50:378–384.

22. Ainamo J, Barmes DE, Beagrie BG, Cutress TW, Martin J, Sardo Infirri J. Development of the World Health Organization (WHO) Community Periodontal Index of Treatment Needs (CPITN). *Int Dent J.* 1982;32:281–291.

23. Bassani DG, da Silva CM, Oppermann RV. Validity of the "Community Periodontal Index of Treatment Needs" (CPITN) for population periodontitis screening. *Cad Saude Publica.* 2006;22(2):277–283.

24. Baelum V, Papapanou PN. CPITN and the epidemiology of periodontal disease. 1996: Commentary. *Community Dent and Oral Epidemiol.* 24;6:367–368.

25. Chaudhry Z., Scully C. Dental manpower: Many questions, weak data and inadequate answers. *Br Dent J.* 1998; 184:432–436.

26. Snoad RJ, Eaton KA. Differences in periodontal complexity assessment between dental hygienists and general dental practitioners during two clinical audits. *Dent Health.* 2006;45:4:5–14.

27. Öhrn K, Crossner CG, Börgesson I, Taube A. Accuracy of dental hygienists in diagnosing dental decay. *Community Dent Oral Epidemiol.* 1996;24:182–186.

28. Öhrn K. The role of dental hygienists in oral health prevention. *Oral Health Prev Dent.* 2004;2(suppl 1): 277–281.

29. Luciak-Donsberger, C. The study of dental hygiene at institutions of higher education. Vienna, Austria; 2003. Report commissioned by the Federal Ministry of Eduction, Science, and Culture.

30. Abbott A. *The System of Professions.* Chicago and London: University of Chicago Press. 1988.

31. US Department of Health and Human Services. *Oral Health in America: A Report of the Surgeon General.* Rockville, MD: US Department of Health and Human Services, National Institute of Dental and Craniofacial Research, National Institutes of Health; 2000.

32. Eaton KA, Newman HN, Widsröm E. A survey of dental hygienists numbers in Canada, the European Economic Area, Japan and the United States of America in 1998. *Br Dentl J.* 2003;195:595–598.

33. Luciak-Donsberger C. Origins and benefits of dental hygiene practice in Europe. *Int J Dent Hyg.* 2003;1:29–42.

34. Luciak-Donsberger C. The effects of gender disparities on dental hygiene education and practice in Europe. *Int J Dent Hyg.* 2003;1(4):195–212.

35. Luciak-Donsberger C. *The Study of Dental Hygiene in Europe: Education and Legal Regulation in Eight Additional Countries. Current Developments in Six Countries.* Vienna, Austria: Federal Ministry of Education, Science and Culture; 2003.

36. McKeown L, Sunell S, Wickstrom P. The discourse of dental hygiene practice in Canada. *Int J Dent Hyg.* 2003;1: 43–48.

37. Cheng YA, Huang ST, Hsieh ST. A predictive study on the role and function of the dental hygienist in Taiwan. *Int J Dent Hyg.* 2007;5(2):103–108.

38. Luciak-Donsberger C, Chan C. Dental hygiene in Hong Kong: A global perspective. *Int J Dent Hyg.* 2003;1(2):84–88.

39. Global goals for oral health in the year 2000: FDI. *Int Dent J.* 1982;32:74–77.

40. World Health Organization. Global goals for oral health. http://www.whocollab.od.mah.se/expl/globgoals20.html. Accessed November 12, 2007.

41. Hobdell M, Petersen PE, Clarkson J, Johnson N. Global goals for oral health 2020. *Int Dent J.* 2003;53:285–288.

42. World Health Organization Sixtieth World Health Assembly, A60/16 Provisional Agenda Item 12.9 22. http://apps.who.int/gb/ebwha/pdf_files/WHA60/A60_16-en.pdf. Accessed March, 22 2007.

43. World Health Organization. WHO collab centres. www.who.int/whocc. Accessed September 30, 2007.

44. Monajem S. Integration of oral health into primary health care: The role of dental hygienists and the WHO stewardship. *Int J Dent Hyg.* 2006;4(1):47–51.

45. Nasry HA, Preshaw PM, Stacey F, Heasman L, Swan M, Heasman PA. Smoking cessation advice for patients with chronic periodontitis. *Br Dent J.* 2006;200(5):272–275.

46. Correa da Fonseca, A. *An Analysis of Mobile Dentistry in Austria in Comparison to International Scenarios* [master's thesis]. Krems, Austria: Danube University; 2007.

47. Chalmers JM. Minimal intervention dentistry: Part 2. Strategies for addressing restorative challenges in older patients. *J Can Dent Assoc.* 2006;72(5):435–440.

48. Phelophepa Train. http://www.mhc.org.za. Accessed November 12, 2007.

49. Nishimura T, Takahashi C, Takahashi E. Dental hygiene residential care in a 3-year dental hygiene education programme in Japan: Towards dysphagia management based on the dental hygiene process of care. *Int J Dent Hyg.* 2007;5(3):145–150.

50. Luciak-Donsberger C, Piribauer F. Evidence-based rationale supports a national periodontal disease screening program. *J Evid Based Dent Pract.* 2007;7(2):51–59.

51. Cobban SJ. Evidence-based practice and the professionalization of dental hygiene. *Int J Dent Hyg.* 2004;2(4): 152–160.

52. Policy Statement—Proceedings of the European Workshop on Oral Care and General Health. Opportunities for the Dental Hygienists in Health Education in the New Century. *Oral Health and Prev Dent.* 2003;1(suppl 1):340.

53. European Federation of Periodontology. Vision. www.efp .net. Accessed November 12, 2007.

54. Dental hygienists' guide to the Internet. www.dhed.net/ guide.html. Accessed November 12, 2007.

55. European Dental Hygienists' Federation. About us. http:// www.edhf.org/. Accessed December 9, 2007.

PEARSON

myhealthprofessionskit™

Multimedia Extension Activities

Use this address to access the interactive Companion Website created for this textbook. Simply select "Dental Hygiene" from the choice of disciplines. Find this book and log in using your username and password. To obtain a username and password, please register using the scratch-off access code on the inside front cover of this book.

Chapter 5

Financing of Dental Care

OBJECTIVES

After studying this chapter, the dental hygiene student should be able to:

- Describe current methods of payment for dental care
- Define and apply terminology associated with financing dental care
- Identify the different insurance plans available for dental care
- Describe the role of the government in financing dental care

KEY TERMS

Barter system
Benefit
Capitation plan
Copayment
Deductible
Dental claim
Dental necessity
Encounter fee plan
Explanation of benefits
Fee-for-service plan
Medicaid (Title XIX)
Medicare (Title XVIII)
Preexisting condition
Premium
Usual, customary, reasonable (UCR) fee

COMPETENCIES

After studying this chapter and participating in accompanying course activities, the dental hygiene student should be competent to do the following:

- Provide quality assurance mechanisms for health services
- Evaluate reimbursement mechanisms and their impact on the patient's access to oral health care

Historically, the financing of dental care was the responsibility of the patient in need of treatment and the dental practitioner involved in managing the dental practice. However, in today's economy, the financing of dental care in the United States involves numerous entities in both the private and public sectors.

Of the total health care expenditures in the United States in 2004, only 7.4% was spent on dental services.[1] Nearly 92% was paid for by private funds whether by the patient (49.3%) or by private insurance (42.2%).[2] (See Table 5-1 ■, pages 74–75.) Approximately 54% of the population had private dental coverage during 2004, 12% had only public dental coverage, and 35% had no dental coverage at all.[3]

Approximately 44% of the population had at least one dental visit during 2004, and of those, 44% the average individual expense was $560. The average number of visits per person was 2.5.[3] (See Figures 5-1 ■, 5-2 ■, and 5-3 ■.) Not surprising, persons from lower income families were less likely to have private dental coverage in 2004 than persons from a family with higher income. Children and adolescents under age 21, persons who were poor, and persons from a family with low income were more likely to have public dental coverage in 2004 than adults age 45 and over or persons from a family with middle or high income.[3]

From 1996 to 2004, no significant change in the percentage of the population who had a dental visit occurred.[3] Average dental expenses increased from $115 ($138 adjusted for inflation) in 1996 to $181 in 2004 and from $142 ($171 adjusted for inflation) in 1996 to $225 in 2004 for preventive/diagnostic procedures and restorative procedures, respectively.[3] (See Figure 5-4 ■.)

What proportion of the community has a dental visit?

- In 2004, there were about 294 million people in the community population of the United States.

- Approximately 44% of the population had at least one dental visit during the year.

- The average expense was $560 per year for persons with a dental visit, and the average number of visits was 2.5 visits per person for persons with a visit (data not shown).

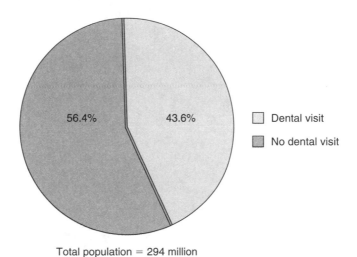

Total population = 294 million

FIGURE 5-1   Proportion of the Community That Had a Dental Visit in 2004

Source: Manski, RJ, Brown, E. *Dental Use, Expenses, Private Dental Coverage and Changes, 1996–2004.* Rockville, MD: Agency for Healthcare Research and Quality; 2007. MEPS Chartbook No.17.

Table 5-1 Dental Service Expenses in the United States, 2000[a]

Population	Population (in thousands)	Percent of Expense	Expense per Person		Total Expenses (in millions)	Percent Distribution of Total Expenses by Source of Payment (percent)				
			Median	Mean		Out of Pocket	Private Insurance[b]	Medicare	Medicaid	Other[c]
Total	278,406	40.1%	$168	$498	$55,551	49.3%	42.2%	0.5%	4.0%	3.9%
Age in Years										
Under 65	243,624	40.2	164	492	48,209	45.2	46.3	0.0[d]	4.6	3.9
Under 6	24,126	20.1	99	193	937	25.4	43.3	0.0[d]	25.6	5.7[d]
6–17	48,405	51.1	155	654	16,172	44.0	47.6	0.0[d]	6.5	1.9
18–44	109,021	36.8	155	404	16,223	42.0	49.1	0.0[d]	4.6[d]	4.3
5–64	62,072	45.4	209	528	14,876	51.2	42.0	0.0[d]	1.1	5.6
65 and over	34,782	39.5	196	534	7341	76.7	15.2	3.6	0.4	4.1
Gender										
Male	135,882	36.9	162	464	23,274	49.8	40.3	0.4[d]	4.6[d]	4.9
Female	142,524	43.2	172	525	32,277	49.0	43.6	0.5[d]	3.6	3.3
Race/Ethnicity										
White and other	209,401	45.0	178	524	49,390	49.8	42.3	0.5	3.6	3.8
Black	35,049	26.0	107	354	3224	40.3	47.4	0.3[d]	7.1	4.9
Hispanic	33,955	24.4	128	354	2936	51.7	35.3	0.6[d]	7.3	5.1
Health Insurance Status[e]										
Under age 65										
Any private	182,658	46.1	174	515	43,411	44.1	51.4	0.0[d]	1.6[d]	2.8
Public only	28,622	27.9	87	287	2290	26.9	0.0[d]	0.4[d]	66.4	6.2
Uninsured	32,344	17.5	151	444	2508	79.8	0.0[d]	0.0[d]	0.0[d]	20.3
Age 65 and Over										
Medicare only	11,515	32.6	195	661	2480	86.8	0.0[d]	5.3[d]	0.0[d]	8.0[d]
Medicare and private	19,570	47.9	200	490	4601	72.6	24.3	1.6	0.0[d]	1.5
Medicare and other public	3568	16.4	—	—	—	—	—	—	—	—
Economic Status[f]										
Poor	32,053	24.8	105	345	2744	44.1	23.3	2.2[d]	22.2	8.2[d]
Near poor	12,196	25.4	150	495	1533[d]	31.0[d]	25.1[d]	0.3[d]	36.8[d]	6.8[d]
Low income	37,059	28.6	144	392	4157	59.5	25.1	0.5[d]	10.5	4.5[d]

(*continued*)

Table 5-1   Dental Service Expenses in the United States, 2000[a]

Population	Population (in thousands)	Percent of Expense	Expense per Person Median	Expense per Person Mean	Total Expenses (in millions)	Out of Pocket	Private Insurance[b]	Medicare	Medicaid	Other[c]
Middle income	90,343	38.6	166	490	17,093	51.1	40.5	0.6[d]	3.3[d]	4.5
High income	106,754	51.6	185	545	30,025	48.3	48.2	0.3	0.2[d]	3.0
Metropolitan Statistical Area (MSA)										
MSA	226,861	40.9	$170	$502	$46 597	48.1	42.9	0.6	4.4	4.1
Non-MSA	51,545	36.5	151	476	8954	56.0	38.7	0.1[d]	2.2	3.1
Census Region										
Northeast	52,636	45.7	185	519	12,469	51.6	39.5	0.7[d]	3.9	4.3
Midwest	64,536	45.0	149	449	13,024	46.7	45.7	0.3[d]	3.3[d]	4
South	97,373	35.4	154	472	16,278	54.1	40.3	0.4[d]	1.3	3.9
West	63,861	37.8	200	571	13,780	44.2	43.6	0.7[d]	8.0[d]	3.5
Perceived Health Status										
Excellent	87,890	42.6	160	477	17,845	45.7	48.3	0.1[d]	3.0	2.8
Very good	93,499	42.8	165	514	20,587	49.2	44.8	0.5[d]	1.9	3.6
Good	67,922	37.5	176	480	12,235	50.6	35.1	0.7[d]	8.4[d]	5.2
Fair	20,666	32.3	200	560	3740	62.3	26.7	0.6[d]	3.8	6.7
Poor	7720	26.4	185	561	1144	53.2	26.9	2.6[d]	12.6[d]	4.7[d]

[a]Includes services provided by general dentists, dental hygienists, dental technicians, dental surgeons, orthodontists, endodontists, and periodontists.

[b]Private insurance includes TRICARE (armed forces-related coverage).

[c]*Other* includes payments from the Department of Veterans Affairs (except TRICARE), other federal sources (Indian Health Service, military treatment facilities, and other care provided by the federal government), various state and local sources (community and neighborhood clinics, state and local health departments, and state programs other than Medicaid), Workers' Compensation, various unclassified sources (eg, automobile, homeowners, other liability insurance and other miscellaneous or unknown sources), Medicaid payments reported for persons who were not identified as being enrolled in the Medicaid program at any time during the year, and private insurance payments reported for persons without any private health insurance coverage during the year.

[d]Relative standard error equal to or more than 30 percent.

[e]*Uninsured* refers to persons without insurance during the entire year. Public and private health insurance categories refer to individuals with public or private insurance at any time during the period; individuals with both public and private insurance and those with TRICARE (armed forces-related coverage) are classified as having private insurance.

[f]*Poor:* persons in families with income less than 100% of the poverty line, including those whose losses exceeded their earnings, resulting in negative income; *near poor:* persons in families with income from 100% to less than 125% of the poverty line; *low income:* persons in families with income from 125% to less than 200% of the poverty line; *middle income:* persons in families with income from 200% to less than 400% of the poverty line; *high income:* persons in families with income at or over 400% of the poverty line.

— indicates fewer than 100 sample cases.

Note: Restricted to civilian noninstitutionalized population. Percents may not add to 100 because of rounding.

Sources: Center for Financing, Access, and Cost Trends, Agency for Healthcare Research and Quality: Medical Expenditure Panel Survey; 2000. Ezzati-Rice TM, Kashihara D, Machlin SR. *Health Care Expenses in the U.S. 2000.* Rockville, MD: Agency for Healthcare Research and Quality; 2004. MEPS Research Findings No. 21. AHRQ Pub. No. 04-0022.

How is dental coverage distributed across the population?

- In 2004, dental coverage varied by age, family income, race/ethnicity, and education.

- About 61% of middle age adults (45–64 year olds) and 24% of older adults (age 65 and over) had private dental coverage during 2004.

- Persons from lower income families were less likely to have private dental coverage in 2004 than persons from a family with higher income.

- Children and adolescents (less than age 21), persons who were poor, and persons from a family with low income were more likely to have public dental coverage in 2004 than adults (age 45 and over) or persons from a family with middle or high income.

Percentage with dental coverage

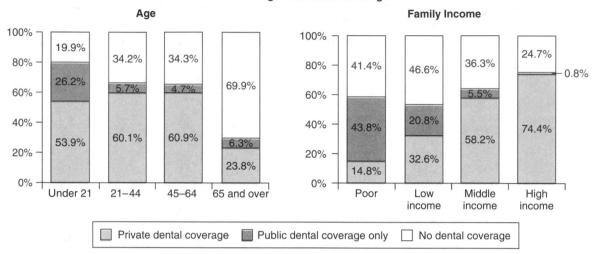

- Black non-Hispanic and Hispanic persons were more likely to have public dental coverage and less likely to have private dental coverage in 2004 than white non-Hispanics or persons of other race/ethnicity categories.

- Persons with some or no school were more likely to have no dental coverage, more likely to have public dental coverage, and less likely to have private dental coverage in 2004 than high school graduates or college graduates.

Percentage with dental coverage

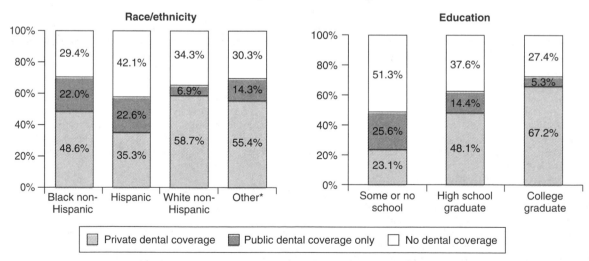

*Other includes non-Hispanics who reported to be of single race other than white or black (i.e., American Indian/Alaska Native, Asian, or Native Hawaiian/Pacific Islander) as well as non-Hispanics who reported to be of multiple races (possibly including black)

FIGURE 5-2 Dental Coverage Across the Population by Age (A), Family Income (B), Race/Ethnicity (C), and Education (D) in 2004

Source: Manski RJ, Brown E. *Dental Use, Expenses, Private Dental Coverage and Changes, 1996–2004.* Rockville, MD: Agency for Healthcare Research and Quality; 2007. MEPS Chartbook No. 17.

Do dental care visits vary by dental coverage status?

- In 2004, 57% of the population with private dental coverage had a dental visit, 32% of the population with public dental coverage only had a dental visit, and 27% of the population without any dental coverage had a dental visit.

- Persons with public dental coverage only had fewer visits on average in 2004 than persons with private dental coverage or no dental coverage.

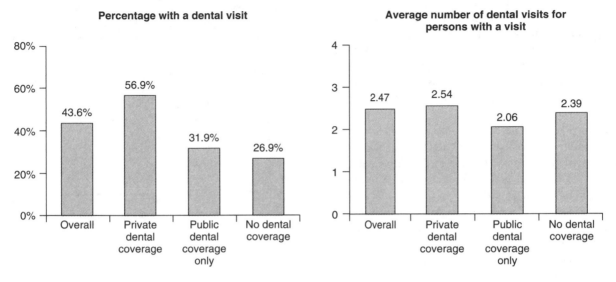

FIGURE 5-3 Dental Care Variations by Dental Coverage Status in 2004

Source: Manski RJ, Brown E. *Dental Use, Expenses, Private Dental Coverage and Changes, 1996–2004.* Rockville, MD: Agency for Healthcare Research and Quality; 2007. MEPS Chartbook No. 17.

How has the percentage of the population with a dental visit changed from 1996 to 2004?

- There was no significant change in the percentage of the population with a dental visit from 1996 to 2004

Percentage with a dental visit

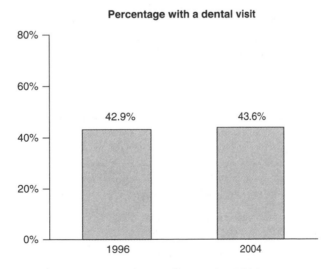

FIGURE 5-4 Dental Care Expense Changes from 1996–2004

Source: Manski RJ, Brown E. *Dental Use, Expenses, Private Dental Coverage and Changes, 1996–2004.* Rockville, MD: Agency for Healthcare Research and Quality; 2007. MEPS Chartbook No. 17.

PAYMENT METHODS

Generally, there are four types of payment methods in dental care delivery. These include the fee-for-service arrangements, capitation plans, encounter fee plans, and the barter system. (See Table 5-2 ▪.) Although these reimbursement mechanisms can be unique to different parts of the country, they have similarities.

The **fee-for-service plan** is based on a fee scale for all covered services, and bills the patient for the services rendered by a dental hygienist, dentist, or denturist. It is the most commonly used payment method in the United States. The patient and/or an insurance company may pay the fee. These set fees are referred to as **usual, customary, and reasonable (UCR) fees,** which are the average dentist fee per service in the immediate local region. *Usual* implies that the fee is what is most often charged by dental providers for a given dental or dental hygiene service. *Customary* refers to a schedule of maximum fees charged by dental providers with similar training and service within a specific and limited geographic area as determined by the administrator of a dental plan based on submitted fees. *Reasonable* indicates that the fee meets the usual and customary definitions and is therefore justifiable.

Some clinics have instituted a sliding-fee scale to make services more affordable for patients with a low income. The fees for services may be decreased depending on the patient's income and family size. This type of reduced-fee program is available through federal grants.

Indemnity plans are traditional fee-for-service insurance plans that operate by a submission and reimbursement method. The dental practitioner provides a service and either bills the patient, who pays the fee and submits the bill to an insurance company for reimbursement, or the insurance company, which makes direct payment to the practice. Usually, patients with an indemnity plan may choose any dentist but may be required to obtain preauthorization for certain procedures. Most indemnity plans require an annual deductible payment, and after the patient has paid that amount, the plan typically pays a percentage of UCR rates for covered services. For example, the insurance company may pay 80% of the UCR and the patient may be required to cover the remaining 20%. Most plans require the patient to make a copayment for a visit, which is deducted from the 20% the patient, not the plan, covers.

Did You Know?

Copayments are often used to discourage the overuse of services.

Many fee-for-service payment methods offer a discounted fee for a target population. For example, a dental office may lower fees by 10% for senior citizens or participants in a prepaid group.

Most dental practices accept fee-for-service plans that provide an incentive for dental practitioners to provide all necessary treatments. Generally, these plans increase the production of an office because it is paid based on the number of services produced. The clinic or provider creates the fee scale, usually similar to the UCR.

Table 5-2 Types of Payment Methods

Payment Method	Definition
Fee for service	Fee scale is developed for all services provided by the dental provider and a payment is then developed for the service(s) rendered. This is the most common payment method used in the United States.
Capitation	Dental provider contracts with a program to provide all or most dental services to the program's subscribers in return for payment on a per capita basis.
Barter system	Dental provider and patient negotiate payment by exchanging goods or services without utilizing money.
Encounter	Payment is based on an office visit and is always the same regardless of the service(s) rendered.

With the **capitation plan,** a dental provider contracts with a third party to provide all or most of the services to a specified group of people in return for a fixed monthly payment, which is determined according to the number of individuals or families in the group. The dental provider receives the payment whether the patients use the care or not. The patients are sometimes charged a copayment for specified treatments. The philosophy behind capitation plans is that it is more cost effective to keep people healthy than it is to treat their disease. The incentive is to keep people well and out of the health care provider's practice. Costs are kept low so the patient benefits and patient demand are also kept low, which benefits the practice.

Dental managed care organizations typically provide capitation plans. Managed care organizations were created in 1973 by the Health Maintenance Organization Act. Participating physicians of a **health maintenance organization (HMO)** provide comprehensive health care to enrolled individuals and families in a specified region and receive fixed periodic payments. Some suggest that because of their primarily preventive care, HMOs actually reduce costs for participants by reducing hospitalization and the use of costly services. Some dental providers do not support dental managed care plans because of the reduction in reimbursement and the decrease in control of treatment that they can recommend. Most HMOs provide medical coverage but do not cover routine dental care.

In some instances, capitation plans may not benefit the patient. For example, a dental practice that receives a set payment each month from a plan has little incentive to provide preventive treatment to the plan-covered patients. In other words, a practice that is paid whether it provides treatment or not may choose not to provide treatment to capitation plan members but instead to schedule as many fee-for-service patients as possible. In this way, the office could collect the monthly stipend from the capitation plan and still collect fees for services provided to fee-for-service patients.

The **encounter fee plan** basically pays for each care encounter regardless of the service provider. For example, if a patient visits a provider on one day for an exam and prophylaxis, on the next day for two amalgam restorations, and the third day for a class-V glass ionomer restoration, each encounter generates the same reimbursement fee.

The encounter fee plan may tend to decrease productivity overall because some dental clinics offer only one service per visit to capitalize on the number of encounters and thus fees paid. This would obviously inconvenience the patient and may subsequently decrease the likelihood of the patient's receiving comprehensive care. Some clinics go so far as to have a new patient appointment take at least three visits by scheduling one visit for radiographs, one for an exam, and another for the dental prophylaxis.

The **barter system,** used only in the private sector, involves exchanging goods and services without using money. The dental provider and the patient negotiate the exchange. For instance, the dental practitioner may provide dental care in return for the patient's carpentry services. Although not common, this payment method is still in place in many US private dental offices, particularly in rural areas.

INSURANCE PLANS

Dental service corporations are legally constituted nonprofit organizations incorporated in a state and sponsored by a dental society to negotiate and administer programs. These programs are contractual agreements with dentists to provide care to eligible beneficiaries using UCR fees. Generally, dental providers accept payment at 90% of fees as payment in full. Their patient charts are regularly audited for fees and inspected. Currently, the largest dental benefits carrier in the United States is Delta Dental Plans Association[4] operated on a state-by-state basis. See Figure 5-5 ■ for a Delta Dental of New Mexico summary of covered dental services.

Health service corporations offer limited dental coverage as part of their hospital-surgical-medical policies. A common health service corporation is Blue Cross/Blue Shield.[5]

Many dental practices in the United States participate in **preferred provider organizations (PPOs).** The practitioners contract with a PPO to provide dental care services for lower than average fees in order to attract patient subscribers who are seeking lower costs. This gives the dental practitioners a competitive edge over nonparticipating practitioners.

Individual practice associations (IPAs) are legal entities organized for individual participating dental practitioners to enter into contracts collectively to provide prepaid dental services to enrolled patients. They may contract directly with a group or an insurance carrier. This is usually referred to as *managed care* and uses the capitation method of reimbursement.

I. SUMMARY OF COVERED DENTAL SERVICES

DIAGNOSTIC & PREVENTIVE SERVICES	UNM Pays: 100%* no deductible	You Pay: 0%*

- Oral Examinations - twice in a calendar year
- Cleanings - twice in a calendar year
- X-rays: Full mouth - once every 3 years / Bitewing - twice in a calendar year
- Topical Fluoride - through age 18, twice in a calendar year
- Emergency Treatment - for relief of pain
- Space Maintainers - through age 15, 5 year limitation
- Sealants - through age 15, permanent molars only, 3 year limitation

RESTORATIVE SERVICES (Fillings)	UNM Pays: 85%* after deductible	You Pay: 15%*

- Amalgam fillings on posterior teeth
- Composite resin fillings for anterior teeth only
- Stainless steel crowns

BASIC SERVICES	UNM Pays: 85%* after deductible	You Pay: 15%*

- Extractions - surgical and non-surgical extractions
- Oral Surgery - maxillofacial surgical procedures of the oral cavity
- Periodontics - nonsurgical and surgical
- Endodontics - pulp therapy and root canal filling
- General Anesthesia - intravenous sedation and general anesthesia, when dentally necessary and administered by a licensed provider for a covered oral surgery procedure

MAJOR SERVICES	UNM Pays: 50%* after deductible	You Pay: 50%*

- Crowns and Cast Restorations - when teeth cannot be restored with amalgam or composite resin restorations
- Prosthodontics - procedures for construction or repair of fixed bridges, partials or complete dentures

ORTHODONTIC SERVICES	UNM Pays: 50%* after deductible	You Pay: 50%*

- Procedures using appliances to treat poor alignment of teeth and/or jaws which significantly interferes with their function
- Coverage is for enrolled adults and dependent children

DEDUCTIBLE	You Pay: $25 per enrolled person $50 aggregate per family

- You pay a deductible for each enrolled person each benefit period up to a maximum aggregate deductible per family.
- The benefit period for your group is July 1 to June 30.
- You do not have to pay a deductible for DIAGNOSTIC AND PREVENTIVE SERVICES or ORTHODONTIC SERVICES. Payments for services described under DIAGNOSTIC AND PREVENTIVE SERVICES or ORTHODONTIC SERVICES will not be credited toward the deductible.

MAXIMUM	Delta Dental Pays: $1500 per enrolled person

- Delta will pay up to a maximum amount for covered services each benefit period per enrolled person.
- The benefit period for your group is July 1 to June 30.
- Any amount for covered dental services that exceed the maximum benefit amount during the benefit period is the responsibility of the enrolled person.

ORTHODONTIC MAXIMUM	Delta Dental Pays: $1000 per enrolled person

- Delta will pay up to a separate maximum per lifetime per enrolled dependent for covered Orthodontic Services.
- Coverage is for enrolled adults and dependent children.

* Applied to the lesser of the Delta Maximum Approved Amount or the Delta Premier dentist's billed amount.

Obtaining services from a nonparticipating dentist may result in higher out-of-pocket expenses.

Please note: You are not eligible for benefits prior to your individual effective date or following your termination date.

This is a summary of benefits. To fully understand the coverage provided, please read the sections of this handbook that describe: How the Plan Works; Eligibility and Enrollment; Benefits, Limitations and Exclusions; Definitions.

FIGURE 5-5 Summary of Delta Dental of New Mexico Covered Dental Services

Concordia Plus Dental Program is an example of a prepaid dental plan that focuses on preventive care and the early diagnosis of dental problems.[6] Under Concordia Plus, members select a primary dental office (PDO) from a contracted and credentialed network of providers. The PDO handles the member's dental care needs, including referrals to specialists when necessary. Members select their own PDO from the Concordia Plus network of participating dentists.

See Table 5-3 ■ for a comparison of the various types of insurance plans.

DENTAL PROVIDER BILLING

Dental providers generally bill insurance companies for dental procedures utilizing a *dental claim form.* (See Figures 5-6 ■ and 5-7 ■ for an example of a fee slip and a claim form, respectively.) These forms generally require the use of five-character, alphanumeric codes to identify and define certain procedures (eg, D2110). See Figure 5-8 ■ for examples of CDT codes and their meanings. The maintenance of these codes is the responsibility of the Council on Dental Benefit Programs with consultation from the Health Insurance Association of America, Blue Cross/Blue Shield, the Health Care Financing Association, National Electronic Information Corporation, and the ADA recognized dental specialty organizations. The *Code on Dental Procedures and Nomenclature* of the American Dental Association (ADA) provides current dental terminology (CDT).[7] The ADA updates the CDT approximately every five years.

A patient who is on a self-pay program generally pays for the dental procedures immediately at the end of the appointment. Many dental offices offer payment plans to patients to make their treatments more affordable, and

Table 5-3 Types of Insurance Plans

Insurance Plan	Definition	Example
Dental service corporations	Not-for-profit organizations that negotiate fees for providing dental care; incorporated on a state-by-state basis and sponsored by a constituent dental society to negotiate and administer programs	Delta Dental Plans Association
Health service corporations	Organizations that offer limited dental coverage as part of their hospital-surgical-medical policies	Blue Cross/Blue Shield
Preferred provider organizations (PPO)	Providers of dental benefits and third-party contractors with employer to offer services to employer's employees at reduced prices	Aetna U.S. Healthcare Dental PPO
Individual practice associations (IPA)	Legal entities organized for dental providers to enter into contracts collectively to provide prepaid dental services to enrolled groups	MD Individual Practice Associates, Inc.
Commercial insurance plans	Operate for profit and designed as an indemnity plan.	Unicare 200
Prepaid group practice	Large group practice that contracts with groups of subscribers	Golden West Dental and Vision
Health maintenance organization (HMO)	Developed in 1973 by the HMO act, organization provides comprehensive health care to enrolled individuals and families in a specified region by participating providers, financed by fixed periodic payments; initially designed to decrease health care costs.	Presbyterian Health Plan
Capitatation plan	Offers per capita payment for a defined population provided by specific dental providers; payment made to provider regardless of use.	Concordia Plus

some use dental credit cards as a financial payment plan for patients.

If a patient is covered by insurance and the office files the claim, it sends the form to the insurance company either electronically or in hard copy. The insurance company decides on payment and sends an *explanation of benefits* (EOB) to the patient and the provider with an accompanying payment to the provider for the allowed amount if the company covers the procedure. (See Figure 5-9 ■.)

Some dental practices prefer to bill patients who pay them for procedures rendered and then the patients submit the charges to their insurance company for possible reimbursement. Many times these practices are referred to as *cash-only* or *no-insurance practices*.

Did You Know?

Dental hygienists are responsible for choosing which code(s) to report and are legally responsible for that choice.

Insurance fraud is committed with the intent to falsely obtain payment from an insurer. Entering a date other than the actual date of treatment and entering a code for a procedure that was not provided are forms of insurance fraud. Even choosing codes incorrectly is considered a form of insurance fraud, so it is important that dental hygienists enter the proper coding and maintain the necessary documentation for all services rendered.

UNIVERSITY OF NEW MEXICO
DIVISION OF DENTAL HYGIENE

I. DIAGNOSTIC SERVICES		
00120	Periodic Oral Evaluation	
00140	Limited Oral Evaluation (Emergency)	
00150	Initial Comprehensive Oral Evaluation	

RADIOGRAPHS		TOOTH	ARCH
00210	Intraoral Comp Series-Inc. BW		
00220	Intraoral Periapical-1st Film		
00230	Intraoral P.A.-Ea. Addl. Film		
00240	Intraoral Occlusal Film		
00270	Bitewing-Single Film		
00272	Bitewing-Two Films		
00274	Bitewings-Four Films		
00330	Panoramic Film		

II. PREVENTIVE SERVICES		TOOTH
01110	Prophylaxis - Adult	
01120	Prophylaxis - Child	
01203	Topical Floride - Child (without Prophy)	
* 01204	Topical Floride - Adult (without Prophy)	
01351	Sealant - Per Tooth (multiple teeth)	
01510	Space Maint-Fixed-Unilateral	
01515	Space Maint-Fixed-Bilateral	
01550	Re-cement Space Maintainer	

III. RESTORATIVE SERVICES		TOOTH	SURFACE
02140	Amalgam-1 Surface, Prim. or Perm.		
02150	Amalgam-2 Surfaces, Prim. or Perm.		
02160	Amalgam-3 Surfaces, Prim. or Perm.		
02161	Amalgam-4+ Surfaces, Prim. or Perm.		
02330	Resin-based comp.-1 Surface, Anterior		
02331	Resin-based comp.-2 Surfaces, Anterior		
02332	Resin-based comp.-3 Surfaces, Anterior		
02335	Resin-based comp-4+ Surfaces or Incisal, Ant.		
02390	Resin-based composite crown, Anterior		
02391	Resin-based composite-1 Surface, Posterior		
02392	Resin-based composite-2 Surfaces, Posterior		
02393	Resin-based composite-3 Surfaces, Posterior		
02394	Resin-based composite-4+ Surfaces, Posterior		

CROWNS		TOOTH	SURFACE
* 02710	Crown Resin (Indirect/Laboratory)		
02740	Crown-Porc/Ceramic Substrate		
02750	Crown-Porc. High Noble Metal		
* 02751	Crown-Porcelain to Base Metal		
* 02752	Crown-Porcelain to Nobel Metal		
02790	Crown-Full Cast. High Noble Metal		
* 02791	Crown-Full Cast. Base Metal		
* 02792	Crown-Full Cast. Nobel Metal		
02910	Recement Inlay		
02920	Re-cement Crown		
02930	Stainless Steel Crown-Primary		
02931	Stainless Steel Crown-Permanent		
02932	Prefabricated Resin Crown		
02940	Sedative Filling		
02950	Crown Buildup, including any pins		
02951	Pin Retention, per tooth, in addt'n to restoration		
02952	Cast Post & Core, in addt'n to crown		
02954	Prefab Post & Core, in addt'n to crown		
* 02960	Crown Repair by report		
06930	Recement Fixed Partial Denture (Bridge)		

IV. ENDODONTIC SERVICES		TOOTH
03220	Therapeutic Pulpotomy	
* 03310	Anterior RCT (Exel. Rest.)	
* 03320	Biscuspid RCT (Excl. Rest.)	
* 03330	Molar RCT (Excl. Rest.)	
03410	Apicoectomy-Anterior	
03421	Apicoectomy/Periadicular Bicuspid	
03425	Apicoectomy/Periadicular Molar	

Con't. ENDODONTIC SERVICES		TOOTH
03426	Apicoectomy/Periadicular ea. Addt'l root	
03430	Retrograde Filling, Per Root	
03450	Root Amputation, Per Root	

V. PERIDONTAL SERVICES		TOOTH	QUAD
* 04210	Gingivectomy Or Gingivoplasty (Per Quad)		
04320	Provisional Splinting, Intracoronal		
04321	Provisional Splinting, Extracoronal		
* 04341	Scaling & Root Planing, 4+ teeth, Per Quad		
* 04342	Scaling & Root Planing, 1-3 teeth, Per Quad		
* 04910	Periodontal Maintenance		

VI. REMOVABLE PROSTHODONTIC SERVICES		
* 05110	Complete Denture-Maxillary	
* 05120	Complete Denture-Mandibular	
* 05130	Immediate Denture-Maxillary	
* 05140	Immediate Denture-mandibular	
* 05211	Maxillary Partial-Resin Base	
* 05212	Mandibular Partial-Resin Base	
* 05213	Maxillary Partial-Cast Metal Framework	
* 05214	Mandibular Partial-Cast Metal Framework	
05410	Adjust Complete Denture-Maxillary	
05411	Adjust Complete Denture-Mandibular	
05421	Adjust Partial-Maxillary	
05422	Adjust Partial-Mandibular	

X. ORAL SURGERY SERVICES		TOOTH	QUAD
07111	Coronal Remnants-Deciduous Tooth		
07140	Extraction, Erupted Tooth or Exposed Root		
07210	Extraction, Surgical Removal-Erupted Tooth		
07220	Extraction-Impacted Tooth-Soft Tissue		
07230	Extraction-Impacted Tooth-Partial Bony		
07240	Extraction-Impacted Tooth-Full Bony		
07241	Extraction-Unusual Tooth-Full Bony w/ compl.		
07250	Extraction-Residual Root-Surgical		
07270	Tooth Reimplantation-Accident (Avulsed)		
07281	Surgical Exposure to Aid Eruption		
07285	Biopsy of Oral Tissue-Hard		
07286	Biopsy of Oral Tissue-Soft		
07320	Alveoloplasty-No Extractions-Per Quad		
07510	I & D Intraoral Abscess		
07520	I & D Extraoral Abscess		
07960	Frenulectomy		

XII. ADJUNCTIVE GENERAL SERVICES		TOOTH
09110	Palliative (Emerg) Treatment-Minor Procedure	
09410	House Call (nursing home visits)	
09420	Hospital Call	
09630	Other Drugs and Medicaments, by report	
0359Y	DD Dental Special Needs	

OTHER SERVICES RENDERED (NOT LISTED ABOVE)

Location: _____ Tax ID#: 00-0000001

Provider: _____

Date of Service: _____ / _____ / _____

PATIENT IDENTIFICATION

Last	First	I.

* Services allowed by Medicaid, but must be pre-authorized

FIGURE 5-6 Fee Slip, University of New Mexico Division of Dental Hygiene

Source: Fee Slip. Albuquerque, NM: University of New Mexico, Division of Dental Hygiene. 2009.

DENTAL CLAIM FORM

1. ☐ Dentist's pre-treatment estimate ☒ Dentist's statement of actual services Provider ID #	2. ☐ Medicaid Claim ☐ EPSDT Prior Authorization # Patient ID #	3. Carrier Name and Address **Fones Dental of New Mexico** **2500 Newman Blvd.** **Bridgeport, CT 06601**

PATIENT COVERAGE INFORMATION

4. Patient Name **Mary Jones**	5. Relationship to employee ☐ Self ☐ Child **Child** ☐ Spouse ☐ Other ____	6. Sex M F F	7. Patient birthdate MM DD YY **07/02/1995**	8. If full time student school city

9. Employee/subscriber name and address **John Jones** **1234 Main St.** **Albuquerque NM 87120**	10. Employee/subscriber dental plan I.D. number **123-45-6789**	11. Employee/subscriber birthdate MM DD YY **02/05/1966**	12. Employer (company)	13. Group number

14. Is patient covered by another dental plan **No** Is patient covered by a medical plan? yes no	15-a. Name and address of carrier(s)	15-b. Group no.(s)	16. Name and address of other employer

17-a. Employee/subscriber name (if different than patient's)	17-b. Employee/subscriber dental plan I.D. number	17-c. Employee subscriber birthdate MM DD YY	18. Relationship to patient ☐ Self ☐ Parent ☐ Spouse ☐ Other ____

19. I have reviewed the following treatment plan and fees. I agree to be responsible for all charges for dental services and materials not paid by my dental benefit plan, unless the treating dentist or dental practice has a contractual agreement with my plan prohibiting all or a portion of such charges. To the extent permitted under applicable law, I authorize release of any information relating to this claim. > **SIGNATURE ON FILE** **09/04/2009** Signed (Patient or parent if minor) Date	20. I hereby authorize payment of the dental benefits otherwise payable to me directly to the below named dental entity. > **SIGNATURE ON FILE** **09/04/2009** Signed (Employee/subscriber) Date

BILLING DENTIST

21. Name of Billing Dentist or Dental Entity **Dental Hygiene DH0000** **University of New Mexico Dental Hygiene**	30. Is treatment result of occupational illness or injury? **N**	No Yes If yes, enter brief description and dates.
22. Address where payment should be remitted **2320 Tucker NE, Novitski Hall**	31. Is treatment result of auto accident? **N**	
23. City, State, Zip **Albuquerque, NM 87131-1391**	32. Other accident? **N**	

24. Dentist SSN or T.I.N. **00-0000000**	25. Dentist License no. **DH-1230**	26. Dentist phone no. **(505)555-4106**	33. If prosthesis, is this initial placement? **N**	(if no, reason for replacement)	34. Date prior placement

27. First visit date current series	28. Place of treatment Office Hosp. ECF Other **X**	29. Radiographs or models enclosed? **N**	No Yes How many? **0**	35. Is treatment for orthodontics? **N**	If services already commenced enter:	Date appliances placed	Mos. treat. remaining **0**

36. Identify missing teeth with 'X'	37. Examination and treatment plan - List in order from tooth no. 1 through tooth no. 32 - Using charting system shown.						For administrative use only
	Tooth # or letter	Surface	Description of service (including x-rays, prophylaxis, materials used, etc.)	Date of service performed Mo. Day Year	Procedure number	Fee	
			Periodic Oral Evaluation	10/26/2001	00120	30.00	
			Prophylaxis, Child	10/26/2001	01120	50.00	
			Topical Fluor.(not proph)Child	10/26/2001	01203	20.00	

38. Remarks for unusual services

39. I hereby certify that the procedures as indicated by date have been completed and that the fees submitted are the actual fees I have charged and intend to collect for those procedures. > **Christine Nathe, R.D.H** **DH-1230** **05/04/2010** Signed (Treating Dentist) License no. Date	41. Total Fee Charged **100.00**
	42. Payment by other plan
40. Address where treatment was performed **2320 Tucker NE, Novitski Hall** **Albuquerque, NM 87131-1391** City, State, Zip	Max Allowable
	Deductible
© American Dental Association, 2008 Claim # 5781	Carrier %
	Carrier Pays
	Patient Pays

FIGURE 5-7 Dental Claim Form

● new procedure code   ▲ revised code   ✖ revised descriptor

D0120 periodic oral evaluation
✖
An evaluation performed on a patient of record to determine any changes in the patient's dental and medical health status since a previous comprehensive or periodic evaluation. This includes periodontal screening and may require interpretation of information acquired through additional diagnostic procedures. Report additional diagnostic procedures separately.

D0140 limited oral evaluation — problem focused
✖
An evaluation limited to a specific oral health problem or complaint. This may require interpretation of information acquired through additional diagnostic procedures. Report additional diagnostic procedures separately. Definitive procedures may be required on the same date as the evaluation.

Typically, patients receiving this type of evaluation present with a specific problem and/or dental emergencies, trauma, acute infections, etc.

▲ D0150 comprehensive oral evaluation — new or established patient
Typically used by a general dentist and/or a specialist when evaluating a patient comprehensively. It is a thorough evaluation and recording of the extraoral and intraoral hard and soft tissues. It may require interpretation of information acquired through additional diagnostic procedures. Additional diagnostic procedures should be reported separately.

This would include the evaluation and recording of the patient's dental and medical history and a general health assessment. It may typically include the evaluation and recording of dental caries, missing or unerupted teeth, restorations, occlusal relationships, periodontal conditions (including periodontal charting), hard and soft tissue anomalies, oral cancer screening, etc.

D0160 detailed and extensive oral evaluation — problem focused, by report
A detailed and extensive problem focused evaluation entails extensive diagnostic and cognitive modalities based on the findings of a comprehensive oral evaluation. Integration of more extensive diagnostic modalities to develop a treatment plan for a specific problem is required. The condition requiring this type of evaluation should be described and documented.

Examples of conditions requiring this type of evaluation may include dentofacial anomalies, complicated perio-prosthetic conditions, complex temporomandibular dysfunction, facial pain of unknown origin, severe systemic diseases requiring multidisciplinary consultation, etc.

FIGURE 5-8   CDT-4 Definitions of Billable Oral Exams

Source: American Dental Association. CDT-4. 2002. Chicago: American Dental Association. CDT-4 Definitions of Billable Oral Exams.

FONES DENTAL

Fones Dental
2500 Newman Blvd.
Bridgeport, CT 06601
555-3161 or 1-555-375-3320

Explanation of Benefits
(THIS IS NOT A BILL)

Check No.:	NO CHECK
Issue Date:	08-25-2010
Receipt Date:	08-20-2010

Patient Name:	MARY JONES
Relationship Code:	03
Subscriber Name:	JOHN JONES
Dentist:	Alfred Fones, DDS

Document No.:	0123
Document Type:	1

Pay To: S=Subscriber
P=Provider

IMPORTANT NOTICE: Payment for these services is determined in accordance with the specific terms of your dental plan and/or Fones Dental's agreements with its participating dentists.

Tooth Code	Date of Service	Procedure Code	Procedure Description	Submitted Amount	Approved Amount	Allowed Amount	Deductible	% Co-Pay	Patient Payment	Plan Payment	Pay To
GROUP NO:	000123		NAME: Dental Hygiene Corp.								
SUBGROUP NO:	0001		NAME: Dental Hygiene Corp.								
	08/05/09	D1120	CLEANING	60.00	60.00	.00	.00		.00	60.00	P
POLICY CODE:	966										
	08/05/09	D1203	FLUORIDE	24.00	24.00	.00	.00		.00	24.00	P
POLICY CODE:	966										
			TOTAL	84.00	84.00	.00	.00		.00	84.00	

THE FOLLOWING POLICIES ARE APPLIED TO EXPLAIN BENEFITS PAYABLE AND ARE NOT INTENDED TO ALTER THE TREATMENT PLAN DETERMINED BY THE DENTIST AND PATIENT:
966. THE PATIENT'S DENTAL COVERAGE WAS NOT IN EFFECT WHEN THIS SERVICE WAS
      PERFORMED OR SUBMITTED FOR PREDETERMINATION. PLEASE VERIFY THE CLAIM
      WAS SUBMITTED TO THE PROPER CARRIER BASED ON THE DATE OF SERVICE AND
      THE CORRECT SOCIAL SECURITY NUMBER WAS PROVIDED.

Payment for these services is determined in accordance with the specific terms of your dental plan and/or Fones Dental's agreements with its participating dentists. For inquiries regarding participating dentists, please call the number above. Fones Dental's payment decisions do not qualify as dental or medical advice. You must make all decisions about the desirability or necessity of dental procedures and services with your dentist.
If your claim was denied in whole or in part so that you must pay some amount of the claim, upon a written request and free of charge, we will provide you with a copy of any internal rule, guideline or protocol or, if applicable, an explanation of the scientific or clinical judgment relied upon in deciding your claim. If you think Fones Dental incorrectly denied all or part of your claim, you may ask to have the claim reviewed. Your written request for a formal review must be sent within 180 days of your receipt of this EOB to the address on the upper-left hand corner. You may submit any additional materials youbelievesupport your claim. A decision will be made no later than 30 days from the date we receive your request. Refer to your Dental Benefit Handbook for a complete description of Fones Dental's Claims Appeal process. You are not required to file a formal appeal to Fones Dental prior to arbitration or taking civil action.

Ilulalulaulllalllillluuullullluullullullluullalulul

#BWNCYPW
#S0041334569NM6#
JOHN JONES
1234 MAIN ST
ALBUQUERQUE NM 87120-6066

Insurance fraud significantly increases the cost of health care. If you are aware of any false information submitted to Fones Dental, you can help us lower these costs by calling our toll-free hotline. You do not need to identify yourself. Only ANTI-FRAUD calls can be accepted on this line.

ANTI-FRAUD TOLL-FREE HOTLINE
1-800-000-0000

PAGE   1 OF 1

FIGURE 5-9 Explanation of Benefits Form

GOVERNMENTAL ROLES IN FUNDING DENTAL CARE

In the United States, the total federal, state, and local governments' share of expenses for dental care is approximately 4%.[8] Basically, the federal government funds dental care delivery through a variety of programs for the express purpose of improving the nation's capacity to provide improved oral health care. The government funds programs that provide research, disease prevention, and control (eg, water fluoridation, fluoride mouth rinse programs—"swish and spit"—and dental sealants in schools); the planning and development of dental programs; regulation by means of quality assurance programs and assessment; and education of dental professionals (via scholarship, loan forgiveness programs, and financial aid). Chapter 19 provides

DENTAL HYGIENIST SPOTLIGHT:
LCDR Karen Sicard, RDH, MPH

As a dental hygienist who works as a US Public Health Service Officer at the Centers for Disease Control and Prevention, Lieutenant Commander Karen Sicard provides training and technical assistance in oral health education and serves as a project officer overseeing three state grantees and three congressional earmarks of approximately $1.3 million per year.

In addition, LCDR Sicard works with a three-member team to provide water fluoridation training to state engineers and water operators. She has spoken to groups across the United States on dental public health treatment modalities and has received numerous dental hygiene awards, public health officer awards, and commendations throughout her career. LCDR Sicard also responded as a PHS officer after Hurricane Katrina. She demonstrates that a dental hygienist has much to offer to the public.

Why did you decide to go into dental hygiene?

It's a long story, but, to sum it up, I was a dental technician in the Navy Reserve—one weekend a month, two weeks a year—and working as a dental practice manager in southern California. The dental assistant in the practice talked constantly about how she wanted to become a dental hygienist because that position pays so much money. The more I checked into it, the more I thought about pursuing it myself.

How did you get into dental public health? Did you need additional education?

I basically stumbled into dental public health by accident. It was 1997 and I was working for a practice in Grand Forks, North Dakota, when we had a flood that closed down the dental office and the city for over eight weeks. I realized that I needed a much more stable income to support my family. Since I had prior military service, I started looking into the Public Health Service. Unlike the military, the PHS offers a commission to dental hygienists with bachelor's degrees.

I went onto the Indian Health Service Web site and contacted the recruiter at the time, Kathy Smith, and entered my information. When all of the paperwork had been completed, I accepted a position as a community/clinical hygienist on a reservation outside of Billings, Montana.

I didn't know where to start because I was coming from private practice without public health experience.

The only public health training I had received was in dental hygiene school when I was given the task of setting up community oral health programs. I was a little lost in the beginning, but things came together fairly rapidly once I got started. I started out with simple things: school oral health education, brushing with fluoridated toothpaste, then sealant programs, fluoride mouth rinse programs, and so on. I read everything related to oral health and the Indian Health Service I could find, and I asked a lot of questions from people already in the field.

I don't think hygienists need additional education to get into public health, but I would strongly recommend getting a master's degree in public health along the way. It offers a broader perspective, provides additional skills and knowledge, and increases the opportunities for advancement.

What is your current position?

My position is Health Education Specialist for the CDC Division of Oral Health, and I have lots of additional duties as assigned.

What do you like most serving in dental public health positions?

I have had lots of great experiences—I love them! I like learning about public health measures, finding out what the science really says. I like the community education and setting up prevention programs.

What advice would you give to a practicing hygienist who is thinking of doing something different?

Do it! Think outside the box! You can do it! Don't limit yourself to private practice dental hygiene. Go to USAJOBS.GOV, and type in program analysis, program manager, communications, administration, and so on.

Think about education. I've never been sorry I had a bachelor's or master's degree even though, to be honest with you, I didn't think when I was pursuing them that they would be much help. I couldn't see the doors that would open up. I kept going for the bachelor's degree because I was only a semester away and thought, "What the heck!" I went for the master's degree because I wanted more at the time and figured this would have to help. I didn't have any idea about the opportunities that would open up each time.

I have never heard anyone say, "I should never have gotten that degree." There are tons of student loan programs, scholarships, loan repayment programs, and so on out there if you want to it make it happen. Life is full of opportunities and you only get one shot at it; you might as well do everything you can to be what you want to be.

Source: Christine Nathe writes the Public Health Column in RDH magazine published by Pennwell Publishing. For more public health spotlights please see RDH magazine online at http://www.rdhmag.com/index.html.

more information on current government incentives for dental hygiene students.

The federal government provides funding to programs concerned with providing dental care services, such as the US Public Health Service and the National Health Service Corps. It also funds dental services for federal prisoners, military personnel, veterans with dental service-connected disabilities, Native Americans via the Indian Health Service, and children enrolled in Head Start and Early Head Start programs.

Did You Know?

Dental hygienists may be eligible for loan repayment programs when practicing in settings defined to provide care for the underserved.

Federal block grants also cover some dental services, especially for children. A *block grant* is an unrestricted federal grant given to a state or local government that does not specify how it is to be spent. The Maternal and Children's Health Services (MCHS) Block Grant Title V and Preventive Health and Human Services are usually used to provide preventive services and may cover dental services for children.

Many dental clinics utilize federal and state grants to help cover their operational costs. Dental treatment for children with craniofacial deformities, cleft lip and palate, and certain other conditions is funded by state and federal governments. In some states, dental hygiene services are offered to individuals participating in the Women, Infants and Children (WIC) program.

State governments generally fund dental services for inmates of state prisons and detention centers. A state often contracts with a private agency to deliver the services. State dental departments also may provide consulting skills for developing and managing dental health programs. Some state dental clinics offer services to a target population, which usually includes children, patients with special needs, older adults, and indigent patients.

Local governments may provide dental care in school or community clinics. In many instances, the funding for these clinics is from federal, state, private, and local entities. Funding for water fluoridation usually falls under the auspices of local government.

Federal and state governments jointly finance the Children's Health Insurance Program (CHIP) initiated in 1997 and is administered by the states. Within broad federal guidelines, each state design its program and determines the eligibile groups, benefit packages, payment levels for coverage, and administrative and operating procedures. In many instances, CHIP finances dental coverage for children whose parents work but have low incomes and do not have health insurance coverage.[9]

Medicaid Dental Coverage

The federal government also funds dental services under the auspices of Medicaid and provides limited funding for medically necessary dental services, such as oral/maxillofacial needs related to a medical condition, through Medicare. As discussed in Chapter 3, Medicaid is the federal program enacted in 1965 that distributes funds to states for providing health care services to the indigent. Dental care is an option that requires additional funding from the state.[10] Each state decides whether to offer Medicaid dental insurance as a traditional fee-for-service plan or a capitation agreement. In many states, private insurance agencies operate Medicaid insurance.

Because of the states' freedom to apply the federal money in various ways, Medicaid dental benefits differ from state to state. Some provide coverage only to children under the age of twenty-one; others choose to insure all low-income individuals regardless of age. A state that limits coverage to children has more money to spend on each child, and the state is able to pay providers UCR rates. This option theoretically motivates more providers to see children covered by Medicaid. However, when only children are covered, many other individuals are left with no dental coverage.

Although many states fund dental care to the indigent population through Medicaid, that population may have difficulty accessing it. Many dental practitioners choose not to enroll as Medicaid providers so that they do not have to accept indigent patients. These providers

BOX 5-1 Terminology of Dental Care Financing

Benefit: Amount that the insurance entity will pay for covered dental services described in its policy.

Children Health Insurance Program (CHIP): Federal program created to cover medical care for children whose families have incomes too high to qualify for state medical assistance but cannot obtain private insurance; all states participate, but some do not cover dental care.

Claims processing: Entering procedures rendered and determining whether payment will be approved or denied.

Commercial insurance plan: Plan that operates for a profit.

Contract: Legal agreement between an insurance entity and a group or individual.

Copayment: Portion of the cost of each service a patient pays.

Deductible: Amount an individual enrolled in an insurance plan must pay for covered services before the insurance entity begins paying.

Dental claim: Patient's formal request for insurance payment for a dental procedure that was rendered.

Dental claim form: Standard dental document used to file a claim or request authorization for a procedure.

Dental necessity: Service provided by a dental provider that has been determined as a generally acceptable dental practice for a specific diagnosis and treatment.

Early and periodic screening, diagnosis and treatment (EPSDT): Service for persons under twenty-one years of age for medical, dental, and vision care paid for by Medicaid.

Exclusive provider arrangement (EPA): Contract between dental care providers and an employer (which eliminates the third party) stating the negotiated fees for services offered to the employer's employees.

Explanation of benefits: Form sent to the patient and provider explaining the approval or denial of payment for procedures rendered.

Fee slip: Form a dental practice uses to detail the services rendered a patient.

Managed care: Integration of health care delivery and financing.

Medicaid (Title XIX): Federal program that distributes funds to states for health care services provided to certain groups including aged, blind, and disabled people; those with low incomes; and certain members of families with dependent children.

Medicare (Title XVIII): Federal insurance program supported by a trust fund; provides limited funding for medically necessary dental services, such as oral/maxillofacial needs related to a medical condition for all people sixty-five years of age and older.

Preexisting condition: Medical condition that exists prior to the person's coverage by an insurance entity.

Premium: Amount a group or an individual pays to the insurance entity for coverage.

Procedure number: Identification given to a specific procedure as designated in the *Codes on Dental Procedures and Nomenclature* published by the ADA.

Provider: Legally licensed dental hygienist or dentist operating within a scope of practice.

Prepaid group practice: Large group of dental providers contracted to provide services to groups of patients.

Single procedure: Specific procedure designated by a specific code.

Sound natural teeth: Either primary or permanent teeth that have adequate hard and soft tissue support.

Three-party system: Program in which a dental provider renders the service for which the patient's sponsor (insurance company or employer) pays.

TRICARE: Health care program serving active-duty service members, National Guard and Reserve members, retirees, their families, survivors, and certain former spouses worldwide; formerly known as Civilian Health and Medical Program of the Uniformed Services (CHAMPUS).

Two-party system: Program in which a dental provider renders the service for which the patient pays.

cite reasons such as frequently missed appointments, difficult treatment issues, low reimbursement rates, and too much bureaucratic paperwork, as well as not wanting Medicaid patients in the waiting room with other patients. This tremendously affects access to care for these patients.

See Box 5-1■ for a list of terms used in financing dental care.

SUMMARY

Most dental care in the United States remains in the private sector, but federal, state, and local governments fund dental care to certain populations. The federal government also funds dental research and education of dental providers. Dental insurance plans have made preventive dental care affordable to many individuals and have focused on prevention as a means to decrease restorative dentistry costs. To become a consumer advocate, dental hygienists must understand dental funding in both private and public organizations.

SELF-STUDY TEST ITEMS

1. Which of the following does financing of dental treatment involve?
   a. Private sector
   b. Dental practitioner
   c. Public sector
   d. Both a and c

2. What payment is based on an office visit and is always the same regardless of the services rendered?
   a. Encounter
   b. Fee-for-service plan
   c. Capitation
   d. Barter system

3. What term refers to a portion of the cost of each service that the patient pays—in other words, the part of the payment not covered by the third party?
   a. Insurance payment
   b. Copayment
   c. Deductible
   d. Exchange

4. What is defined as the number given to a specific procedure as designated in the *Codes on Dental Procedures and Nomenclature* published by ADA?
   a. Premium number
   b. Procedure number
   c. Contract number
   d. Benefit number

5. What form is sent to the patient and provider explaining the payment or denial for procedures rendered?
   a. Explanation of benefits
   b. Managed care
   c. Exclusive provider arrangement
   d. Dental claim

REFERENCES

1. Sommers, JP. *Dental Expenditures in the 10 Largest States, 2003.* Rockville, MD: Agency for Healthcare Research and Quality; 2007. Statistical Brief 156.
2. Ezzati-Rice TM, Kashihara D, Machlin SR. *Health Care Expenses in the U.S. 2000.* Rockville, MD: Agency for Healthcare Research and Quality; 2004. MEPS Research Findings No. 21. AHRQ Pub. No. 04-0022.
3. Manski RJ, Brown E. *Dental Use, Expenses, Private Dental Coverage and Changes, 1996–2004.* Rockville, MD: Agency for Healthcare Research and Quality; 2007. MEPS Chartbook No.17.
4. About Delta Dental plans. http://www.deltadental.com/Public/AboutDeltaD/AboutDeltaDental.jsp?DView=About Home. Accessed August 22, 2008.
5. BlueCross BlueShield of Illinois. http://www.bcbsil.com/member/dental/. Accessed August 22, 2008.
6. Concordia Plus. http://ptc.hroffice.com/common/benefits/dental/dental0006.asp. Accessed August 22, 2008.
7. *Current Dental Terminology.* Chicago: American Dental Association; 2008.
8. US Department of Health and Human Services. *Oral Health in America: A Report of the Surgeon General.* Rockville, MD: US Department of Health and Human Services, National Institute of Dental and Craniofacial Research, National Institutes of Health; 2000.
9. State Children's Health Insurance Plan. http://www.cms.hhs.gov/home/schip.asp. Accessed August 22, 2008.
10. Medicaid overview. http://www.cms.hhs.gov/home/medicaid.asp. Accessed on June 8, 2009.

PEARSON
myhealthprofessionskit™

Multimedia Extension Activities

Use this address to access the interactive Companion Website created for this textbook. Simply select "Dental Hygiene" from the choice of disciplines. Find this book and log in using your username and password. To obtain a username and password, please register using the scratch-off access code on the inside front cover of this book.

Chapter 6

Federal and State Legislation Affecting Dental Hygiene Practice

OBJECTIVES

After studying this chapter, the dental hygiene student should be able to:

- Explain the legislative process in the United States
- Identify the major bodies of law in the United States
- Describe the entity responsible for regulation of the dental hygienist
- Advocate for the utilization of a dental hygienist without restrictive barriers
- Describe the legislative initiatives affecting dental hygienists in the United States

KEY TERMS

Bodies of law
Common
Statutory
Constitutional
Administrative
Government branches
Executive
Judicial
Legislative
Legislature
Regulation
Statute

COMPETENCIES

After studying this chapter and participating in accompanying course activities, the dental hygiene student should be competent to do the following:

- Adhere to state and federal laws, recommendations, and regulations in the provision of dental hygiene care
- Promote the values of oral and general health and wellness to the public and organizations within and outside of the profession
- Facilitate client access to oral health services by influencing individuals and/or organizations for the provision of oral health care

Many legislative initiatives affect the practice of dental hygiene. Legal changes to practice can impact dental hygienists' treatment of the public more or less effectively. Most states make changes to dental hygiene rules and regulations annually. These changes can be accessed at any time at www.adha.org, which updates the changes throughout the year.

Public health and the law have always been interdependent. Public health law focuses on issues in public health practice and how they affect practice. Generally, three major areas of public health law are police power, disease and injury prevention, and populations. *Police power* includes laws enforced by governmental agencies, such as dental boards or emergency health operations. *Disease and injury prevention* includes legal activities such as prevention initiatives and Occupational Safety and Health Agency regulations. Population law uses epidemiology to analyze health issues, such as the environment and community water.

HISTORICAL PERSPECTIVE OF PRACTICE ISSUES

The first statutes pertaining to dental hygiene were written in Connecticut based on the legislative initiative of Dr. Alfred Fones.[1] Since then, all states have added statutes that define dental hygiene practice. Historically, many state dental hygiene associations have worked to expand the settings and the scope of dental hygiene practice. Additionally, dental hygiene organizations have worked to allow the regulation of dental hygienists by dental hygienists.[2] In contrast, many state dental organizations had worked to permit the practice of on-the-job-trained personnel (preceptorship).[3,4] Resolutions passed by the American Dental Association (ADA) support this alternative education model of preceptorship.[5]

Within the past decade, New Mexico passed a statute giving dental hygienists the freedom to provide dental hygiene in any setting without the supervision of dentists.[6] The state's health policy commission, not the dental hygiene association, brought about the impetus for the change. The reason for the change, which is termed *collaborative practice,* was to increase access to care for underserved populations. This initiative created a precedent, and most states have made similar changes to their practice acts so that dental hygienists can treat patients without the physical presence of dentists.[7] (See Figure 6-1 ∎.)

Changes in policy and even terminology can impact the legal aspects of dental hygiene practice. Within the past decade, the *Current Dental Terminology* (*CDT*) published by the ADA redefined oral prophylaxis as a dental prophylaxis performed on transitional or permanent dentition that includes scaling and/or polishing procedures to remove coronal plaque, calculus, and stains. In other words, a dental assistant could provide a polishing, which would be legal in many states, and then bill it as a cleaning. Fortunately, the ADA unanimously rescinded this decision after the American Dental Hygienists' Association (ADHA) explained the significance of this wording change.[8] The dental insurance industry would not want to fund preventive services such as prophylaxis when a polishing was done without the necessary scaling to remove plaque and calculus.

Did You Know?

Although legislative action is not required for changing billing definitions, it can directly affect the provision of patient care. Policies, rules, and regulations are other initiatives that affect practice.

Regulations by state boards concerning the delivery of dental hygiene services are not always in accord with the law. In 2003, the South Carolina Board of Dentistry passed an emergency regulation that restricted dental hygienists from providing preventive dental services—including cleanings, sealants, and fluoride treatments—to children who had not previously been examined by a dentist in state schools. The Federal Trade Commission (FTC) issued a complaint, stating that the regulation violated federal laws, and in 2007, the FTC issued a consent order that upheld the law, which allowed a hygienist to provide services without a previous dentist exam of the child if conducted in a public health setting. It also required the board of dentistry to publicly announce its support of the law and to notify the FTC if it considered altering any policies related to preventive dental care services in the future.[9]

In 2009 in California, new legislation gave a dental hygiene committee of four consumers, one general practice or public health dentist, and four dental hygienists the authority to regulate the licensure, education, and

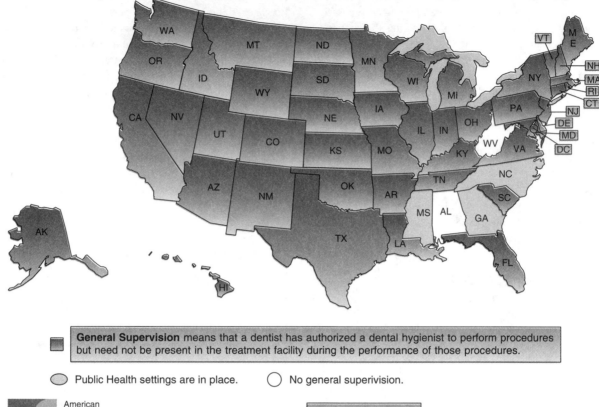

STATES WHERE DENTAL HYGIENISTS MAY PERFORM SOME SERVICES IN AT LEAST ONE SETTING UNDER GENERAL SUPERVISION

General Supervision means that a dentist has authorized a dental hygienist to perform procedures but need not be present in the treatment facility during the performance of those procedures.

Public Health settings are in place.   No general superivision.

American Dental Hygienists' Association

TOTAL STATES: 47
February, 2008

www.adha.org

FIGURE 6-1   Legislative Activity

regulatory enforcement of the profession of dental hygiene. One of the dental hygienist members will be a dental hygiene educator and another will be a Registered Dental Hygienist in Alternative Practice (RDHAP), a dental hygienist allowed to practice independently in California. The legislation in California marks the first time a state dental hygiene committee has been granted the power to make rules and regulations that apply to the profession.[10]

The US Surgeon General's 2003 *Call to Action* requested an increase in the diversity, capacity, and flexibility of the oral health workforce.[11] The ADHA House of Delegates, recognizing the need to increase the organization's efforts to address the public's unmet oral health needs, approved the development of the advanced dental hygiene practitioner (ADHP), a mid-level provider. As a result, the ADHP will extend primary oral health care to all while improving the health of underserved groups by providing access to early interventions, quality preventive oral health care, and referrals to dentists and other health care providers.[12] This new position will move the profession one step closer to meeting the changes the Surgeon General's report requested.

DENTAL HYGIENIST SPOTLIGHT:
Pamela Myers, RDH, CCHP

Pamela Myers has worked as a dental hygienist in the Texas Prison System for more than twenty years. She worked in private practice before going into public health. She is a member of Phi Theta Kappa National Society for Junior Colleges and Alpha Chi National Honor Society.

Ms. Myers was instrumental in adding a referral for dental evaluations to the Disease Management Guidelines for Diabetes and Coronary Artery Disease of the University of Texas Medical Branch–Correctional Managed Care (UTMB–CMC). She presented the paper "Diabetes Disease Management and Dental Care: A Transdisciplinary Approach" at the National Commission on Correctional Health Care Conference in Orlando, Florida.

Ms. Myers answered some questions about her career.

Why did you go into dental hygiene?

In 1970, I worked at a local dental office as a part-time dental assistant. I really loved working in dentistry and discovered I enjoyed working with people. My husband was drafted into the Army later in the year. I moved back home with my parents and went to work for my previous dentist as an assistant. The dentist's wife was his hygienist, and they both encouraged me to pursue a career in dental hygiene.

I applied to Wharton County Junior College Dental Hygiene Program in 1972 after my husband returned from the armed services and graduated in 1974 with an associate's degree in dental hygiene. The first dental office I practiced in was in

An interior view of a dental operatory (top) and an exterior view of the Texas Department of Criminal Justice Estelle Regional Medical Facility in Huntsville, Texas. The facility houses offenders who have serious chronic health problems and the prison system's dialysis program.

Huntsville, Texas. I was blessed to practice with an excellent dentist who was highly motivated and truly believed in the preventive philosophy.

How did you get into dental public health?

Huntsville, Texas, is the headquarters for the Texas Department of Criminal Justice. Some of the local private general dentists, including the practitioner I worked with, practiced at the prison a couple of hours each morning. I heard stories, learned about interesting cases, and was very curious about the care provided. In 1981 as a result of a federal court case, the state was required to make numerous changes in the prison operations, including health care. Before then, nursing care, mid-level care, and all dental hygiene care were provided by unlicensed inmates, and all dental assistants and clerical support personnel were incarcerated individuals. The court ruled that no inmate could provide care, handle health records, or in any way be involved in the delivery of health care.

I applied for and was offered a vacant position at the Wynne Unit in Huntsville. I worked 7 AM to 3:30 PM, Monday through Friday. I had every holiday off and received twelve days of paid sick leave per year plus more than two weeks of vacation. The vacation increased over the years, and I now receive more than four weeks paid vacation and still have holidays off and paid sick leave. After more than twenty years, I'm still behind the walls, barbed wire, and fences, and it has been the most rewarding career I could have ever dreamed.

What positions do you currently hold?

In 1986 I was named the Dental Hygiene Coordinator for the Texas Department of Criminal Justice. At that time, the Department of Corrections had more than twenty-four facilities, nine of which were located within a 20-mile radius of Huntsville. The incarcerated population was about 32,000. The state still had a case in federal court and was undergoing many changes. More than half of our dental hygiene positions were vacant, and the courts were going to fine the state a specific amount each day the positions remained open. So I became a recruiter overnight. My position is still evolving.

My official job description requires a current Texas dental hygiene license, a minimum of five years of correctional dental hygiene experience, and a bachelor's degree can be considered in lieu of three years of the correctional experience. When I retire, the position will be posted with similar requirements. When applying for a position with a prison, a hygienist with a bachelor's degree would be preferred over a hygienist without a bachelor's degree, but that would not be the only consideration for employment. The majority of our hygienists have two-year degrees. I believe that will change in the future.

Most incarcerated individuals come from a low socioeconomic background, have less than a high school education, and are at risk for developing serious health problems. The majority of inmates come from the population that has the least access to care.

Currently, I am also employed by the UTMB–CMC as manager of the dental hygiene program. In this position, I wear a number of different hats. For many years, we provided care only to an adult incarcerated population, but then we assumed the health care of the Texas Youth Commission, the juvenile correctional system. UTMB-CMC also provides care in the Federal Bureau of Prisons complex in Beaumont, Texas, so I have learned about the differences in the federal and state prisons.

The change from a population of 32,000 to one of more than 125,000 in the UTMB sector has been challenging. I coordinate all of the continuing education programs for the entire dental staff and manage the preventive care provided by UTMB-CMC. I make decisions regarding materials, instruments, and equipment used in our clinics, develop policies, and participate on the dental utilization quality review committee. We operate the largest electronic medical record system in the world. This electronic health network has been recognized at the state and national levels for innovation in technology.

Can you discuss any particularly interesting experiences you have had in your dental public health position?

Security is paramount in a correctional institution, and some days I feel like a correctional officer. We must maintain a continual count of all instruments, needles, and blades. All of our cabinets and drawers must be locked. Products such as antimicrobial mouthwash must be issued in a unit dose, and the offender must be observed while swishing and expectorating.

We do not send the patient "home" with a bottle of chlorhexidine or even disclosing tablets. We evaluate preventive and home care products such as toothbrushes and dental floss and can make recommendations to the DOC, but each product has to be evaluated for security risks. The offenders cannot have regular floss; instead they can purchase a floss pick in the commissary. The toothbrushes are about 3.5 inches long and have a spoon-shaped handle because a long handle can be sharpened on a concrete floor and made into a weapon.

What type of advice would you give practicing hygienists who are thinking of doing something different?

Hygienists who are interested in doing something different should explore all available opportunities. They should pursue a bachelor's or master's degree because most opportunities other than private practice require one or the other. They need to learn and grow as much as possible, participate in state or national dental hygiene conventions, and network with providers in public as well as private health sales. They need to read as much as possible because knowledge truly is power.

Source: Christine Nathe writes the Public Health Column in RDH magazine published by Pennwell Publishing. For more public health spotlights please see RDH magazine online at http://www.rdhmag.com/index.html.

STATE GOVERNMENT OVERVIEW

Although the federal laws discussed in Chapter 14 affect dental hygiene *science,* the laws that affect dental hygiene *practice* are enacted and enforced by individual states. The federal government does not play a major role in governing the dental hygiene practice, but it is the model after which each state's system of government is fashioned. See Table 6-1 ■ for a comparison of the branches of federal and state governments.

Did You Know?

The federal government has no responsibility or authority for the regulation of dental hygiene in states.

The governments of the United States and its individual states have three sections, or **branches of government:** legislative, executive, and judicial. Each branch has a specific function and limited areas of authority, which is exclusive to that branch. (See Table 6-2 ■.) The **legislature,** or legislative branch, of each state makes its laws, including the licensure and practice of the dental hygienist. The **executive branch** executes, or carries out,

Table 6-1 Comparison of State and Federal Governments

Branch	Federal Government	State Government
Legislative	Congress	State legislature
Executive	President	Governor
Judicial	Federal courts	State courts

Table 6-2 Function of State Government Branches

Branch of Government	Function
Legislative	Create laws
Executive	Enforce laws
Judicial	Interpret laws

Table 6-3 Major Bodies of Law

Body	Definition
Common	Created and changed only by courts
Statutory	Created and changed by legislature
Constitutional	Created and changed by people through their legislators
Administrative	Delegated legislative power to an administrative agency

the laws passed by the legislature. The **judicial branch** composed of courts interprets the laws the legislature passes, but it does not make them.

A **body of law** refers to the rules of conduct or action prescribed or formally recognized as binding or enforced by a controlling authority. In the United States, the major bodies of law are common, statutory, constitutional, and administrative. (See Table 6-3 ■.) Courts create **common law** through judicial decisions that in many cases other courts can change. It contains notions of common sense and precedent. **Statutory law** is the legislature-enacted, written law, which serves to promote justice. Only the legislature can change statutory law. **Constitutional law** deals with the interpretation and implementation of a government's codified constitution. The people through their legislators created it, and the people, also through their legislators, have the power to change it. It takes precedence over both common and statutory law. The fourth body of law is **administrative law,** which refers to the body of rules, regulations, orders, and decisions created by a government's administrative agencies. Agencies such as state dental boards fall within this law. The legislature has the authority to say whether and when administrative agencies can develop rules and regulations.

Generally, a state legislature includes two legislative bodies, the Senate and the House of Representatives, sometimes referred to as the Assembly or House of Delegates. In most states, the legislature meets each year for up to six months.

STATE LAWS AND THEIR PASSAGE

To become a state law, a concept (or bill) must be reviewed by specific committees within each house of the legislature, which may amend, or change, it. If the

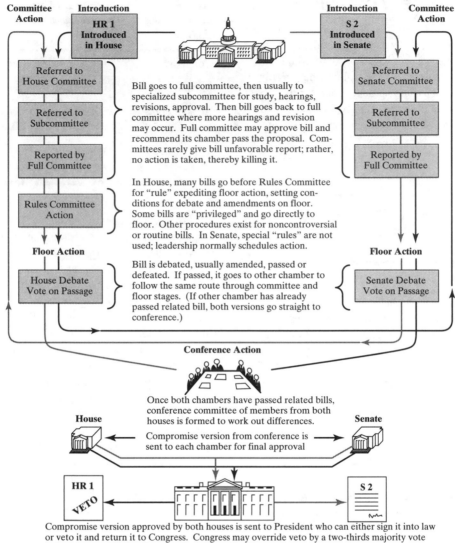

Bill goes to full committee, then usually to specialized subcommittee for study, hearings, revisions, approval. Then bill goes back to full committee where more hearings and revision may occur. Full committee may approve bill and recommend its chamber pass the proposal. Committees rarely give bill unfavorable report; rather, no action is taken, thereby killing it.

In House, many bills go before Rules Committee for "rule" expediting floor action, setting conditions for debate and amendments on floor. Some bills are "privileged" and go directly to floor. Other procedures exist for noncontroversial or routine bills. In Senate, special "rules" are not used; leadership normally schedules action.

Bill is debated, usually amended, passed or defeated. If passed, it goes to other chamber to follow the same route through committee and floor stages. (If other chamber has already passed related bill, both versions go straight to conference.)

Conference Action

Once both chambers have passed related bills, conference committee of members from both houses is formed to work out differences.

House   Compromise version from conference is sent to each chamber for final approval   **Senate**

Compromise version approved by both houses is sent to President who can either sign it into law or veto it and return it to Congress. Congress may override veto by a two-thirds majority vote in both houses; bill then becomes law without President's signature.

FIGURE 6-2 How a Bill Becomes a Law

committees accept it, both houses must vote to approve it. (See Figure 6-2 ■.) Although a bill often "dies" in committee, its most vital provisions may be incorporated in a totally different bill. If either house fails to pass the bill, it will not become a law. If both houses pass it, the governor must sign it. If the governor vetoes the bill, both houses may override the veto by a two-thirds majority vote.

Laws pertaining to dental hygiene are generally found in the state dental hygiene law(s) regarding its

practice. However, policies enacted at the federal level pertaining to dental insurance and Medicaid may impact state dental hygiene practice. For instance, if federal Medicaid law allows dental hygienists to be reimbursed for performing oral examinations, oral prophylaxis, and other procedures, states must ensure that their laws and rules do not conflict with it in order to receive Medicaid funding. These funds can support dental hygiene care delivered in schools or practice settings other than private dental offices and to the underserved. In this case, the state may even push for the passage of a **statute**—a law enacted by a government's legislature—to allow dental hygienists to be reimbursed for providing such care.

Dental hygienists lobby for the support of bills that could impact dental hygiene care delivery. *Lobbying* is the act of educating legislators and promoting specific bills that would benefit the lobbyists; for dental lobbyists, this could involve supporting legislation to enhance dental care or opposing bills that are detrimental to dental care delivery.

Did You Know?

Some dental hygiene associations hire professional lobbyist to promote legislative initiatives and educate legislators about them.

STATE DENTAL BOARDS

A state's laws pertaining to dental hygiene practice describe its allowable scope, supervision and licensure requirements, and procedures for suspension and revocation of license. Aiding in the interpretation of practice laws are regulations and rules. **Regulations** are orders imposed by an executive authority or government agency governing practice, which in this case could be a state dental board.

Rules implement and interpret the law or define the practice and procedure requirements of a state government's agency; an example is a state dental board's interpreting and implementing a law concerning educational requirements. Thus, a mandatory rule establishes a requirement, fee, or fee rate; sets a standard; provides a set procedure; pronounces how a law will be implemented; gives guidance for compliance with a law; describes the structure of an organization; or instructs members of the public how they must deal with any agency. The rule-making process is ongoing. State dental boards may promulgate rules at any time provided they follow state law and, by applying the rule-making process, can change a rule it believes should be changed or in response to a petition.

The state dental board is responsible for regulating dentistry and dental hygiene, usually by interpreting or further defining the law as well as granting and suspending or revoking licenses. Some states have dental hygiene committees or advisory boards that have a role in governing but do not have full authority to regulate practice. Most state dental boards are composed primarily of dentists, one or two dental hygienists, and one or two public members. This representation on the board means that dental hygienists in the state are basically governed by dentists. The dentists, usually the majority board members, can interpret the law to limit the practice of dental hygiene while increasing the functions of on-the-job trained dental personnel. Unfortunately, in many instances, the profession of dental hygiene has not had power to affect its own practice. With recent legislation allowing self-regulation by its dental hygiene committee, California became the exception to this. (See Figures 6-3 ■ and 6-4 ■.)

SUPERVISION OF DENTAL HYGIENISTS

Many states have requirements dictating the situations in which dentists are to supervise dental hygienists. In more than thirty states, dental hygienists may provide services in certain settings under various forms of unsupervised practice. Moreover, in fifteen states, dental hygienists may enroll as Medicaid providers, billing and collecting for services rendered.[13] Supervision is a major problem because it usually restricts the practice of dental hygiene to dental offices and decreases the effectiveness of public health efforts.[6] See Table 6-4 ■ for the definitions of different forms of supervisions of dental hygienists.

DENTAL HYGIENISTS ON STATE DENTAL BOARDS

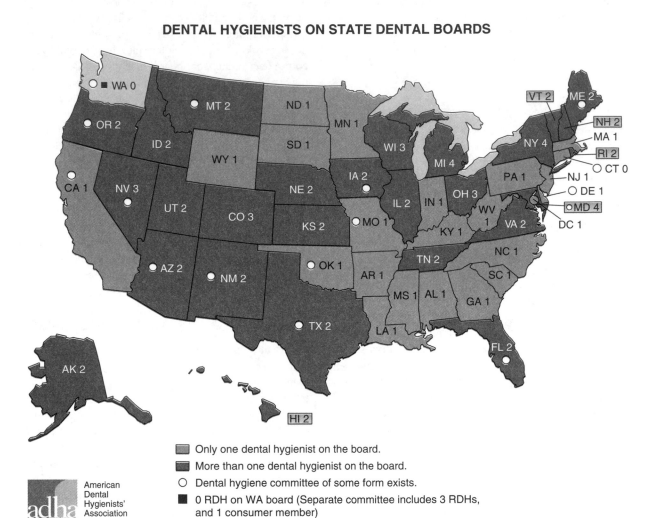

WA 0 · ○ ■
OR 2 ●
MT 2 ●
ND 1
MN 1
VT 2
ME 2
NH 2
MA 1
NY 4
RI 2
CT 0 ○
NJ 1
DE 1 ○
MD 4 ○
DC 1
ID 2
WY 1
SD 1
WI 3
MI 4
PA 1
IA 2 ●
NE 2
OH 3
CA 1 ●
NV 3 ●
UT 2
CO 3
KS 2
IL 2
IN 1
WV 1
VA 2
MO 1 ●
KY 1
AZ 2 ●
NM 2 ●
OK 1 ●
AR 1
TN 2
NC 1
SC 1
MS 1
AL 1
GA 1
TX 2 ●
LA 1
FL 2
AK 2
HI 2

⬛ Only one dental hygienist on the board.

⬛ More than one dental hygienist on the board.

○ Dental hygiene committee of some form exists.

■ 0 RDH on WA board (Separate committee includes 3 RDHs, and 1 consumer member)

adha American Dental Hygienists' Association

FIGURE 6-3 State Dental Board Representation

The following states have dental hygiene advisory committees or varying degrees of self regulation for dental hygienists.

1. **Arizona** The Arizona advisory committee consists of one dentist and one dental hygienist from the board, plus four additional dental hygienists and one public member. The committee serves as a forum for discussion of dental hygiene issues and advises the board on rules and proposed statute changes concerning dental hygiene education, regulation and practice. In addition the committee evaluates CE classes for expanded functions and monitors dental hygienists' compliance with CE requirements.

2. **California** The Committee on Dental Auxiliary (COMDA) of the dental board consists of the public member of the board, two dentists (only one of whom can be a board member), three dental hygienists and three registered dental assistants. Duties include evaluating dental hygiene and dental assisting education programs, advising the board on discipline and recommending regulations concerning dental hygiene and dental assisting. The new Dental Hygiene Committee of California will go into effect on January 1, 2009.

3. **Connecticut** Connecticut is unique. Dental hygiene is directly under the health department, and although there is no standing dental hygiene committee, if there is a need to address rules or disciplinary matters, the department director has the ability to appoint an ad hoc committee of dental hygienists.

4. **Delaware** Delaware's advisory committee is appointed by the governor and consists of three dental hygienists. During a recent sunset review of the board the committee was granted enhanced authority and now writes the examination for dental hygiene licensure (in conjunction with the dental board). Committee members also vote with the board on issues of dental hygiene licensure by credentials, disciplinary decisions and continuing education requirements for dental hygiene licensure.

5. **Florida** Florida has both dental hygiene and dental assisting councils. The dental hygiene council is composed of four dental hygienists, one of whom sits on the board, and one dentist member of the board. The council is expected to develop all dental hygiene rules to submit to the board for its approval.

6. **Iowa** Beginning in 1999, both dental hygienists on the dental board and one of the dentists became a dental hygiene committee of the board. This committee has the power to make all rules pertaining to dental hygiene. The board will be required to adopt those rules and enforce the committee rules.

7. **Maine** Maine has a subcommittee on dental hygiene. The subcommittee consists of five members: one dental hygienist who is a member of the board; two dental hygienists appointed by the governor; two dentists who are members of the board and appointed by the president of the board. The duties of the subcommittee are to perform an initial review of all applications for licensure as a dental hygienist, submissions relating to continuing education of dental hygienists, and all submissions relating to public health supervision status of dental hygienists.

8. **Maryland** Maryland's committee consists of three dental hygienists, one dentist, and one public member, all of whom are full voting members of the dental board. The committee was created during sunset review as a compromise to the creation of a separate dental hygiene regulatory board. According to statute, all matters pertaining to dental hygiene must first be brought to the committee for its review and recommendation.

9. **Michigan** A five member advisory committee, comprised of four dental hygienists and one dentist, considers matters related to the dental hygiene profession and makes recommendations to the full board of dentistry. All members of the advisory committee are voting members on the board. The existence of the advisory committee is not mandated by state rules or statutes, but

FIGURE 6-4 State Dental Hygiene Committees

instead is a committee appointed by the chairperson of the board.

10. **Missouri** A five member advisory commission, composed of the dental hygienists on the board and four dental hygienists appointed by the governor was created by the state legislature in 2001. The commission will make recommendations to the board concerning dental hygiene practice, licensure, examinations, discipline and educational requirements

11. **Montana** In 2002 the board assigned both dental hygienist members and one dentist member to be a standing committee to consider and address dental hygiene issues in a timely fashion. The committee will formulate specific recommendations to bring to the entire board for action.

12. **Nevada** Legislation in 2003 added a third dental hygienist to the board, who together with a dentist appointed by the board, will constitute a dental hygiene committee that may formulate recommendations on dental hygiene rules for the board and be assigned additional duties by the board.

13. **New Mexico** New Mexico has a board of dental health care comprised of five dentists, two dental hygienists and two public members. There is a dental hygiene committee comprised of five dental hygienists, two public members and two dentists. The committee selects two of its dental hygiene members to serve as the dental hygienists on the board. The board's public members and two of its dentist members are the dentist and public members of the committee. The committee adopts all the rules pertaining to dental hygiene and is also responsible for the discipline of dental hygienists. The board enforces the dental hygiene committee's rules.

14. **Oklahoma** The dental hygiene advisory committee is comprised of the dental hygiene board and four additional dental hygienists appointed by the board.

15. **Oregon** Under its authority to create standing committees, the Oregon dental board has appointed a committee comprised of three dentists, three dental hygienists, and one non-dental healthcare provider to advise the board concerning dental hygiene issues.

16. **Texas** In 1995 a dental hygiene advisory committee comprised of three dental hygienists and two public members appointed by the governor and one dentist appointed by the board was established. All rules relating to the practice of dental hygiene must be submitted to the committee for review 30 days prior to board adoption. The committee has been responsible for researching and developing recent rules for licensure by credentials and the application of tetracycline fibers. Legislation in 2003 gave the committee the authority to propose specific rules for board action.

17. **Washington** The state of Washington has a uniform disciplinary code which applies to all health professions and creates the regulatory bodies to implement each practice act. Dentistry and dental hygiene have separate practice acts. Dentists are regulated by the Dental Quality Assurance Commission (an independent dental board with no dental hygiene members). Dental hygienists are regulated by the Dental Hygiene Advisory Committee (comprised of three dental hygienists and one public member appointed by the department). Created in the early eighties, its original charge was to develop rules for dental hygiene education and licensure. Now, the committee has authority to originate all dental hygiene rules. Although nominally advisory, it meets and deliberates like a board. The department of health has consistently implemented rules as proposed by the committee.

FIGURE 6-4 (continued)

Source: www.adha.org. Revised August, 2008

Table 6-4 Types of Supervision of Dental Hygienists

Supervision Type	Generally Accepted Definition
Unsupervised, independent, collaborative practice	Dental hygiene practice without any supervision required from a dentist. Dental referral is necessary. In many states, a dental hygienist may practice only in certain public health settings.
General supervision	Dental hygiene practice without a dentist's "physically present" supervision. The patient must be a patient of record of a dentist in some states. Many states have additional stipulations, such as the patient must have had an exam within 30 days prior to or 30 days after dental hygiene treatment.
Indirect supervision	The dentist must be in the facility during dental hygiene treatment.
Direct supervision	The dentist must be in the treatment operatory during dental hygiene treatment.

SUMMARY

Dental hygienists must understand the function of governmental entities in order to make legal changes benefiting the public and the profession. Dental hygiene organizations continually strive to increase access to dental hygiene care. The profession supports the concept that to effectively prevent dental diseases, dental hygienists must become empowered in the political process and act as the voice for underserved populations who currently face barriers to care.

SELF-STUDY ITEMS

1. State agencies such as dental boards fall within which type of law?
   a. Common
   b. Statutory
   c. Constitutional
   d. Administrative

2. Which branch of government makes laws for the state?
   a. Legislative
   b. Executive
   c. Administrative
   d. Judicial

3. Laws which explain what services dental hygienists can provide are found in
   a. Medicaid rules
   b. State law
   c. Federal Law
   d. Health care regulations

4. Judges do not make laws, but they interpret them.
   a. The first statement is true, but the second statement is false.
   b. The first statement is false, but the second statement is true.
   c. Both statements are true.
   d. Both statements are false.

5. Because federal laws regulate dental hygiene practice, federal senators are involved with state regulation.
   a. The first statement is true, but the second statement is false.
   b. The first statement is false, but the second statement is true.
   c. Both statements are true.
   d. Both statements are false

REFERENCES

1. Motley WE. *History of the American Dental Hygienists' Association 1923–1982.* Chicago, IL: American Dental Hygienists' Association; 1983:39.
2. American Dental Hygienists' Association. *Governmental Affairs.* Chicago, IL: American Dental Hygienists' Association; 2008.
3. Alabama Dental Hygiene Program. *2006–2007 Dentist Instruction Manual.* Hoover, AL: Board of Dental Examiners of Alabama; 2006.
4. American Dental Hygienists' Association. *On-the-Job Training: A Dangerous Proposition.* Chicago, IL: American Dental Hygienists' Association. N.d. Professional Issues Paper. http://www.adha.org. Accessed August 26, 2008.
5. American Dental Association House of Delegates. Resolutions, 139th Annual Session. San Francisco, CA: 1998. Chicago: American Dental Association.

6. Nathe C, Posler, B. Collaborative practice: A form of independence. *RDH*. 1999;20:16–19.

7. American Dental Hygienists' Association. *Direct Access to Care by a Dental Hygienist*. Chicago, IL: American Dental Hygienists' Association; 2008.

8. American Dental Hygienists' Association. Prophylaxis Definition Restored in CDT-4 [presss release]. Chicago: American Dental Hygienists' Association. http://www.adha.org/profissues/cdt.htm. Accessed December 9, 2008.

9. Federal Trade Commission. South Carolina Board of Dentistry settles charges that it restrained competition in the provision of preventive care by dental hygienists: FTC complaint alleged conduct limited needy children's access to care. http://www.ftc.gov/os/adjpro/d9311/070911decision.pdf. Accessed October 16, 2007.

10. California Self Regulation Signed into Law. http://www.cdha.org/downloads/FINALSB853-6-13-08.pdf. Accessed August 27, 2008.

11. US Department of Health and Human Services. *A National Call to Action to Promote Oral Health*. Rockville, MD: US Department of Health and Human Services, Public Health Service, Centers for Disease Control and Prevention, National Institutes of Health, National Institute of Dental and Craniofacial Research; 2003. NIH Publication No. 03-5303.

12. *Competencies for the Advanced Dental Hygiene Practitioner (ADHP)*. Chicago, IL: American Dental Hygienists' Association; 2008:1–32.

13. States which directly reimburse dental hygienists services under the Medicaid program. http://www.adha.org/governmental_affairs/downloads/medicaid.pdf. Accessed on June 8, 2009.

PEARSON

myhealthprofessionskit™

Multimedia Extension Activities

Use this address to access the interactive Companion Website created for this textbook. Simply select "Dental Hygiene" from the choice of disciplines. Find this book and log in using your username and password. To obtain a username and password, please register using the scratch-off access code on the inside front cover of this book.

Chapter **7**

Advocacy for Dental Care

Shari Peterson, RDH, MEd

OBJECTIVES

After studying this chapter, the dental hygiene student will be able to:

- Identify four roles that the dental hygienist can assume as an agent of change
- Describe the various levels of change agent performance
- Utilize tools and resource models to implement change
- Identify the role of the change agent in policy making
- Promote partnership and coalition development
- Identify components of grant writing

KEY TERMS

Change agent
Collaboration
Empower
Ethics
Facilitator
Grantsmanship
Lobbying
Networking
Partnerships
Policy
Request for proposals
Stakeholder

COMPETENCIES

After studying this chapter and participating in accompanying course activities, the dental hygiene student should be competent to do the following:

- Promote the profession through service activities and affiliations with professional organizations
- Promote the values of oral and general health and wellness to the public and organizations within and outside the profession
- Assess the community's oral health needs and the quality and availability of resources and services
- Facilitate client access to oral health services in a variety of settings

The concept of *social advocacy* spans many disciplines but is predominantly associated with the business and legal worlds. A social advocate is frequently referred to as a **change agent,** an individual who intentionally or unintentionally causes social, cultural, or behavioral change. A change agent proactively bases action not only on a vision but also on well-defined goals and measurable objectives.

A change agent is not as effective without the collaboration of others motivated by both external and internal factors to pursue change. Rarely is a sole person entirely responsible for a total evolution, and rarely does a true change agent take credit as the sole individual responsible for change. Often a person is considered a change agent because of specific abilities to coordinate change or **empower** others to take action or make a change.

An important part of the art of being a change agent is to know what resources are available and the position that those who oppose changes take. *Change* is a process of evolution and is better facilitated when the change agent follows a pathway that allows for professional growth and increased ability to perform.

This chapter explains the process of change and how dental hygienists can recognize and effect change in dental public health. To help dental hygienists develop as agents of change, the chapter discusses the roles and responsibilities of change agents, the significant actions that change agents must perform, and ways to apply these skills. As dental hygienists develop an understanding of these components and abilities, they can become competent social advocates and be more effective in the community and in public health programs.

UNDERSTANDING CHANGE AND ITS AGENTS

Social advocates for dental public health are needed to implement change in regard to delivering dental care and ensuring program sustainability for various populations. In fact, dental public health would not be readily available if it were not for individuals empowered to change the existing systems and provide alternative concepts and pathways.

A basic understanding of the link between change and dental public health is critical to the dental hygiene profession. The number of dental hygienists entering the field of dental public health and involved with pol-icy making and networking with other health care providers continues to increase. Changing dental public health should be a primary concern and interest of dental hygienists. They must advocate for patients' health by affecting changes in their behavior, in dental office protocols, in products used in practice, and in dental hygiene practice through the legislative and regulatory systems.

> **Did You Know?**
>
> The dental hygiene profession originated in a public health setting and then was removed from public health because of legal restrictions. This resulted in limiting dental hygiene positions to private dental services. In the past decade, however, the presence of dental hygienists and dental hygiene advocates in the public health sector has increased, and a movement by the profession to return to its roots has occurred.

Change is recognized as an evolution or transformation from one state to another state. It can be abrupt or happen slowly over time. It can be only one person's decision impacting that person or large numbers of people uniting for a particular cause with decisions that affect many or all of them. For an idea to evolve into an action, many things must occur, but interaction is first. For change to take place, the individual must engage others through interaction. To understand how individuals behave in certain situations is sound preparation for managing barriers to change and achieving success. The key to successful change is to understand others and resolve to work with them regardless of whether they share the change agent's goals or interests.

Understanding programs or policies that need change and identifying the people responsible for bringing about change is necessary. A person acting on behalf of a particular group has a responsibility to represent its best interests regardless of personal opinion. This can create a conflict if the change agent does not have a vested interest in the desired change or if the change agent is not completely sold on doing things differently.

To create policy change, it is necessary to create change in individuals who govern that policy. A policy is the outward manifestation of a collective opinion.

Because people create policies, advocates of change must devote a significant amount of time convincing the policies' creators of the need for change. The receptiveness of the target individual(s) must be determined.

Roles and Responsibilities

Four roles have been identified for the dental hygiene change agent: catalyst, solution giver, resource linker, and process helper.[1]

A *catalyst* is defined as an agent that provokes or speeds significant change or action; to be one, a person must understand what needs to change and motivate others to transform their opinions and actions. Positive dental hygienists motivate patients to invest in themselves as a priority. The change agent can facilitate change by brainstorming of ideas, projecting excitement in the process of change, maintaining a positive disposition, and encouraging others to be positive during oral health education.

The *solution giver* is a problem solver who is vital to establishing or maintaining rapport among a group of individuals such as a dental office. A solution giver is often a person or a group who can "think outside the box," offer creative problem solving, and break a problem into individual components that can then be examined and addressed. A community dental hygienist, for example, may assemble a group of stakeholders to develop solutions to the oral health disparities seen in specific populations.

The *resource linker* is a facilitator. For example, dental hygienists can bring together individuals who share interests, abilities, monetary support, and common goals. There is strength in numbers, and change agents recognize the abilities of others and link together people who are suited to similar tasks or have similar abilities. Linking people with different perspectives on a problem is often crucial to the success of an endeavor, but balancing groups is also important. A dental hygienist may act as a resource linker by scheduling social services for prospective patients to help them find dental funding for specific needs. Individuals who have been involved in the organization or cause for a significant time period can mentor, and inexperienced individuals can draw wisdom from veterans.

The *process helper* understands all aspects of the change process and provides help where it is needed, focusing on goals rather than stumbling blocks or obstacles. The process helper often jumps into roles that have been abandoned or neglected or convinces others to assume those roles.

Actions

Change as a verb implies action. The actions of modifying, altering, and transforming imply a movement from one state or condition to another. To *modify* something means to make basic or fundamental changes without losing essential components. A modification is usually a more acceptable form of change as a starting point. To *alter* is to deviate from what is normal or expected or to make different without changing into something else. In some cases, an alteration may prevent returning to the original status or method. Alterations should be carefully weighed and considered before they are made. To *transform* is to change something from one state to a completely different one. For example, it results in abandoning one concept or procedure for a completely different one. This is a substantial change that cannot be taken lightly. Change agents must foresee the impact of a transformation and make plans to address problems that result from it. This process usually occurs over a period of time to allow for responsible changes.

Procedures and Applications

The process of change becomes tangible when it is incorporated into specific procedures. Planned changed can be integrated into the dental hygiene process. (See Box 7-1 ■.) The familiarity and versatility of the model described in Box 7-1 makes it easy for dental hygienists see how to become involved in the process of change. The concepts of assessment, diagnosis, planning, implementation, and evaluation are identified with procedures to incorporate into an action plan. Action plans become "recipes" for carrying out procedures.

The cyclic nature of the dental hygiene process of care allows for continual change. During the various stages of the process, regular meetings between all involved should be held to allow for immediate changes in procedures. Additionally, a final evaluation of outcomes helps to establish a need for future change. In dental public health settings, dental hygienists can easily adapt a model similar to that just discussed to their communities or create their own model within the parameters of their state laws and regulations; doing so is essential for clarifying how a dental hygienist practices. As scopes of practice change, models will need to be adapted.

BOX 7-1   Components of a Planned Change

Assessment

- Recognize when a change is needed.

- Collect data to verify the problem to be solved through change, and identify the desired situation that will result from the change.

Diagnosis

- Identify the problem that has created a need for change.

Planning

- Plan solutions/approaches and alternatives to the problem for which change is needed. Analyze the alternative approaches in terms of advantages, disadvantages, consequences of each, resources needed, cost, and level of support. Decide on a course of action from the alternatives analyzed.

- Design a plan for change: state objectives, outline methods, develop timetable, involve people,

assign responsibilities, assign resources, and monitor stability.

Implementation

- Implement the plan for change.

- Monitor for unforeseen problems.

Evaluation

- Determine whether the desired outcome and stated objectives have been achieved as a result of the implemented change.

- If necessary, reassess the situation and modify the plan for change.

- Stabilize the change by directing human and material resources to make the change permanent. Rewards and incentives should meet the human needs of the people involved.

Modified from: Darby M, and Walsh M. 2010. *Dental hygiene theory and practice.* 3rd edition Canada: Saunders.

DENTAL HYGIENIST SPOTLIGHT:
Shari Peterson, RDH, MEd

Professor Shari Peterson, RDH, MEd, is a dental hygiene educator who epitomizes the word *mentor* for dental hygienists interested in the public health path. She has great enthusiasm for community health and has educated hundreds of students about public health. Professor Peterson serves on numerous state and national committees that focus on community oral health endeavors and continually strives to improve the dental care delivery system in Nevada. She is the recipient of the Student American Dental Hygienists' Faculty Advisor Award from the American Dental Hygienists' Association, the Outstanding Dental Hygienists' Award from the Southern Nevada Dental Hygienists' Association, and a Letter of Commendation for Community Water Fluoridation from Dr. David Satcher, US PHS Surgeon General.

I asked her some questions regarding her career.

Why did you decide to go into dental hygiene?
I was always interested in biological sciences, but my mother is the one who convinced me to seek a career in dental hygiene. She felt it was important to pursue a career that was flexible and would allow me to work my schedule around motherhood. My mother had always taken me to dentists who did their own cleanings. When I was in high school, she worked as a dental receptionist, and I enjoyed watching the dentist work, but dentistry as a profession didn't interest me. When my mom left her job, she looked for another dentist closer to our home to take our family to for care. She decided on Dr. Robert Racine in Grass Valley, California. His wife, Rue, was his dental hygienist, and I have to credit her with inspiring me to pursue dental hygiene as a career. She let me sit by her chair for an afternoon while she

worked with her patients. I loved the fact that she could provide care directly to the patients in her own operatory, and I was really impressed by how she educated her patients: She connected with them on a personal level and made the appointments pleasant for them. All of my previous cleanings had been very rough, but she was gentle.

Watching her that day, I knew that I wanted to be just like her. She gave me the phone number for ADHA; I called and requested information and a list of programs. I was accepted at Idaho State University and headed to school with only $500 to my name. The program director, Denise Bowen, was fantastic in setting me up with grants, loans, and scholarships. I would not have been able to go to school otherwise.

How did you begin to educate hygienists about public health? Did you need additional education?

Well, I was always interested in teaching. My mother had taught elementary school too. After working for ten years in private practice, I returned to college and obtained a master's degree in education from the University of Nevada–Las Vegas. I thought that maybe someday I would pursue a teaching career, but someone at the local dental hygiene school (College of Southern Nevada) found out I was working on my master's degree and asked if I would accept a part-time teaching position there. Several years later, I applied for a full-time position in the program.

I became passionate about dental public health after being invited to participate in a prophy/sealant clinic for homeless children organized by my local dental hygiene component. It was a fantastic event, but I was frustrated with the lack of organized dental public health opportunities that existed in Nevada at that time. A friend, Cathy Lytle, kept me in the loop about opportunities to serve and help with the programs we did have. We worked together on many projects over the years. Chris Wood with the Nevada State Health Division also became a mentor for me on developing programs and grant writing. She helped me understand the intricacies of government and legislation.

What are your current positions?

Currently, I am on sabbatical leave from teaching to write a textbook on public health dental hygiene practice for hygienists who want to transition from working in private practice into the field of dental public health. Prior to my leave, I was Community Outreach/Community Dental Health Course Director and adviser to the American Dental Hygienists' Association Student Chapter at the College of Southern Nevada. I teach many of the public health track courses in our online baccalaureate completion program.

Can you discuss any particularly interesting experiences you have had in your dental public health and/or educational positions?

Wow, there are so many! Most of my inspiring experiences have happened as a result of being a member of ADHA and advocating returning public health dental hygiene back to the scope of practice for dental hygienists in my state. With these changes, dental hygienists are allowed to practice unsupervised in public health settings with a public health endorsement from our Board of Dental Examiners.

My most interesting and memorable experiences have occurred when working with our statewide dental sealant program. Most of the time, we see rampant decay in the second grade children; however, this last year I have seen a dramatic drop in the amount of decay our children are experiencing. I believe this can be attributed to the combination of sealant placement and community water fluoridation that was established in Clark County around 2001. It is awesome to have visible results.

What advice would you give to a practicing hygienist who is thinking of doing something different?

I would say serve your community first. There is so much to offer in your own community. The feelings you get from helping others are incredible. The reality check of working in dental public health puts into focus the true nature of prevention that dental hygienists committed to when they pledged their oath. And service is free; giving of yourself has tremendous value to others. Pursuing a career in public health also increases your leadership abilities and your capacity for changing the profession to make it more beneficial for the public.

Source: Christine Nathe writes the Public Health Column in RDH magazine published by Pennwell Publishing.
For more public health spotlights please see RDH magazine online at http://www.rdhmag.com/index.html.

Having teams of change agents at various levels of experience increases the likelihood that a dental hygienist will manage change effectively. In participating in the change process, the dental hygienist gains self-confidence and accepts additional roles and responsibilities, thus increasing competence. Competency is directly related to understanding and experience. It is inherent in the dental hygienist to strive to attain competency in all abilities. The key competencies for dental change agents identified in Box 7-2 ■ can be used as a dental hygienist's personal standard.

Did You Know?

The competent change agent has refined abilities of vision, collaboration, communication, and negotiation.

The most important contributions of a competent change agent are those that sustain an organization's current performance and ensure its future performance. Competency enables people to work effectively as they plan, implement, and experience change; it also increases their ability to manage future change.

Barriers to Change

The process of change frequently must overcome impediments for various reasons. Typical barriers are unexpected changes in external conditions, lack of commitment to implementation, resistance of the people involved, and lack of resources.

Unfortunately, the implications of failed change go well beyond the unmet objectives. Because of the many problems and risks associated with change projects, the change agent affects not only the success or failure of the project but also the extent of negative outcomes, which can result in a lack of motivation among those involved. As a result, some may never again be willing to commit to change initiatives. Some will become skeptical of any future change project and consider the process to be just another elaborate idea from leadership bringing much work and few benefits.

The change agent can become competent by acknowledging and adapting the concepts presented in various models. The multifaceted road to competence can be visualized as a road map. See Table 7-1 ■ for the roles of the change agent, concepts of change and the change model, and the significance of each in the change process. The table indicates the reciprocal relationship of change and competency.

BOX 7-2   Key Competencies of Dental Change Agents

Vision

- Sensitivity to changes in dental care delivery, professional perceptions, technology, and in the way in which each impacts the health of the public

- Ability to develop clearly defined, realistic goals for a project of change

- Generalized perspective of priorities

Collaboration

- Ability to bring together key stakeholders and establish effective partnerships

- Networking skills to establish and maintain appropriate contacts within and outside the organization

- Management skills to establish working groups and to define and delegate respective responsibilities clearly

Communication

- Effective interpersonal skills, predominantly listening to and recognizing the concerns of others

- Ability to express enthusiasm in partnership ideas and stimulate motivation and commitment in others

- Ability to convey effectively the need for adaptation to colleagues and partners

Negotiation

- Skills to influence others to commit to plans and ideas by creating a desirable and challenging vision of the future

- Tolerance of uncertainty about the causes and effects of change

- Fosters cohesiveness

- Political awareness in identifying potential hazards and balancing conflicting goals and perceptions

Table 7-1   PAUSE: A Collaborative Style for Reaching an Agreement

Prepare

Acquire facts.	Plan an alternative to a negotiated agreement.
Identify issues and interests.	Select an appropriate time and place to meet.
Use ethical principles.	Plan opening remarks.
Develop options.	Seek counsel.
Anticipate reactions.	

Affirm Relationships

Courteously communicate.	Seek solutions that satisfy all.
Acknowledge personal issues.	Confront in a gracious manner.
Respect leaders' authority.	Allow face-saving.
Seek to understand others' position(s).	Praise valid points.
Discuss participants' responses.	

Understand Interests

Focus on interests rather than positions.	Determine coinciding or conflicting points.
Seek to fully understand interests.	Use caution in revealing personal interests.

Search for Creative Solutions

Invent solutions based on need.	Expand the topic with additional interests.

Evaluate Options Objectively and Reasonably

Keep an open and fair mind.	Identify concession points for both sides.
Use rules of reason, laws, ethics, and culture.	Identify unbendable points for both sides.
Discover reasons behind objections.	Identify and focus on agreeable points.

Source: Sande K. *The Peacemaker.* Baker Books: Grand Rapids, MI, 1997.

Dental hygienists as agents of change have made substantial contributions in the field of dental public health. The remaining sections of this chapter discuss factors related to making change.

The scope of practice for dental hygienists varies significantly from state to state, so it is imperative that public health dental hygiene be practiced according to the specific state's governing and regulatory agencies.

Becoming acquainted with policy making, collaboration and partnership, coalition building, and grant writing in the dental hygienist's state is essential. Whether directly involved with managing these processes as a change agent or as an active participant, the dental hygienist must have a clear picture of how these processes occur.

MAKING GOVERNMENTAL POLICY

In the field of health care, research is conducted and technology is explored to find better ways to do things. The results of these findings are used to create **policy,** a written description of rules, regulations, and stipulations to govern individual actions and procedures. Policies can be as formal as laws or rules with accountability and consequences or as loosely structured as guides or advisory opinions with no binding legality. Policy in the form of a practice act can be open to interpretation by a body of peers recognized in their field.

In the regulatory environment that governs licensed health care providers, a set of ethics is assumed to be the standard of professionalism. **Ethics** are guiding principles for individuals or groups based on what is right and what is wrong. In policy related to health care, ethical behavior has no legal binding. However, ethical standards can be adopted or utilized to assess the degree to which policies are followed or ignored, and a breach of these standards can result in disciplinary action imposed by a regulatory body.

In the evolution of society, government—persons elected or appointed to represent society—has predominantly set policy. The scope of governments and the policies they enact affect dental care, specifically dental public health.

National Health Policy

The federal government has adopted national policies on behalf of and in the best interest of the public as a whole. It does this through federal agencies that have been delegated the authority to research and record the status of health in the country and to determine guidelines and set goals to affect change in the nation's health. In addition to policy development, the federal government allocates funds through initiatives to the states so that national policies can be implemented.

Examples of federal health initiatives that impact dental care are Healthy People 2010 and the Surgeon General's *A Call to Action to Promote Oral Health.* Both of these issued benchmarks of achievement in dental care that are essential to public health. These benchmarks, such as the increase in the use of dental sealants and community water fluoridation, should become the goals of all entities that advocate for quality dental care.

State Health Policy

The federal government manages policies and funds; the states are the change agents that develop and implement programs supported by those funds. State health divisions bear the responsibility of carrying out federal policy as well as developing protocols for implementation. In regard to oral health, each state has a designated dental director or representative who manages the state's oral health programs, which are extremely varied in composition, functions and, goals.

Some states implement clinical programs and services directly, using state personnel; others execute programs indirectly by subcontracting nonstate agencies, such as professional associations, community advocates, private partnerships, and local governments. Subcontracting usually comes as a response to a request for proposed work.

Some policies at the state level may need to be changed to implement these programs effectively. State regulatory practice acts governing dentistry and dental hygiene need to be reviewed to ensure that programs comply with practice standards and to be evaluated for change opportunities.

Local Health Policy

Local health departments or city or county governments develop health policy. Professional associations with financial support from local businesses, private foundations, and educational institutions represent a growing presence in local policy establishment and enactment. The success of these partnerships has brought together experts and advocates to create an environment in which to consider and create change agents. These partnerships will be discussed in more detail in another section.

Did You Know?

Examples of local oral health programs are community clinics, professional association–sponsored oral health programs, and the activities of individual practitioners, such as a direct access dental hygienist who works in public health settings.

To change policy at the national, state, or local level, change agents must thoroughly understand the organization and be persistent. Government policy is not easily changed. When Surgeon General Richard Carmona wrote *A Call to Action to Promote Oral Health,* public forums were held in various locations for individuals to provide input for his consideration. The administration identified the workforce as the experts in their field with valued comments. Many states hold oral health summits of stakeholders to facilitate strategic planning. This active process brings together varied viewpoints to determine strategies for a state's office of oral health to pursue and extend resources. By participating as an agent of change, each individual's voice can be heard in helping to establish legislative policy. Change agents are broadly used to implement and monitor programs in addition to proposing legislation.

Lobbying for Policy Change

The act of **lobbying** is attempting to influence or sway others to take or support a desired position or action. In simple terms, it is the "art of the sell." Lobbying formally seeks to influence legislators to enact desired legislation and informally to persuasade others. A lobbyist can be a representative of an association or organization, a government employee, a corporation, or a public interest group. Lobbyists can be paid or unpaid and are typically members of the organization they represent. Professional lobbyists are paid for their services on a fee-for-service or contract basis.

Lobbyists' most valued assets are their established relationships, which provide access to those whom the change agent wants to influence, but they do not guarantee success in securing change. The lobbyist is a tool to provide advice on strategies, tactics, and procedures to maximize effectiveness. An organization's professional or other lobbyist should be considered the expert in understanding the dynamics and motivation for change. The "sell" ultimately comes from agents of change who have done their homework, invested themselves emotionally, and perservered.

WORKING IN COLLABORATION AND THROUGH PARTNERSHIPS

When it comes to change, there is strength in numbers. Individuals can join partnerships, collaborations, and teams to express their beliefs on a subject to effect a greater change through synergy.

Collaboration

Collaboration is the process of working with others toward a common goal.[2] It occurs when two or more individuals or organizations work together on a task of mutual interest and benefit. The sum of the collaboration is greater than the value of the individual contributions. The predominant factor is cooperation, in which organizations or individuals work in association on tasks. Collaboration can occur without a formal agreement or partnership.

Collaborative efforts are strengthened by **networking,** or sharing resources or services to cultivate productive relationships. Networking enables an individual or group to draw on multiple resources and build a consensus to accomplish desired objectives. An important networking skill is the ability to identify resources, both financial and human, available within the community and to contact them.

In the book *The Peacemaker,* Sande discusses "the collaborative style" as a tool for affecting change.[3] The method of PAUSE found in Table 7-1 stands for *prepare, affirm relationships, understand interests, search for creative solutions,* and *evaluate options objectively and reasonably.* This collaborative style helps to balance the principles and interests of all parties.

Partnerships

A **partnership,** which can be viewed as an intense form of collaboration, is the state or condition of associating or participating with others regularly in pursuit of a joint interest. Each member brings a unique perspective to the partnership. The need for partnerships between health care professionals within geographical communities is becoming increasingly important as new health care needs, practice changes, and issues are identified.[4] The health care system and delivery of services to the public are improved when health-related disciplines share and borrow from one another. Successful partnerships recognize that each partner may contribute different ideas and that flexibility is the key to success.

Formal partnerships have legal documents outlining each member's responsibilities, contributions, and boundaries. Partnerships created specifically to render services generally require a contract; one organization signs an agreement with another to complete services for one of them, each other, or a third entity. A partnership agreement can be a measurement tool to evaluate the partnership's effectiveness.

A *partnership agreement* does not have to be a legal document. Community-Campus Partnerships for Health, a nonprofit organization that promotes health through partnerships between communities and higher educational institutions, recommends its use. The organization establishes and promotes collaboration, health through service learning, community-based participatory research, broad-based coalitions, and other partnership strategies.[5]

> **Did You Know?**
>
> Formal partnerships commonly use documents stating affiliation agreements or memorandums of understanding (MOUs).

A *memorandum of understanding* (MOU) is an agreement that some formal partnerships use, but because it is not a legal document, it is not enforceable in court. In most cases, the signers of an MOU indicate that they do not intend to try to enforce its terms, although the document expresses a convergence of will between the parties, indicating an intended common line of action rather than a legal commitment. Changes or amendments to the MOU often occur during formal evaluation or the end of a fiscal cycle.

Educational institutions sometimes use an affiliation agreement, a legally binding contract made between one entity such as a clinic, hotel, or hospital and an educational institution to allow students to participate in an internship or other educational experience at the entity's location. The affiliation agreement states the terms and conditions under which the educational institution and entity agree to furnish education, training, and/or clinical experience integral to the specific institution's academic degree or course objective. Most affiliation agreements are standardized documents and very rarely amendable.

BUILDING COALITIONS

A **coalition** is an alliance of distinct organizations or persons to take a joint action. It represents an array of interests and brings together organizations and individuals to build a power base that works to accomplish change in response to a mutual concern. A well-organized, broad-based coalition can increase the potential for success in creating policy change, educating the public, creating a network, and developing innovative solutions to complex problems. **Stakeholders,** individuals in organizations who have a particular vested interest in a specific topic, issue, or initiative, usually compose coalitions.

When community problems or issues are too large and complex for any one agency or organization to address, forming a coalition of representatives of numerous segments can be an effective strategy to move everyone in the same direction to reach a common goal. That goal could be as narrow as obtaining funding for a specific intervention or as broad as trying to permanently improve the overall quality of life for most people in the community.

Common goals of coalitions follow:

- **Influencing or Developing Public Policy.** Such policy usually involves a specific issue.
- **Changing Behavior.** Reducing the incidence of smoking or caries is an example of behavior that might be changed.
- **Building a Healthy Community.** This generally involves strengthening both the community's physical health (such as performing oral prevention services, community planning, curbing substance abuse) and its social and psychological health (for example, encompassing diversity; improving education, culture, and the art; preventing violence).

Consistency can be particularly important in addressing a community issue, especially if a number of organizations or individuals are already working on the same issue. Having significantly different approaches and/or failing to cooperate or collaborate can lead to a chaotic situation in which very little is accomplished. If, on the other hand, the organizations or individuals work together and agree on common goals and ways to reach them, they are much more likely to be successful.

It is important to be aware of and anticipate barriers to creating a coalition to be able to prevent or overcome them. (See Box 7-3 ■.)

A broad membership is advantageous for coalitions, but the involvement of these people and groups are absolutely essential: stakeholders, community opinion leaders, and policy makers. In addition, virtually any coalition can benefit from the membership of at least some concerned citizens who may have no direct connection to the issue at hand. Such people can act as barometers of community attitudes and provide information about the coalition's work. Media groups should be involved to publicize the coalition and its efforts. People from the media who are members of the coalition, however, may be ethically limited as to the amount of coverage they can provide.

Bringing all these entities together requires the efforts of a coalition **facilitator.** This person conducts meetings, brings diverse ideas together, and helps the group work to reach goals. The most important role of the facilitator, however, is to lay the groundwork for creating trust as the coalition develops. The facilitator should be perceived as trusted and neutral by coalition participants.

BOX 7-3 Barriers to Creating a Coalition

Turf Issues. Organizations are often very sensitive about sharing their work, their target populations, and especially their funding. Part of creating a coalition may be to convince a number of organizations that working together will in fact both benefit all of them and better address their common issues.

Negative History. Organizations, individuals, or the community as a whole may have had experiences in the past that have convinced them that working with certain others is simply not possible. A new coalition may have to contend with this history before it can actually start the work it needs to do.

Domination by "Professionals" or Some Other Elite. All too often in their rush to solve problems or to "help the disadvantaged," agency people with advanced degrees, local politicians, business leaders, and others neglect to involve the people most affected by the issue at hand and other effected community members. Creating a participatory atmosphere and reining in those who believe they have all the answers are almost always required when starting a coalition.

Poor Links to the Community. A first step may have to be the development of hitherto nonexistent relationships among agencies and the community at large.

Minimal Organizational Capacity. It might be necessary to find a coordinator or one or more individuals or organizations to seek a way to share the burden with the new group if it is to develop beyond a first meeting.

Funding. The difficulty of finding funding is an obvious obstacle. Less obvious are the dangers of available funding that push the coalition in the wrong direction or requires it to act too quickly to address the issue effectively. New coalitions should be alert to funding possibilities from all quarters and be vigilant about the kind of funding they apply for and accept.

Failure to Provide and Create Leadership Within the Coalition. Coalitions demand a very special kind of collaborative leadership. It may be necessary to bring in an outside facilitator and/or training someone in collaborative leadership to salvage the situation.

Failure to Show Benefits of Perceived—or Actual—Costs of Working Together. The task may be to find ways to increase benefits and decrease costs for individuals and organizations if the coalition is to survive.

Source: The Community Tool Box. http://ctb.ku.edu/about/en/index.jsp. Accessed June 8, 2009.

WRITING GRANTS

This brief overview of the grant-writing process is intended to identify the various processes involved and the essential functions of change agents in grant writing. **Grantsmanship** the art of obtaining grants for funding projects. It is also a technical skill that requires hard work, a state of readiness, information, and sometimes trial and error before having a successful outcome.[6]

A *grant* is a financial resource given to an agency, organization, or individual to address a problem or need. The grant writer prepares a written document (*grant proposal*) that requests support (funding). The grant writer also researches the availability of funds and the criteria that apply to petitioners.

Did You Know?

A request for proposals (RFP) by groups or agencies is also called *request for applications, notice of funding availability,* or *program announcement.*

An organization usually notifies the public about the availability of funding through its announcement of a **request for proposals (RFP).** The deadline for proposal submission can be as little as one month after an REP is issued. Good grammar, accurate spelling, and cohesion are critical to a well-written proposal. The grant writer can be creative in presenting substantive elements (such as identifying the need for funding for the topic or population of interest). In some cases, innovative or creative approaches can enhance a grant proposal's likelihood of success. A grant proposal should adhere to standard guidelines. (See Table 7-2 ■.)

Features of a strong proposal that enhance the likelihood of receiving funds include:

- Well-organized proposal sections
- Well-researched and documented statement of the problem
- Creative or innovative strategies for addressing the need or problem
- Statements of *feasible* goals and objectives
- Identification of *measurable* objectives
- Inclusion of a sound evaluation plan

Table 7-2 Standard Components of a Grant Proposal

Component	Description
Cover letter	Includes the project title, name of the agency submitting the grant, agency address, name of the prospective funder, beginning and ending project dates, and total amount of funds requested. Title page and abstract, which briefly describes the major points of the proposal.
Needs statement or statement of problem	Documents present the problem to be addressed with text, statistics, graphs, and or charts. It should also describe the causes of the problem creating the need and identify approaches or solutions that have already been attempted.
Project description	Contains three main parts: goal(s) and objective(s), methods to address the identified problem or need, and a time line for the completing each component.
Evaluation plan	Shows how the organization will measure the success of the project and outcome objectives; should include details about how information will be collected, analyzed, and shared with the funder.
Budget request and budget justification	Should contain details regarding salaried individuals, direct and indirect costs of supplies and equipment, administrative costs, and any matching donations of money or supplies.
Applicant qualifications	Should convince grant reviewers of the validity of the requesting organization's project.
Future funding or sustainability plan	Shows a continued effort to ensure the program's security and longevity.
Appendices	Provides supplemental materials that do not belong in the body of the proposal but are important data that should be shared with the funder.

SUMMARY

Change in dental care can be accomplished as the result of the efforts of an individual, collaboration, partnership, or coalition. Understanding how change occurs, using effective tools that facilitate change, and preparing for common barriers to its occurrence can greatly enhance the change agent's success. Studying the various attributes of vision, communication, collaboration, and negotiation required for being a successful and competent change agent can help that person recognize existing qualities and areas to be developed. As technology and health care evolve, so do opportunities for new ways to practice. The dental hygienist is a valued member of the dental team and can make a difference in changing the policies of a dental practice, local coalition, state strategic organization, and even a national agency. With other stakeholders, the dental hygienist can contribute to the change process by advocating for a specific agenda such as increasing Medicaid coverage, providing community water fluoridation, or obtaining state funds for oral health programs. Understanding how policy is created on a national, state, and local level can help the change agent focus on realistic expectations of change.

SELF-STUDY TEST ITEMS

1. Which of the following is an individual or group who causes a social, cultural, or behavioral change, be it intentional or unintentional?
   a. Coalition
   b. Change agent
   c. Lobbyist
   d. Grant writer

2. Which of the following is *not* a way in which social advocates initiate change in dental public health?
   a. By delivering dental care
   b. By helping to sustain dental public health programs
   c. By determining the type of dental treatment rendered
   d. By determining who receives dental care

3. What is necessary to create change?
   a. Influencing individuals who govern policy
   b. Increasing an organization's financial status
   c. Redesigning a public health facility
   d. All of the above

4. What are the roles identified for the dental hygiene change agent?
   a. Catalyst
   b. Solution giver
   c. Resource linker
   d. All of the above

5. Making basic changes without losing the essential components is termed?
   a. Modification
   b. Competency
   c. Application
   d. Networking

REFERENCES

1. Parker E. The dental hygienist: Change agent for the future. *Dent Hyg.*1984;58(8):362.
2. *Merriam-Webster Online Dictionary.* www.m-w.com. Accessed June 8, 2009.
3. Sande K. *The Peacemaker.* Baker Books: Grand Rapids, MI, 1997.
4. Boswell C, Cannon S. New horizons for collaborative partnerships. *Online J Issues Nur.* 2005;10(1). www.nursingworld.org/ojin/topic26/tpc26_2.htm. Accessed June 8, 2009.
5. Community Campus Partnerships for Health. http://www.ccph.info/. Accessed June 8, 2009.
6. Gitlin L, Lyons K. *Successful Grant Writing: Strategies for Health and Human Service Professionals.* New York: Springer; 1996.

PEARSON
myhealthprofessionskit™

Multimedia Extension Activities

Use this address to access the interactive Companion Website created for this textbook. Simply select "Dental Hygiene" from the choice of disciplines. Find this book and log in using your username and password. To obtain a username and password, please register using the scratch-off access code on the inside front cover of this book.

Dental Hygiene Public Health Programs

Dental hygienists practicing in public health settings strive to ensure that a given population attains oral health. As in private practice, one of the dental hygienist's most important roles is to motivate patients to change values and influence behaviors aimed at attaining oral health. When dental hygienists treat a target population, an important strategy is to provide group education.

Educating individuals in a group setting is as vital for the dental hygienist as is providing that same education to individual patients in private practice. For example, dental hygienists practicing in a prison strive to improve the oral health of the inmates they treat through education; those consulting for a Head Start program focus on helping the children in it to attain oral health. Therefore, it is important for dental hygienists to understand the differences, similarities, and diversities of various populations and know how to effectively promote oral health for each through planning, implementing, and evaluating effective programs.

Chapter 8

Dental Health Education and Promotion

OBJECTIVES

After studying this chapter, the dental hygiene student should be able to:

- Define dental health education and promotion
- Describe health education and promotion principles
- Outline the different learning and motivation theories

KEY TERMS

Behavior change
Habit
Health education
Health promotion
Healthy behavior
Values

COMPETENCIES

After studying this chapter and participating in accompanying course activities, the dental hygiene student should be competent to do the following:

- Communicate with individuals and groups from diverse populations both verbally and in writing
- Promote the values of oral and general health and wellness to the public and organizations within and outside the profession
- Provide screening, referral, and education to bring consumers into the health care delivery systems

Dental hygienists frequently are asked to present information to groups regarding dental health education. Generally, these groups have underlying similarities and are referred to as *target populations,* which are discussed in Chapter 10. Although fundamental differences affect educating a group of individuals as opposed to an individual patient, many of the concepts are similar.

Dental health education presented to groups can be an effective, productive, and inexpensive way to provide preventive dental care. For these reasons, all dental hygienists need to be skilled in providing such presentations to the community.

Health education historically has been paternalistic in nature. Dental hygienists typically prescribed a regimen and dictated behavior to patients. The dental hygienist was considered an expert who imparted knowledge to the patient who in turn was expected to change behaviors accordingly.[1] Today, patients are considered participants in their health care, and their social environments are important for the dental hygienist to consider when providing health education. Empowerment models that emphasize provider and patient working collaboratively toward treatment have become more common in recent years and are practiced routinely by dental hygienists when instructing patients on brushing and flossing. Patients become active learners during the demonstration of skills.

> **Did You Know?**
>
> Patient autonomy gives a patient the right to control the course of medical treatment and participate in the treatment decision-making process.

PRINCIPLES OF HEALTH

Health has been defined as a state of physical, mental, and social well-being that involves more than just absence of disease.[2] A *wellness scale* is basically a continuum of total health to death, or a state of being from optimal health and wellness to serious illness or disease with areas between for quality of life indicators.[3]

Five-Dimensional Health Model

Today, the accepted view is that a person is a multidimensional being consisting of five dimensions: physical, mental, social, spiritual, and emotional.[4] (See Figure 8-1 ■.) It is helpful to look at the dimensions as five need systems,

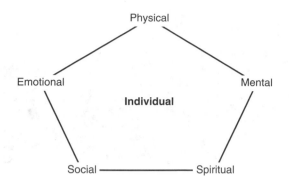

FIGURE 8-1 Five-Dimensional Health Model

each requiring specific input from the environment for an individual's complete development. (See Table 8-1 ■.) The term *input* refers to phenomena that feed each dimension in positive ways. Basically, if a dimension receives an adequate amount of input, it will have the maximum potential for efficient function; conversely, if the input is lacking, the likelihood that a detriment to health may develop increases.

Maslow's Hierarchy of Needs

It is advantageous to keep in mind Maslow's Hierarchy of Needs (see Figure 8-2 ■) when contemplating the meaning of health. Maslow arranged needs in lowest to highest levels. He theorized that when the needs at one level are met, those of the next higher level can be subsequently

Table 8-1 Five-Dimensional Health Model

Dimensions	Positive Input	Negative Input
Physical	Food, toothbrush, floss	Poor nutrition, inadequate dental care
Emotional	Trust	Mistrust, fear of dental provider
Mental	Knowledge	Ignorance
Social	Interaction with people	Withdrawal, inadequate communication skills
Spiritual	Values, morality	No value for dental health, no morality

Source: Eberst R. Defining health: A multidimensional model. *J Sch Health.* 1084;54:100.

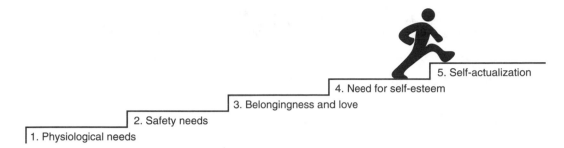

FIGURE 8-2 Maslow's Hierarchy of Needs

Source: Maslow AH. *Motivation and Personality.* 3rd ed. New York, NY: Harper and Row; 1987.

addressed in a linear, stair-step approach. In Maslow's hierarchy, the more advanced needs are not addressed until lower ones have been met. In addition, when lower needs such as hunger reappear, all higher needs momentarily vanish.[5] When adapted to dental health, this theory assumes that when individuals have not met a basic need, such as getting relief from a toothache, they cannot attain the next level, which might be flossing regularly.

HEALTH EDUCATION AND MOTIVATION THEORIES

A **healthy behavior** can be defined as an action, such as daily flossing to remove plaque, that helps prevent disease and promotes health for the individual or population. **Health education** can be defined as instruction regarding health behaviors that bring an individual to a state of health awareness, such as teaching a population the proper flossing technique. **Health promotion,** a process that informs and motivates people to adopt healthy behavior to enhance their health and prevent disease, occurs, for example, when a dental hygienist provides samples of floss at a local health fair. Health promotion is similar to health education but is geared more toward motivating people to adopt healthy behaviors. In contrast, the intention of health education is to have the learner gain accurate knowledge about healthy behaviors and lifestyles. Both promotion and education are methods to modify detrimental behaviors and promote healthy ones.

One example of dental health promotion is the local dental hygiene association's work to ban sugary snacks and beverages from vending machines in schools in the district. The goal of this promotional activity is not to teach the effects of a sugary diet but to increase awareness of such foods' availability in the schools and to promote actions to decrease children's access to them.

The primary goal of dental health education is the prevention of disease using appropriate dental health interventions. Dental health education is a planned activity that utilizes the population's knowledge, attitudes, culture, and values to promote proper oral health practices.[6] If the local dental hygiene association held classes on dental health prevention modalities for middle school teachers who passed a test qualifying them to teach dental health to students, the dental hygiene association would have performed a dental health educational activity.

Dental health education theory suggests that although a person may be educated on a particular health behavior, that knowledge will not impact dental health until the person positively changes the behavior, which then becomes a habit. A **behavior change** simply is changing a behavior, such as decreasing the amount of sugar in ones' diet, whereas a **habit** is a behavior that becomes automatic, such as daily brushing. Although dental hygienists may make an effective dental health presentation that those who observe it understand, they will not necessarily practice dental health behaviors discussed. Therefore, it is necessary to change a person's values regarding the behavior before the behavior is changed. **Values**—the ideas and beliefs a person possesses that influence behavior—give meaning to our lives. A person may develop values early in life from parents, grandparents, older siblings, teachers, or other influential people from whom that person seeks love and acceptance.[7] Values generally must first be changed if behavior is to change. See Figure 8-3 ■ for the steps in changing behavior. If dental hygienists could change values that the population holds toward dental health, they could dramatically decrease if not totally eliminate suffering from dental diseases. Unfortunately, changing values is a bit of a challenge.

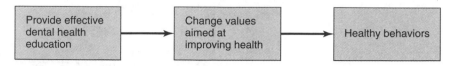

FIGURE 8-3 Goals of Dental Health Education

Did You Know?

The dental hygiene student must be aware that education is the basis for any dental hygiene treatment.

Theories on Methods to Change Values

Dental health education is based largely on the scientific principles of psychology and sociology that facilitate learning and behavioral change in the individual.[6] The following theories offer ideas on possible methods to use when attempting to change values.

Theory of the Health Belief Model

The theory of the *health belief model* suggests that in order to display a readiness to take action to avoid a disease or act in preventive manner, an individual needs to believe that he or she is susceptible or vulnerable, the disease has serious consequences, the behavior is beneficial, and it is important.[8] This theory is based on the premise that when individuals have accurate information, they will make better choices including those pertaining to health. The US Public Health Service uses the health belief model for health interventions. See Table 8-2 ■ for an example of the health belief model in dental hygiene practice.

Theory of Stages of Learning

Understanding the increments in which a person actually learns information is important. The learning ladder in Figure 8-4 ■ depicts an individual's natural progression from knowledge absorption to value adoption. This ladder

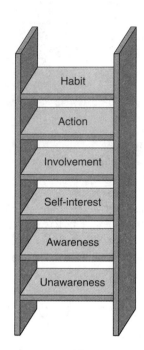

FIGURE 8-4 Learning Ladder

Source: Harris NO, Garcia-Godoy F. *Primary Preventive Dentistry.* 6th ed. Upper Saddle River, NJ: Prentice Hall, 2004.

has six rungs that begin with *unawareness* of the topic. *Awareness,* which occurs when education is provided, is second followed by the *self-interest* rung characterized by the recognition of desire and involvement. The next stage, *involvement,* occurs when the person becomes involved in the learning process. *Action* is when the individual makes a change and then a *habit* can be formed.

Table 8-2 Example of Health Belief Model in Dental Hygiene Practice

1. Susceptibility	Individual believes he or she is susceptible to oral cancer because he or she chews tobacco
2. Serious consequences	Individual believes that oral cancer can be disfiguring and fatal
3. Benefit	Individual believes that to decrease the risk of disfigurement, illness, and possibly death, it would be beneficial to stop chewing tobacco
4. Salience	Individual makes the cessation of chewing tobacco top priority in life and stops the practice

Theory of the Transtheoretical Model

The transtheoretical model is similar to the stages of learning and includes five stages of change through which a person travels before achieving a desired state. Each stage of readiness is characterized by certain behaviors and attitudes. These stages of change are pre-contemplation, contemplation, preparation, action, maintenance and termination. A person at the precontemplation stage has no intention of taking action soon whereas someone at the preparation stage does. Action is followed by maintenance. A person who never relapses from the overt behavior is said to be at the termination stage.

Assessing an individual's stage allows educators including health care workers to tailor the appropriate instruction[9] and is key to applying the transtheoretical mode. Individuals may skip stages or lapse to previous stages, but an awareness of the individual's current stage allows the teacher, perhaps a dental hygienist, to provide appropriate assistance in meeting the stated goal. An example of this theory could be as simple as an individual contemplating daily flossing and finally taking action to do it.

DENTAL HYGIENIST SPOTLIGHT:
Mary Foley, RDH, MPH

Mary Foley is the project director for the Perinatal and Infant Oral Health Project and Oral Health Consultant for Head Start's Region I. She is the former state dental director in Massachusetts, a position she held for approximately five years. She is a graduate of the Quinsigamond Community College dental hygiene program and has a bachelor of science degree, magna cum laude, from Worcester State College. She earned a master's degree in public health from the University of Massachusetts School of Public Health and Health Policy. Ms. Foley's career epitomizes the variety of opportunities in dental public health. She has used her creative and educational skills to help further dental hygiene, which has ultimately benefited society!

I asked her several questions about her career.

Why did you decide to go into dental hygiene?

I had a good friend whose father was a dentist. One day during our sophomore year, she and I explored potential careers and colleges. In those days, men were doctors and dentists, and women were nurses and dental hygienists.

My dentist's office had no dental hygienist, so the notion of becoming a health professional in this capacity intrigued me. After investigating the courses that dental hygiene students must take, I was sold. I was strong in the sciences, and the will to help and serve others had been instilled in me from youth. The fact that it was a good-paying job—one that a woman could fall back on if something were ever to happen to her husband—made it all the more perfect a choice.

How did you get into dental public health? Did you need additional education?

When I entered the public health workforce after more than twenty years in private practice and clinical dental hygiene instruction, I went back to school to obtain a master's degree in public health (MPH). Actually, a college adviser pulled me aside the day I completed the last course of my bachelor's degree. Just when I thought I had finished, he said to me, "You have to get an MPH." He went on to say that it was a powerful degree. At the time, I didn't know what he meant, but his seriousness and intentions were so genuine that I took his wise advice. I attended the University of Massachusetts School of Public Health and Health Sciences where I earned an MPH degree in epidemiology and biostatistics with a subspecialty in cancer prevention. I loved this program. It took me nearly four years to complete on a part-time basis.

I actually entered the public health workforce as program coordinator upon graduation. I was hired to run a school-based fluoride mouth rinse program and a community water fluoridation program. On my first day of work, I was given a stack of books about eighteen inches high and was told to start reading so that I could become a fluoridation expert—so I did.

Two years later, I was appointed the state dental director, a position I never aspired to or even in my wildest dreams thought I could ever attain. I accepted it and took the position very seriously, assuming a very high level of responsibility for the broad array of constituents. I knew I had to serve the residents of the Commonwealth, my dental hygiene colleagues in Massachusetts and across the country, the dental community of Massachusetts, and a host of other groups. It was quite an opportunity as well as a distinct privilege for me to serve so many. It just goes to show one never knows what life has in store.

What are your current positions?

In late July 2007, I stepped down from my position as the Massachusetts' state dental director to move to Washington, D.C., where I am currently serving as the project director for the new project Improving Perinatal and Infant Oral Health. It focuses on improving perinatal and infant oral health by providing increased access to dental care services for pregnant women and their very young children.

In addition, I am the Oral Health Consultant for Head Start's Region I (New England). In this position, I provide education and technical assistance to the eighty-four Head Start grantees/programs, the Head Start regional office staff, and others interested in improving oral health among our region's most vulnerable children.

Can you discuss any particularly interesting experiences you have had in your dental public health positions?

My dental public health experiences have been incredibly interesting and varied. I will share one that has particularly moved me. I had the wonderful opportunity of meeting Betty at 3 PM on the Friday of the 2001 Memorial Day weekend. I was sitting at my desk when the call came in from a woman who identified herself as "Betty." She told me that she was calling me because she had reached a dead end and had nowhere else to turn. She went on to say that she had a painful toothache and needed immediate care but was unable to access it because of a condition from which she suffers. Her physician had made calls to local dentists, but none was willing to make a home visit.

At age 64, Betty said that she had not left her home in more than thirty years because of the anxiety that she experienced in the outside world. She shared with me the suffering that she had encountered as a result of this condition, including the emotional pain of being unable to attend her father's funeral. Despite years of attempted therapies, hypnosis, and other medical treatments, she continued to be a prisoner in her home. Compelled by her story and the impending urgency of needed treatment, I immediately located a dentist who lived on the other side of the state to travel on the holiday weekend to care for this woman's dental infection. Dr. Doherty, whom I consider a true saint among us, provided Betty's necessary treatment with portable dental equipment.

These qualities observed in a woman who has clearly been shortchanged on many levels have been inspirational to me and has helped me realize the many challenges that people live with. Her existence, which she may think insignificant, really reaches more people than she knows. Her way of life signifies the need for compassion by those of us who are more fortunate. Since my meeting with Betty, we have been able to establish routine home-care dental services for her. Nancy Johnson, a dental hygienist who works for the Tufts University's community outreach program, visits her regularly to provide routine oral assessment and preventive services.

What type of advice would you give to a practicing hygienist who is thinking of doing something different?

Dental hygiene is about promoting oral health for all Americans so that they may fully achieve their overall health and well-being. I have practiced dental hygiene for nearly thirty years. I have been fortunate to grow in the profession and experience a variety of practice roles. Every step of my journey has been critical, and I would not trade one day of it. In all aspects—private practice, education, and in public health—I have faced adversity. But each time, I have grown from it and became a better person. When we are young, adversity and challenge have a way of making us fearful, and we often back away. It is only through these tough times that we come to realize who we are, what our needs are, the needs of others, the potential we have to help others, the gifts we can offer others, and the opportunity to experience a richer and more meaningful existence.

Advancing my education was key. Some believe that advanced education is about getting a better job. I would argue it is really about personal growth. When I was in school, many people asked me what I was planning do with my master's degree in public health. Surprisingly, I had no answer. I'm not one to plan. I just knew that I loved to learn and what I was learning was of particular interest to me. I knew that the right opportunity would present itself and that I needed to be watchful, ready, and willing when it did.

Source: Christine Nathe writes the Public Health Column in RDH magazine published by Pennwell Publishing. For more public health spotlights please see RDH magazine online at http://www.rdhmag.com/index.html.

Theory of Reasoned Action

Reasoned action focuses on the belief that people make rational decisions based on *behavioral intention.* A *behavior intent* is a combination of a person's *attitudes* and is therefore the most immediate and relevant predictor that the person will indeed take the intended action. Few actions that produce a healthy outcome happen without ample knowledge of and the full intention to practice the healthy behavior.[1] Two cognitive processes are at work to develop healthy behaviors: belief about what significant others think is important, *social norms* and personal motivation to comply with the beliefs of those significant people. Other external variables that influence attitudes and, thus, behaviors are internally processed depending upon its importance to an individual.[10] Social norms formed in families, local communities, or larger societal communities and the actions or experiences of celebrities may influence social norms and, thus, behaviors, such as maintaining a healthy, white smile, which may influence others to want a healthy, white smile.[1]

The following excerpt exemplifies the theory of reasoned action.

Example: Behavior/Cessation

Attitude: You know what? I think smoking is dangerous for my health.

Social Norm: I wonder if my wife would like me to quit smoking.

Behavioral Intention: I want to quit smoking right now!

Theory of Reasoned Action Outcome: As you can see, I'm not smoking anymore. Instead of taking a cigarette, when I get the cravings, I crumble paper now.[6]

Social Cognitive Theory

Social cognitive theory (SCT), also known as *self-efficacy theory,* postulates that knowledge, behavior, and environment act in a reciprocal manner to continually affect each other.[11] *Self-efficacy,* the main SCT construct, is the belief that one's personal actions will have an impact on a desired outcome. Individuals with high self-efficacy practice forethought and planning, develop contingency plans, and put effort into overcoming obstacles. Self-efficacy is gained as information, behavior, and environment interact in a reciprocal manner. Lapses are a part of the learning process as the individual uses personal choices to develop behaviors consistent with individual choice and lifestyle.[12–13]

> **Did You Know?**
>
> The tenet of social cognitive theory behavior is conditioned by knowledge, environment, and behavior. It was expanded from the social learning theory, which was a product of Skinner and other behaviorists. Bandura added the focus on personal action, which led to the social cognitive theory.

SCT reinforces the belief that social pressure is the most powerful factor in influencing social norms. It emphasizes the power that social leaders have in influencing values and behaviors. An application of this model is the celebrity "Got Milk?" promotional campaign that shows celebrities with a milk mustache. It suggests that "social pressure" will cause people to emulate the celebrities and drink milk. See Figure 8-5 ■.

Theory of the Sense of Coherence

Antonovsky took a very different tact in health promotion and disease prevention. His central premise is that it is more useful to study health than to study disease,[14] which he termed *salutogenesis,* the beginnings of health. Antonovsky's objection to the study of pathogenesis, which focuses on the origin of disease, is that it tends to classify people into either a healthy or ill state. He contends there is a continuum from "ease," or perfect health with no limitations, to *dis-ease,* or severe

FIGURE 8-5   Social Cognitive Theory

disease or disability resulting in severe limitations of daily life. Most individuals exist somewhere between these two extremes.[14]

Antonovsky's sense of coherence (SOC) theory is a method of seeing the world and one's specific place in it. Individuals who have a strong network of resistance resources will develop an overall SOC that can be used in any situation to deal with various stressors. Individuals with this type of SOC find problems manageable, comprehensible, and meaningful. If they have sufficient resources to handle the situation and the means to use those resources, these individuals can manage stressors, which are comprehensible if they are predictable or make sense and are meaningful if the individuals are willing to expend time and energy to deal with those stressors.[14]

For example, suppose that a thirty-five-year-old female patient presents with multiple carious lesions. She says her family has "soft teeth," so she thinks her decay rate is completely out of her control. Through questioning, the dental hygienist discovers the patient has very good oral hygiene skills but lacks knowledge about nutrition related to oral health. She had the habit of slowly sipping on a sugar-sweetened soft drink throughout the day. The dental hygienist identifies resources available to the patient for improved health, thereby increasing her SOC. By identifying resources, the dental hygienist has helped make oral health manageable. When the patient understands that decay is the result of personal behavior, the oral health becomes comprehensible. Through conversations with the patient, the dental hygienist learned that oral health is very important to the patient who believed that tooth loss was inevitable. She now believes that she can save her teeth; therefore, she now believes that her oral health is meaningful and is willing to expend time and effort needed to ensure good oral health.[1]

Theories of Motivation

Motivation, or the will of the individual to act, is an important factor in learning. It is a drive that propels an individual to satisfy a need.[6] Remember that the individual must be aware of the need before he or she can be motivated.

Motivational models generally identify the considerations that must be present for values to change.[8–18] Dental hygienists initiating a change must be aware of their own values and must recognize and understand those of the patient. It is important to determine what motivates the patient and to understand his or her knowledge of dental care; hygienists must not thrust their own values on patients.

A *need* must exist for changes to be considered. *Attitude* is a powerful influence on human behavior and motivation because it determines the learner's investment in the desired outcome. *Stimulation* is an experience that makes a learner active when affect is a major influence on the learner's emotion, because of the actual experience. *Competence* occurs when an individual masters a skill.[15]

Behavior Modification Theories

Changing behavior requires more than education; behavior modification also is necessary. In fact, at one time or another, most if not all people have considered taking some type of action for change, often to improve health. Some may have started exercising or dieting at the beginning of the year or before an important event, and many may have promised themselves to get more sleep or stop smoking.

Psychologists have theorized that behavior modification is accomplished by classical conditioning, operant conditioning, or modeling. *Classical conditioning* as by Pavlov described in the late 1920s maintains that animals become conditioned to act in a specific way in response to specific stimuli. An example of classical conditioning applied to oral hygiene might be the inclination of a patient who is praised at an appointment for flossing to maintain the practice to receive the same praise at subsequent appointments.[16] *Operant conditioning,* described by Skinner, is based on the concepts of rewarding good behavior and punishing bad behavior. It suggests, for example, that a dental hygienist who gives a pediatric patient treats following good behavior while being treated is reinforcing positive behavior; a parent's discipline of a child exhibiting bad behavior during treatment may prevent that behavior at subsequent appointments.[17] *Modeling* behavior can facilitate learning through imitation. For example, if a child is present when an older sibling receives a treat for exhibiting good behavior, that child may imitate the good behavior.

The behavior modification model suggests that it is necessary to travel through different stages in order to have behavior changed. It is important to note that all of these theories suggest that behaviors can indeed be changed.

These health theories can help dental hygienists understand human motivation to change behaviors and work to improve health. (See Table 8-3 ■.) No single

Table 8-3 Summary of Health Behavior Models

Theory	*Major Elements*
Health belief model	1. Perceived susceptibility 2. Perceived seriousness 3. Beneficial 4. Salience
Transtheoretical model	Behavior changes move through a predictable set of stages including: 1. Precontemplation 2. Contemplation 3. Preparation 4. Action 5. Maintenance 6. Termination
Theory of reasoned action	1. People make rational decisions based on behavioral intent (combination of knowledge, values, and attitudes). 2. Intentions and behavior changes are affected by attitudes and social norms.
Stages of Learning	1. Unawareness 2. Awareness 3. Self-interest 4. Involvement 5. Action 6. Habit
Social cognitive theory (SCT)	1. Extension of social learning theory that emphasizes personal actions 2. Self-efficacy is the belief that personal actions will affect outcomes. 3. Self-efficacy is gained as information, behavior, and environment interact in a reciprocal manner. As self efficacy increases, individuals plan for contingencies, and persevere through difficulties.
Theory of the sense of coherence (SOC)	1. Health lies on a continuum of ease to disease. 2. Stressors move an individual to the disease end of the continuum. 3. Individuals develop a network of general resistance resources that reduce stressors. 4. Individuals with high SOC find stressors manageable (they have the resources to cope), comprehensible (stressors make sense), and meaningful (willing to spend resources to deal with the stressor).

Modified from: Hollister M. Health Education and Promotion Theories. In: Nathe C. *Primary Preventive Dentistry*. 7th ed. Upper Saddle River, NJ: Pearson; 2008. Modified from original.

theory applies to all situations or is effective for all people. Combining pertinent elements of several theories often produces the best results.[1] Researchers have suggested that multidimensional models may prove to be the most effective, particularly for conditions with multiple risk factors, such as early childhood caries.[18]

Before deciding on a course of behavior modification for an individual, the dental hygienist must consider the patient's values and beliefs, readiness to change, perception of control, perception of the effectiveness of personal actions, behavioral and social norms, and available resources. If the dental professional is considering proposing a change of policy for a community, school, or other group of people, the primary considerations may be social norms, community resources, and level of knowledge.[1]

SUMMARY

Dental hygienists should be able to conduct effective presentations to successfully transform knowledge into positive behaviors. The key word here is *successfully*. The ultimate goal of a presentation should be to instill the value of dental health and thus change an individual's behavior.

Dental health educators must remember that education involves much more than simply relaying information. Effective dental health education should develop positive values toward dental health and cause behavior changes. Therefore, it is necessary for dental health educators to fully understand a specific population's knowledge level and to be aware of its values.

SELF-STUDY TEST ITEMS

1. Empowerment models that focus on patient autonomy and collaborative relationships are paternalist regimens. These regimens are led by patients whose knowledge of health and disease increases the likelihood that healthy behaviors are attained.
   a. The first statement is true, the second statement is false.
   b. The first statement is false, the second statement is true.
   c. Both statements are true.
   d. Both statements are false.

2. Which of the following aspects is part of the multidimensional model of health?
   a. Spirituality
   b. Knowledge
   c. Behavior
   d. Values

3. The local dental hygiene association worked on policy change that banned sugary beverages from school vending machines. This is an example of
   a. Healthy behavior
   b. Health action
   c. Health education
   d. Health promotion

4. For behavioral change to occur, an individual must reach what milestone?
   a. Value the change
   b. Understand the healthy behavior
   c. Understand unhealthy behavior
   d. Understand why a behavior was chosen

5. A patient who receives praise for having healthy gums during two routine dental hygiene appointments will be more likely to maintain good home care to ensure that the praise will continue at subsequent appointments. This theory is called
   a. Classical conditioning
   b. Operant conditioning
   c. Modeling
   d. Empowerment

REFERENCES

1. Hollister, M. Health Education and Promotion Theories. In: Harris NO, Garcia-Godoy F, Nathe C. *Primary Preventive Dentistry.* 7th ed. Upper Saddle River, NJ: Pearson; 2008.
2. *Constitution of the World Health Organization—Basic Documents.* 45th ed. (suppl); 2006. Switzerland: World Health Organization.
3. World Health Organization. WHOQOL measuring quality of life. Introducing the WHOQOL instruments [Internet site]. http//www.who.int/msa/mnh/mhp/ql.htm. Accessed September 2000.
4. Meeks-Mitchell L, Heit P. *Health: A Wellness Approach.* Columbus, OH: Merrill Publishing; 1987:6.
5. Maslow AH. *Motivation and Personality.* 3rd ed. New York, NY: Harper & Row; 1987.
6. DeBiase CB. *Dental Health Education Theory and Practice.* Philadelphia, PA: Lea & Febiger; 1991:6.
7. Seaward BL. *Managing Stress Principles and Strategies for Health and Well-Being.* Sudbury, MA: Jones and Bartlett; 1999:83–90, 181–190.
8. Becker MH. *The Health Belief Model and Personal Health Behavior.* Thorofare, NJ: Charles B. Slack; 1974.
9. Prochaska JO, Norcross JC, DiClemente CC. *Changing for good.* New York: Avon Books; 1994.
10. Ajzen I, Fishbein M. *Understanding attitudes and predicting social behavior.* Upper Saddle River, NJ: Pearson; 1980.
11. Bandura A. *Social Foundation of Thought and Action: A Social Cognitive Theory.* Englewood Cliffs, NJ: Prentice Hall; 1986.
12. Bandura A. Social cognitive theory: An angentic perspective. *Annu Rev Psychol.* 2001;52:1–26.
13. Bandura A. *Self efficacy: The exercise of control.* New York: Freeman; 1997.

14. Antonovsky A. *Health Stress and Coping.* San Francisco: Jossey-Bass; 1979.

15. Chopoorian K. How adults learn: The dental hygienist as an educator. *Dental Hygienist News.*1996;9:3–6.

16. Pavlov IP. *Conditional Reflexes.* New York: Dover Publications; 1960. This edition is an unaltered republication of the 1927 translation by Oxford University Press.

17. Skinner BF. *About Behaviorism.* New York: Dover Publications; 1974.

18. Freire MC, Hardy R, Sheiham A. Mothers' sense of coherence and their adolescent children's oral health status and behaviours. *Community Dent Health.* 2002; 19:24–31.

Multimedia Extension Activities

Use this address to access the interactive Companion Website created for this textbook. Simply select "Dental Hygiene" from the choice of disciplines. Find this book and log in using your username and password. To obtain a username and password, please register using the scratch-off access code on the inside front cover of this book.

Chapter 9

Lesson Plan Development

After studying this chapter, the dental hygiene student should be able to:

- Explain the dental hygiene process of care
- Describe the process of lesson plan development
- Identify and describe teaching methods
- Identify the characteristics of an effective teacher
- Develop a lesson plan

KEY TERMS

Dental hygiene process of care
Lesson plan
Teaching methods

COMPETENCIES

After studying this chapter and participating in accompanying course activities, the dental hygiene student should be competent to do the following:

- Promote the profession through service activities and affiliations with professional organizations
- Communicate effectively with individuals and groups from diverse populations both verbally and in writing
- Promote the values of oral and general health and wellness to the public and organizations within and outside the profession
- Provide screening, referral and educational services that allow patients to access the resources of the health care system

DENTAL HYGIENE PROCESS OF CARE

Planning an effective presentation of dental hygiene principles to a target group involves understanding the **dental hygiene process of care.** This process can be described as the assessment, dental hygiene diagnosis, planning, implementation, and evaluation of dental hygiene care of a target population. (See Figure 9-1 ■.) Utilizing the dental hygiene process of care enables the dental hygienist to follow logical steps in developing an effective lesson. Never underestimate the importance of planning the presentation. Although dental hygienists frequently educate individual patients on the importance of oral health care, when presenting to a group, planning is crucial.

The best way to ensure that a presentation will be effective and successful is to be prepared. Preparation and strong organization decrease the initial nervousness some dental hygienists feel when asked to present to a group. Use of the steps in the dental hygiene process of care as outlined in Table 9-1 ■ can ensure an effective lesson plan and aid in making an effective presentation.

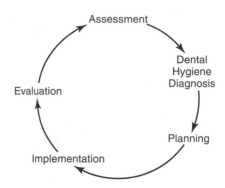

FIGURE 9-1 Dental Hygiene Process of Care

ASSESSMENT

Before the planning phase begins, the dental hygienist must assess the audience population. Assessment entails identifying its needs, interests, and resources. If this stage is skipped, the presentation may not be pertinent to the target audience.

It is important never to assume things about a target population. Consider this example. A long-term care facility asks a dental hygienist to present dental health information to its nurse's aides. Without assessing this population, the dental hygienist decides to discuss periodontal diseases based on the assumption that nurse's aides would find that information valuable because older adults generally have periodontal diseases. However, the most pressing issue in this facility is difficulties with dentures: The residents keep losing them and have trouble keeping them clean. Consequently, the nurse's aides are hoping to learn more about denture identification and care. The nurse's aides—the target population—leave the presentation feeling disappointed that only during the last three minutes, when they were able to ask questions, were their specific needs addressed. To have avoided this situation, the dental hygienist could have talked with the head nurse regarding the group's particular needs, interests, and abilities *before* planning the presentation. Doing so would have better prepared the dental hygienist to answer questions.

Assessment also includes defining the target population's level of dental knowledge. Many groups have similar levels of dental health knowledge, but some do not. Although dental knowledge can be assessed at the beginning of a presentation, researching before the presentation is a better way to plan for the group's knowledge

Table 9-1 Lesson Plan Development Using Dental Hygiene Process of Care

Stage	Action
Assessment	Assess target populations' needs, interests, abilities, and resources Assess dental status
Dental hygiene diagnosis	Formulate findings from assessment Prioritize goals
Planning	Select broad goal formulation Identify specific objectives Select teaching method(s)
Implementation	Prepare for various scenarios Demonstrate effective teacher characteristics
Evaluation	Use qualitative measurement Use quantitative measurement Provide information to appropriate parties

level. Discussing the topics the specific population is interested in with a contact person is one assessment method; providing a brief survey to the group prior to planning the presentation is an excellent one. The presenter can use the survey to question the group about topics that interest them.

Another important assessment goal is to learn what resources are available at the site. The dental hygienist should ask about the availability of a screen or a projector before planning a PowerPoint feature. Not having the expected resources can sabotage the presenter's confidence and effectiveness.

DENTAL HYGIENE DIAGNOSIS

After a thorough assessment of the target population has been conducted, the diagnosis phase can begin. When diagnosing a group, the dental hygienist does not need to

talk with each member but can identify the topic after speaking to one or two contacts about the group's particular needs, interests, and capabilities. Specifically, dental hygiene diagnosis requires analyzing and identifying dental needs that can be fulfilled through dental hygiene education.

An example of a dental hygiene case presentation with corresponding diagnosis follows. Before giving a presentation to a support group for patients with diabetes, the dental hygienist contacted the group leader and staff nurse regarding this group's needs, interests, and capabilities. The dental hygienist learned that many members complained of bleeding and sore gums and wanted to learn more about gum disease associated with diabetes. The dental hygiene diagnosis for this group was periodontal disease associated with diabetes. Basically, the diagnosis is the step that describes the primary need found during the assessment phase.

DENTAL HYGIENIST SPOTLIGHT:
Christine Murphy, RDH, BS

Christine Murphy graduated with a bachelor of science degree in dental hygiene in 1997. She received numerous awards in college and has been inducted as a member of Sigma Phi Alpha, the National Dental Hygiene Honor Society. Since graduation, she has been busy! She has held various positions as an officer in the local dental hygienists' association, worked in private practice, and teaches part-time at the University of New Mexico.

Ms. Murphy is currently the dental director at Pueblo of Isleta Dental Clinic. She started at Isleta as a staff dental hygienist shortly after graduation. Within a year, she had taken the managerial role of dental director. The clinic has grown from having one part-time hygienist and one full-time dentist to one full-time and one part-time hygienist, two full-time dentists, several contract dentists, two dental specialists, and five dental assistants.

Her efforts have allowed the clinic to treat more patients and enhance dental care for the Pueblo. In addition, she wrote the proposal to allow the Pueblo of Isleta to run the program separately from the Indian Health Service, thereby dramatically increasing the budget.

I asked her some questions about her career.

Why did you decide to go into dental hygiene?

I had four small children and my husband's back went out. He suggested I go back to school to become a dental hygienist because he knew I could not support our family as a dental assistant. It was a difficult decision because I had been out of high school for fifteen years at that time. I wasn't a great student in high school, but age does wonders. I graduated from dental hygiene school with a 3.98 GPA summa cum laude and have realized that I love dental hygiene!

How did you get into dental public health? Did you need additional education?

I didn't need additional education because I graduated from University of New Mexico with a bachelor's degree in dental hygiene. I got into public health slowly but surely.

When I graduated from UNM, I wasn't sure exactly what I wanted to do. I worked in private practice one day a week, taught at UNM two days a week, and worked for a temp service one day a week. I answered an advertisement for a full-time hygiene position at the Isleta Dental Clinic but informed the dentist that I was available only part-time because of my teaching commitment. I started out at the clinic two days a week. Within six months, I had quit temping and private practice and was working three days a week with the tribe. Eventually, the tribe offered me the position of dental director, and I currently work four days per week.

What is your current position?

I am the dental director for the Pueblo of Isleta, and I see patients in the clinic two days per week. Additionally, I serve as an adjunct faculty member for the University of New Mexico dental hygiene students who rotate through my clinic.

Can you discuss any particularly interesting experiences you have had in your dental public health career?

Not long after starting here, I began trying to learn some of the Pueblo language. It is beautiful but not written, so each person must learn from another. I quickly learned that you should be very careful whom you ask to teach you the language. I asked one patient how to say a particular phrase, but when I repeated it, the meaning was definitely not what I intended. It could have been quite embarrassing, but the person I repeated the phrase to was very understanding.

What advice would you give to a practicing hygienist who is thinking of doing something different?

Try anything and everything. In school I never even considered public health as an option. I had been a dental assistant in private practice for years, so I just assumed that's where I would practice dental hygiene. When I got into public health, I realized how much I loved being able to practice hygiene to the best of my ability without any other factors involved. I don't have to worry about whether or not the patient can afford scaling and root planing or anyone making me sell dentistry.

Working in public health has been such a great experience. I have met the most fantastic people—not just the patients I see but also the providers whom I work with...and not just in my clinic but across the nation.

Source: Christine Nathe writes the Public Health Column in RDH magazine published by Pennwell Publishing. For more public health spotlights please see RDH magazine online at http://www.rdhmag.com/index.html.

PLANNING

After assessing and developing a dental hygiene diagnosis for a group, the dental hygienist begins the planning phase by determining a goal for the presentation and identifying several objectives. This activity helps the hygienist plan the specific information to present to the group and how to present it effectively. Carefully preparing the lesson organizes the teacher's thinking process and builds confidence in presenting the material. The process includes gathering and organizing the information and developing the presentation of this information. Effective planning should include rehearsing the presentation that has been developed and timing it to make sure

it fits within the given time limitations. In addition, consider and prepare for the questions the audience is likely to ask; having the opportunity to ask questions will increase audience participation.

First, it is necessary to prioritize the groups' particular needs. Consider, for example, the situation in which a parent teacher association (PTA) has asked the dental hygienist to come to its meeting to discuss dental care for fifteen minutes. After questioning contacts, the dental hygienist learns that the PTA group's primary interests in this presentation were access to dental care for families with Medicaid insurance, motivating their children to brush, and helping parents find quick and easy nutritional food choices. In addition, some parents were interested in learning more about periodontal surgery, implants, and bleaching. The dental hygienist realized that comprehensive dental health education on all of these topics could not be delivered in only fifteen minutes and therefore prioritized the most beneficial and important topics for inclusion in the presentation. The next step is to prepare a **lesson plan,** which is a written document used in planning a presentation.

Lesson Plan Preparation

Goals

The first step in writing a lesson plan is to identify the presentation's goal, which is a broad statement of the final outcome that the instructor expects from the target group upon completing the presentation.[1–5] It is important to write only one or two broad goals to expect the group to accomplish. After setting the overall goal, the instructor identifies the specific outcomes that are intended to result.

Objectives

An objective includes a specific, observable action or behavior that a learner will perform or exhibit.[6] Many times objectives include a target group, a condition, and measurement. The *audience* is the target group. The *condition* entails relevant factors affecting the actual performance, such as time or environment, and the *measurement* is the way to evaluate the level of achievement the audience is to attain or the acceptable performance. For example, consider the objective "following the presentation, the physician's assistants will be able to describe the dental caries process according to the presented information." The audience is physician's assistants; the condition is that following the presentation, they can describe the dental caries process. The measurement could be how many audience members can describe it according to the presented information.

Did You Know?

Writing objectives allows the dental hygienist to plan in detail the information that will be presented and discussed.

When writing an objective, it is important to be aware of three learning domains.[7] (See Table 9-2 ■.) The *psychomotor domain* describes actions. The behaviors in

Table 9-2 Domains of Learning

Domain of Learning	Example
Psychomotor	To describe actions
Cognitive	To describe behavior
Affective	To describe feelings
Levels of Learning	
Knowledge	To know
Application	To apply
Problem solving	To problem solve

this domain are the easiest to identify with precise verbs. An example of an objective written for the psychomotor domain would be "Following the dental health presentation, the nurse's aides will clean dentures effectively." This behavior is concrete and observable, and the verbs that refer to them denote a neurophysical activity. See Box 9-1 ■ for a list of verbs commonly used in the psychomotor domain.

The *cognitive domain* represents intellectual skills. The verbs used to describe behavior in this domain (presented in Box 9-2 ■) are slightly more abstract than those in the psychomotor domain. An example of an objective in this domain is "Following the presentation, the first grade students will identify three healthy snacks from the chart."

Finally, the domain that includes feelings, attitudes, values, and interests is referred to as the *affective domain*. See Box 9-3 ■ for verbs used in this domain. Although it can be measured by qualitative assessment, the affective

BOX 9-1 Verbs Used in the Psychomotor Domain

- Brush
- Clean
- Detect
- Disinfect
- Demonstrate
- Eat
- Exercise
- Experiment
- Floss
- Identify
- Irrigate
- Measure
- Probe
- Screen
- Sterilize

BOX 9-2 Verbs Used in the Cognitive Domain	
• Collect	• Indicate
• Contrast	• Label
• Classify	• List
• Compare	• Show
• Describe	• Recognize
• Diagnose	• Record
• Design	• Solve
• Explain	

BOX 9-3 Verbs Used in the Affective Domain	
• Advocate	• Evaluate
• Assess	• Judge
• Believe	• Lead
• Challenge	• Live out
• Debate	• Persuade
• Defend	• Suggest
• Discuss	• Value
• Deduct	

domain is not directly observable and not as easily measured as the behaviors in the other two domains. For those in the dental hygiene profession, however, the affective domain is extremely important. An objective for this domain is "Following completion of the current issues course, the dental hygienist will be able to defend, in writing, the dental hygienist's role in consumer advocacy with a passing grade."

See Box 9-4 ■ for a list of verbs whose meanings are open to interpretation and should be avoided when writing objectives.

BOX 9-4 Verbs Whose Meaning as Objectives Can Be Unclear	
• Appreciate	• Interpret
• Comprehend	• Know
• Empathize	• Like
• Familiarize	• Realize
• Grasp	• Think
• Have Faith	• Understand

The levels of learning should also be considered when identifying objectives. The three levels are *knowledge, application,* and *problem solving.* (Refer to Table 9-2.) The knowledge level is the lowest and simply requires that knowledge be gained. The application level requires applying the new knowledge. Being able to solve a problem implies that the learner has mastered the problem-solving level.

Understanding the domains and levels of learning will enable the dental hygienist to adequately define and plan the lesson.

Teaching Methods

Another important aspect of planning is deciding which teaching strategies or methods to use. A **teaching strategy** is the approach or method used in instruction. The instructor must decide which method(s) to use to obtain the desired outcome. Furthermore, the method(s) should be appropriate for the activities involved and resources available. Most important, the method should be interesting and motivate the audience.

Lecture is probably the most well known and traditional method of teaching. It is effective if a formal presentation of information is needed and the information is appropriate for the audience's knowledge level. Lecturing is also effective when the intention is to create awareness of various ideas, issues, and beliefs. The lecture method is best used in conjunction with other methods.

Did You Know?

The drawback to using the lecture method is that it does not involve the audience, which decreases motivation and learning.

The *discussion* method involves interaction between the students and the instructor and more easily arouses interest, which helps students to develop reasoning abilities. *Presentation* is defined as employing the lecture and discussion methods together. *Demonstration* can be used with lecture, discussion, or presentation methods when the desired outcome is learning a behavior, such as the proper way to brush.

The *inquiry* method, sometimes referred to as *problem-based* learning, uses case studies in which the teacher acts as a facilitator and the student is responsible for gaining the correct information.[4] Group or individualized games and activities usually increase motivation and learning. Examples are CD-ROM– or Internet-based interactive activities or puzzles including playing a version of dental health Jeopardy as a group. Role-play and simulation activities can also be utilized as a group.

Did You Know?

Interactive methods can increase student comprehension and problem-solving skills when presenting information by affording everyone an opportunity to participate.

Visual Aids

The use of visual aids can add a great deal to a presentation by engaging the learners and contributing an organizing aspect to the lesson. They include PowerPoint slides, DVDs, and flip charts. If used improperly, however, visual aids can be a distraction. For instance, instructors often pass a tooth model around the class during a presentation, but this can be disruptive to the learning process because the students must listen to the instructor and inspect the tooth. By planning the presentation well, effective integration of a tooth model can be useful. See Table 9-3 ■ for more information on using visual aids effectively.

Table 9-3 Using Visual Aids

There are effective and ineffective ways to use visual aids in presentations. Ineffective use is very common in both academia and industry. Good visuals used in the right way can help your audience stay attentive and retain information. The tips below will help you decide when and how to effectively use overhead projectors and slides, blackboards, handouts, and computer programs like PowerPoint. You may also wish to see the Teachings Tips sheet called "Designing Visual Aids."

1) *Use visuals when they will help your audience*

To make visuals effective, use them to:

- focus the audience's attention
- reinforce the key components of your verbal message
- stimulate and maintain interest
- illustrate complex concepts that are difficult to visualize
- aid the audience's comprehension
- increase retention

Avoid using them to:

- impress your audience with overly-detailed text, charts, or animations—avoid information overload
- limit interaction with your audience
- present simple ideas that are easily stated verbally
- serve as your cue cards

2) Select appropriate visual aids and equipment

Elaborate does not necessarily mean effective. It can be tempting to spend more time preparing visual aids than presentation content. The result may be insubstantial and distracting—and the higher the technology, the more things can go wrong. The following tips will help you choose appropriate visual aids and equipment:

- consider giving your audience context via a handout before the presentation
- have a "plan B" visual aid: bulbs burn out, screens fall down, and computers crash
- weigh the pros and cons before using computer programs like PowerPoint:

PowerPoint pros:

- potentially inexpensive
- attractive designs
- smooth transitions between slides
- possible to add/subtract material (parts of charts, graphs) from slides

PowerPoint cons:

- complicated equipment required
- hassle to set up
- special effects often distracting
- time-consuming to prepare except for experienced users

(continued)

3) *Interact with your audience and make sure YOU remain their focus*

Presenters may be tempted to hide behind (or lose themselves in) their visual aids. It is important to maintain contact with your audience and remember that you, not your visual aids, are giving the presentation. At best, visual aids are an accessory—you should remain the center of attention. The following tips will help:

- remember to ask questions, stimulate discussions, and use other interactive methods as appropriate
- maintain eye contact with your audience
- watch out for facial cues of boredom, confusion, falling behind, etc.
- remember that visual aids are aids *for your audience;* lecture notes are aids for you
- assume that your audience will copy everything from your visual aids: keep information on visual aids minimal, and keep it visible for long enough
- if possible, position overhead projectors and screens diagonally to the front of the class; thus, you can occupy the room's focal point instead of having to stand aside.

4) *Prepare and be organized*

Preparation and organization can make the difference between a successful and a frustrating presentation. The following tips can help:

- computers may be ruined in areas of excessive chalk dust
- before the presentation, check lines of sight to your visual aids from all parts of the seating area: use only those areas that will be visible to all audience members
- before the presentation, experiment with arrangements of furniture and visual aids
- place overhead slides in a pile in order, right side up before the presentation
- test overhead projectors and screens in advance to focus and find the right distance for the projector to fill the screen
- turn off overhead projectors when you've finished with a slide if you don't intend to present another one shortly—the fan and glaring white screen are distracting
- you're better off without any visual aid about which you think you will say, "You don't need to worry about this material," "Ignore this," "This probably doesn't make sense to you," or, "You probably can't see this at the back."

Source: http://cte.uwaterloo.ca/teaching_resources/teaching_tips/tips_activities/using_visual_aids.pdf. Accessed June 9, 2009.

Refer to Box 9-5 ■ for an example of a lesson plan prepared to teach eighth grade students about dental hygiene careers during a career month at school when they were preparing to register for high school classes. More than fifty different individuals presented information about possible careers during the month.

IMPLEMENTATION

The most important aspect of implementation is preparation. By completing the first three phases—assessment, dental hygiene diagnosis, and planning—the dental hygienist should be well organized and feel confident about the presentation.

Classroom Management

An instructor who feels prepared and confident can effectively manage many different situations that may occur when making a presentation. Surprisingly, managing a classroom of adults can be as challenging as managing children. Signals such as frequent talking, shuffling, or sleeping indicate that the presentation is not being well received. Staying calm and conveying your enthusiasm, knowledge, and expectations can stop these signals. Moreover, being well organized will increase instructor confidence and decrease the likelihood of losing control of the class.

Characteristics of an Effective Teacher

Effective teaching involves motivating the students to learn the information presented and apply it. To accomplish this, communication skills are vital for an educator. Teachers needs to be able to effectively communicate to groups of students and students on an individual basis. Being available before and after a course is

BOX 9-5 Sample Lesson Plan

Dental Hygiene Presentation

Audience
24 eighth grade students

Time
15 minutes

Goal
To promote the career of dental hygienist

Objectives
Following this presentation, the students will be able to:

1. Describe the functions of a dental hygienist
2. Describe the settings in which dental hygienists work
3. Identify careers available in the dental field

Teaching Methods
Lecture
Discussion
Role-playing

Audiovisual Aids
Dental Hygiene Career DVD (5 minutes)
PowerPoint slide series
Dental hygiene career pamphlets

Introduction
Today we will be discussing the career of dental hygienists, their functions in dental care delivery, and other careers available in the dental field.

Rationale
It is important for you as eighth graders to be aware of career opportunities available so that next year when you begin taking classes in high school, you can identify courses that will help prepare you for college course work pertaining to the career that interests you.

Dental Hygienists Defined
A dental hygienist is a health care provider who practices the art and science of preventive oral health. (Give examples.)

Educational Preparation
The University of New Mexico in Albuquerque offers a dental hygiene program. All neighboring states offer dental hygiene programs in university and community college settings. Dental hygienists can receive associate's, bachelor's, and master's degrees in dental hygiene.

When preparing for a dental hygiene career in high school, remember that dental hygienists must have a strong background in basic health and social sciences. Recommended subjects include biology, chemistry, physics, anatomy, physiology, algebra, geometry, calculus, English, and social science courses.

Roles of the Dental Hygienists
The six roles of dental hygienists are manager, clinician, educator/health promoter, researcher, consumer advocate, and change agent. (Provide examples.)

Practice Settings
Dental hygienists work in private dental offices; public schools; nursing homes and hospitals; military, state, and federal public health programs; the dental industry; and business and research facilities. They provide oral health services through preventive, educational, diagnostic, and therapeutic sciences.

View DVD and answer questions concerning the material it presents.

Careers Available in the Dental Field
Additional roles in the dental field include dentist, dental assistant, dental technician, consultant, and dental office manager/receptionist. (Provide examples of these careers.)

Conclusion
Today we discussed the dental hygiene career, education needed to become a dental hygienist, and other careers available in the dental field.

BOX 9-6 Characteristics of Effective Teachers

- Ability to interact with students, their families, and colleagues
- Enthusiasm
- Flexibility
- Broad knowledge
- Organization skills
- Patience
- Pleasant personality
- Willingness to learn

important for those students who have questions or ideas. See Box 9-6 ■ for a list of some characteristics of effective teachers.

Did You Know?

Being prepared is definitely the best way to increase the likelihood that a presentation will be effective.

Effective teachers are prepared and organized. By carefully preparing a lesson, the teacher will have an organized thinking process and should be confident in presenting the material. Other important attributes of a teacher are flexibility and fairness. Being flexible with student learning is key to motivating students to learn. Fairness is important in all aspects of life, which of course, includes learning and teaching by example.

Fear of Public Speaking

Many people, including dental hygienists, may initially be nervous when speaking to an audience. The best way to prevent this nervousness is to practice. A presenter should practice in front of an audience, even if it is only one other person, until feeling completely confident. Fear of public speaking should be improved by repeated presentations. Public speaking can actually become close to a habit if done consistently. In other words, the more a dental hygienists presents to groups, the easier it should become.

EVALUATION

Evaluation is an ongoing process and should be considered in the planning phase when objectives and goals are developed. Writing effective, measurable objectives ensures that the dental hygienist can accurately evaluate the presentation's effectiveness. Its smoothness and audience interest and participation can also help to evaluate it. Teachers should be well aware of the motivation level of a class. Remember that the more interested the students are and the more they participate, the more likely it is that the objectives will be met. Students who are motivated are more likely to adapt these effective dental health behaviors promoted during the presentation.

Refer to Box 9-7 ■ for a pretest/posttest evaluation for seventh grade students. In this example, a dental hygienist is presenting a lesson plan on the prevention of oral cancer and is planning to evaluate the

BOX 9-7 Self-Evaluation Example

Oral Cancer Prevention Strategies Pretest

1. Smokeless tobacco products do less harm to oral tissues than cigarettes.
   True
   False
2. Alcohol use increases the risk of oral cancer.
   True
   False
3. Regular dental hygiene examinations include oral cancer examinations.
   True
   False

Oral Cancer Prevention Strategies Posttest

1. Smokeless tobacco products do less harm to oral tissues than cigarettes.
   True
   False
2. Alcohol use increases the risk of oral cancer.
   True
   False
3. Regular dental hygiene examinations include oral cancer examinations.
   True
   False

BOX 9-8 Lesson Plan Evaluation Checklist

- Displays organization
- Demonstrates evidence of research of topic
- Presents effective introduction
- Presents lessons on level of target population's understanding
- Presents expected behavioral objectives
- Asks appropriate questions
- Material is covered in appropriate length of time
- Develops and utilizes appropriate visual aids
- Presents effective conclusion
- Implements self-evaluation strategies

BOX 9-9 Presenter Evaluation Checklist

- Shows evidence of research of topic
- Includes instruction on level of target population's understanding
- Indicates appropriate teaching methods
- Includes the use of effective visual aids
- Timed to meet requirements
- List appropriate probing questions to ask
- Presents professional appearance
- Maintains proper eye contact
- Projects voice meaningfully
- Demonstrates a prepared, organized manner

---

lesson with the pretest/posttest evaluation. The same questions are asked before the presentation and afterward to assess the degree of learning. Other methods of evaluation can include games, activities, computer games and quizzes, or simply group questioning of the information presented.

Evaluating the dental hygienist's effectiveness as an information conveyor is imperative. See Boxes 9-8 ■ and 9-9 ■ for evaluation criteria for lesson plans and presentations. By following the phases of creating effective presentations, the dental hygienist increases the likelihood of meeting those criteria.

SUMMARY

The dental hygiene process of care involves assessment, dental hygiene diagnosis, planning, implementation, and evaluation of dental hygiene care of a target population. The dental hygienist should thoroughly assess the target population's needs to develop an appropriate lesson and determine an appropriate dental hygiene diagnosis. Thorough planning, including developing goals and objectives with an emphasis on identifying measurable outcomes, should follow. Being prepared is the most important step in providing effective dental health education to groups.

SELF-STUDY TEST ITEMS

1. The best way to ensure an effective presentation is to:
   a. Decrease the number of participants
   b. Utilize audiovisual aids
   c. Have at least ten objectives for each presentation
   d. Be prepared

2. "Following the presentation, the audience will be able to compare ten healthy and unhealthy snack choices" is an example of a(n)
   a. Goal
   b. Lesson plan
   c. Objective
   d. Healthy behavior

3. Lecturing is always an effective way to teach dental health education. Lecture always includes the inclusion of the problem-based method of learning.
   a. The first statement is true; the second is false.
   b. The first statement is false; the second is true.
   c. Both statements are true.
   d. Both statements are false.

4. Which verb pertains to the psychomotor domain?
   a. Demonstrating
   b. Comparing
   c. Advocating
   d. Defending

5. When used in an objective, the verb *understand*
   a. Is easily measured
   b. Is open to misinterpretation
   c. Always requires skill
   d. All of the above

REFERENCES

1. Fodor JT, Dalis GT. *Health Instruction: Theory and Application.* 4th ed. Philadelphia, PA: Lea and Febiger; 1989.

2. DeBiase CB. *Dental Health Education: Theory and Practice.* Philadelphia, PA: Lea and Febiger; 1995.

3. Dignan MB, Carr, PA. *Program Planning for Health Education and Health Promotion.* Philadelphia, PA: Lea and Febiger; 1987.

4. Smith TC. *Making Successful Presentations: A Self-Teaching Guide.* New York: Wiley; 1984.

5. The Difference Between Goals and Objectives. South Dakota State University. http://edweb.sdsu.edu/courses/edtec540/objectives/Difference.html. Accessed September 8, 2008.

6. Gagliardi L. *Dental Health Education: Lesson Plan and Implementation.* 2nd ed. Upper Saddle River, NJ: Pearson; 2006.

7. Tolle L. Dental Hygiene 400/500 Oral Health Promotion Course-Pak. Copytron: Anaheim, California; 1988.

PEARSON
myhealthprofessionskit™

Multimedia Extension Activities

Use this address to access the interactive Companion Website created for this textbook. Simply select "Dental Hygiene" from the choice of disciplines. Find this book and log in using your username and password. To obtain a username and password, please register using the scratch-off access code on the inside front cover of this book.

Chapter **10**

Target Populations

OBJECTIVES

After studying this chapter, the dental hygiene student should be able to:

- Define target populations to whom dental hygienists may provide services.
- Describe faith-based initiatives
- Define target profiles
- Identify barriers to dental hygiene care

KEY TERMS

Barriers to care
Faith-based initiatives
Target populations
Target population profile

COMPETENCIES

After studying this chapter and participating in accompanying course activities, the dental hygiene student should be competent to do the following:

- Promote the profession through service activities and affiliations with professional organizations
- Promote the values of oral and general health and wellness to the public and organizations within and outside the profession
- Respect the goals, values, beliefs, and preferences of the patient/client while promoting optimal oral and general health
- Provide screening, referral, and education to bring consumers into the health care delivery system

The term **target population** refers to a clearly identified segment of the population. A target population can be broad or narrow; for example, it can represent all three-year-old children, a group of youths involved in a local church group, or elderly people in an assisted living community. Age can be a factor of a target population, but it usually has other common characteristics as well. For instance, the three-year-old children mentioned may be further identified by other shared characteristics, such as attending the same Head Start program, living in the same geographic area, or coming from families with similar incomes.

TARGET POPULATIONS

Dental hygienists provide service and education to many different groups and frequently are asked to present dental health information to these groups, which can be referred to as *target populations*. Dental hygienists should consider what type of information is appropriate to present to the target population.

> **Did You Know?**
>
> In the community setting, dental hygienists frequently treat a population rather than an individual patient, but the concept of dental hygiene treatment does not change.

Dental Hygienists' Colleagues

In their professional capacities, dental hygienists serve a number of different populations. They work with individuals as colleagues in advisory capacities, providing advice and acting as resources.

Family Caregivers

Family caregivers provide daily care to their family members. These caregivers may be parents, grandparents, children, other relatives, or close friends. The care may be as comprehensive as dispensing medicine, both orally and intravenously to a family member, helping the member with hygiene and sanitary functions, cooking, and feeding. These individuals usually assume some responsibility specifically pertaining to oral hygiene care. Many hospitals and health care organizations provide this group with health education and caregiving classes, which

should include oral hygiene care. For instance, dental hygienists could present information to this population on how to care for the oral cavity during cancer treatments.

Health Care Workers

This target group provides direct patient care and/or treatment. It includes nurses, physicians, physician assistants, physical and occupational therapists, speech pathologists, and nurses aides. This group has considerable knowledge about the diseases of the population they treat but may need additional information on the impact that the disease or condition has in relation to oral health. Dental hygienists should be knowledgeable about diseases and ask health care workers about their experiences treating and caring for individuals suffering from the diseases. Integrating an oral health component into health care is an excellent way to promote oral health.[1,2]

Hospice Workers

This group includes a variety of professionals who work together to make terminal illness more tolerable and comfortable for the patients and their families. Dental hygienists can alleviate oral pain by educating hospice workers, providing dental hygiene treatment, and referring them to a dentist if needed. Dental hygienists may coordinate dental care for the hospice program.

Teachers

Teachers can influence students a great deal and are particularly important to dental hygienists. Theorists suggest that teachers' discussion of dental health is more influential for students than is information provided by a dental hygienist once a year during dental health month. For this reason, teachers must have proper dental knowledge and be motivated to instill positive dental health behaviors in their students. Teachers should be able to recognize noticeable dental disease and know a dental hygienist within the community to contact. Dental hygienists can be effective in changing dental behavior by educating and collaborating with teachers.

Social Workers

A *social worker* is a professional who helps individuals, groups, and communities to enhance or restore their capacity for social functioning and to create societal conditions favorable to reaching the goals they set.[3] Social workers influence the populations they serve, and dental hygienists can work with them to provide access to dental care and education for many people in need. Dental hygienists should instruct social workers in proper oral hygiene and serve as a liaison between the social worker and patient.

┌─ **Did You Know?** ─────────────────┐

Social workers are great resources for dental hygienists. They have invaluable information about local and state social services that are available to the people they serve.

└──────────────────────────────────┘

Dental Hygienists' and Their Target Populations

The relationship of oral health to overall health is most important to remember in working with this population. A patient afflicted with a medically compromising condition such as cardiovascular disease, respiratory disease, metabolic and endocrine disease, immune-compromising diseases including HIV infection, liver and kidney disorder, arthritis, physical disabilities, joint prostheses, or cancer, may also present with many symptoms, conditions, and diseases in the oral cavity.[4] Table 10-1 ■ provides

Table 10-1 Medical Conditions and Their Descriptions, Oral Manifestations, and Preventive Strategies

Condition	Description	Oral Manifestations	Preventive Strategies
Alcohol abuse	Excessive consumption of ethanol	Oral cancer Poor oral hygiene Xerostomia Petechiae Ecchymoses Increased bleeding Candidiasis Tooth erosion	Individualized oral hygiene instruction Saliva stimulants and substitutes Self-care fluoride treatments Antifungal agent Diphenhydramine rinse
Arthritis	Group of diseases that damage joints	Poor oral hygiene Temporomandibular joint disorder (TMJ) issues	Individualized oral hygiene instruction Short appointment times Oral appliance Alternative positioning during appointments
Asthma	Abnormal function of the lungs	Candidiasis Increased caries Increase gingivitis	Antifungal agent Diphenhydramine rinse
Bulimia	Binge eating followed by purging	Tooth erosion Increased caries and periodontitis Tooth sensitivity	Individualized oral hygiene instruction Self-care fluoride treatments
Cancer	Out-of-control growth of abnormal cells	Mucositis Candidiasis Xerostomia Loss of taste Trismus Cervical caries Sensitive teeth Excessive, spontaneous bleeding Poor healing Increased susceptibility to infection	Antifungal agent Individualized oral hygiene instruction Saliva stimulants and substitutes Self-care fluoride treatments Antimicrobial rinse Mouth exercises Tongue depressors to open mouth
Cardiac arrhythmias	Abnormal heart beat or rate	Xerostomia Ulceration Petechiae	Diphenhydramine rinse Saliva stimulants and substitutes Self-care fluoride treatments

(continued)

Table 10-1 Medical Conditions and Their Descriptions, Oral Manifestations, and Preventive Strategies

Condition	Description	Oral Manifestations	Preventive Strategies
Cocaine use	Use of addictive stimulant drug	Ulceration of mucosa Palatal perforation Necrosis of gingiva Bruxism Cervical tooth abrasion Tooth erosion	Individualized oral hygiene instruction Mouth guard Diphenhydramine rinse
Congestive heart failure	Inability of heart to pump enough blood to the body's other organs	Infection Bleeding Petechiae Ecchymoses Xerostomia	Saliva stimulants and substitutes Self-care fluoride treatments
Depression	Illness of mind, body, and thoughts	Poor oral hygiene Xerostomia Damage to tissues due to overcleaning	Saliva stimulants and substitutes Self-care fluoride treatments
Diabetes	Metabolic disorder resulting in abnormal blood glucose levels	Impaired healing Increased susceptibility to infections Candidiasis Accelerated periodontal disease Xerostomia Ulcerations Numbness/burning/pain of oral tissues	Antifungal agent Diphenhydramine rinse Baking soda and water rinse Saliva stimulants and substitutes Self-care fluoride treatments
Epilepsy	Neurologic disorder causing seizures	Gingival hyperplasia Fractured teeth Injury to lips and tongue	Individualized oral hygiene instruction Surgical reduction of gingiva
Hemophilia	Bleeding disorder	Spontaneous bleeding Prolonged bleeding Hematomas	Individualized oral hygiene instruction
HIV/AIDS	Immune system failure	Candidiasis Kaposi sarcoma Hairy leukoplakia Linear gingival erythema NUG/NUP	Antifungal agent Individualized oral hygiene instruction Antibiotics Corticosteroid therapy
Hypertension	Elevated blood pressure	Xerostomia Ulceration Lichenoid reactions Decreased healing Increased bleeding Gingival hyperplasia	Diphenhydramine rinse Saliva stimulants and substitutes Self-care fluoride treatments
Hyperthyroidism	Excessive release of thyroid hormone	Progressive periodontal disease Extensive caries Tumors on tongue Osteoporosis of alveolar ridge Premature loss of teeth Early eruption patterns Burning sensation	Baking soda and water rinse Individualized oral hygiene instruction

(continued)

Table 10-1 Medical Conditions and Their Descriptions, Oral Manifestations, and Preventive Strategies

Condition	Description	Oral Manifestations	Preventive Strategies
Hypothyroidism	Thyroid failure	Increased tongue size Delayed eruption of teeth Delayed wound healing	Individualized oral hygiene instruction
Liver disease	Inflamed liver	Bleeding, lichenoid eruptions	Individualized oral hygiene instruction
Marijuana use	Smoking plant *Cannabis sativa*	Xerostomia Oral cancer Poor oral hygiene Candidiasis Increased gingivitis and periodontitis	Individualized oral hygiene instruction Antifungal agent Saliva stimulants and substitutes
Methamphetamine use	Addictive stimulant drug use may cause rapid weight loss, carelessness, mental impairment and rapid tooth decay	Poor oral hygiene Xerostomia Rampant decay	Individualized oral hygiene instruction Saliva stimulants and substitutes Self-care fluoride treatments
Organ transplants	Solid organ/tissue or hematopoietic cell transplantation	Candidiasis Herpes (simplex and zoster) Hairy leukoplakia Kaposi sarcoma Aphthous stomatitis Spontaneous bleeding Increased infection Ulceration Petechiae Ecchymoses Gingival hyperplasia Salivary gland dysfunction Xerostomia	Individualized oral hygiene instruction Antifungal agent Saliva stimulants and substitutes
Renal disease	Complete or near failure of the kidneys	Mucosal pallor Xerostomia Metallic taste Ammonia breath Stomatitis Loss of lamina dura Bone radiolucencies Increased bleeding Ulcerations Candidiasis	Antifungal agent Diphenhydramine rinse Saliva stimulants and substitutes Self-care fluoride treatments Individualized oral hygiene instruction
Tobacco use	Use of plants in the genus *Nicotiana* compromises the immune system	Oral cancer Leukoplakia Xerostomia Alveolar bone damage Gingival damage Hairy tongue Nicotine stomatitis Increased caries	Saliva stimulants and substitutes Self-care fluoride treatments

Source: Sanchez Dils EM. In: Harris NO, Garcia-Godoy F, Nathe C. *Primary Preventive Dentistry*. 7th ed. Upper Saddle River, NJ: Pearson; 2008.

specific information about oral health and systemic diseases and conditions.

Persons with Medical Conditions/Diseases

Dental education for patients with a systemic disease can be complicated but help to alleviate many infections and also may improve overall health. When making presentations to groups with systemic diseases or their caregivers, dental hygienists should have information available on oral manifestations of the disease, specific drugs that are commonly prescribed and their effects on dental health as well as premedication coverage information.

People Who Are Developmentally Disabled

Developmental disability is either present at birth, occurs during the developmental period, or is not present at birth but appears years later. The major disorders in this category are mental retardation, cerebral palsy, epilepsy, and autism.[5,6] Education directed to this group may consist of interventions aimed at reducing high rates of periodontal disease and caries as well as the care of teeth that may be rotated and/or crowded. Specific drug interactions and appointment scheduling issues common to this group should be assessed.

People Who Are Hearing Impaired

Hearing impairment is hearing that is functional but not effective, and hearing aids may be utilized to improve it. *Deafness* refers to an inability to understand speech even with the use of a hearing device. Please see the Web site that accompanies this text for figures that illustrate sign language to use when educating this population. The use of visual aids and hands-on learning in which the entire group participates are helpful when addressing it.

People Who Have Visual Impairments

Limitations in sight range from a slight impairment to complete blindness with no perception of light.[6] Education for individuals who are blind should focus on descriptions. When speaking to this group, dental hygienists can utilize audio (tapes) and manual aids, allowing individuals to feel the teeth, brush, and floss while discussing proper oral hygiene care. Few resources are available for blind individuals regarding dental health. Therefore, it may be helpful to work with an individual who is blind when creating teaching aids for a presentation.

Individuals Who Live in Poverty

In the United States, poverty affects more than 10% of the population, and children are consistently considered to be the age group it most afflicts.[7] In fact, the United States spends about 12% of its gross national product on public assistance and social insurance programs such as Social Security, Medicare, Aid to Families with Dependent Children (AFDC), food stamps, and Medicaid.[8] Some researchers believe that the growth of an urban underclass locked in a cycle of welfare dependency, joblessness, crime, and out-of-wedlock birth has contributed to the persistence of poverty.[9] However, some researchers propose that the culture of poverty, which can be explained as individuals living in poverty and assuming their own culture, has not developed in the United States.[9] An important role for dental hygienists is to help these individuals gain access to their care and find dental providers who accept Medicaid insurance as payment. Dental hygienists may need to work with a social worker or case manager to locate funding for dental care if the individual or group is not enrolled or eligible for Medicaid insurance. Barriers to care for this population may include transportation and language issues. As with all groups, these people need to become aware of dental diseases and dental disease prevention.

Inmates

This target population lives in a state or federal prison. In the United States, inmates have a right to health care, thus creating the need for dental hygiene services. Basically, dental hygienists working in a correctional institution can help decrease dental diseases and restorative and emergency dental conditions and subsequently decrease dental care costs within this group. Many inmates previously have had minimal if any prior dental hygiene treatment, so dental hygienists working with them need to focus on the etiology of dental disease and oral health behaviors designed to prevent or control disease. During the time they spend in prison, many inmates live a healthier lifestyle than they had previously and do not practice from substance abuse and unhealthy behaviors. This is the ideal time to emphasize the value of optimum oral health on general health.

Specific Age Groups

Dental hygiene care for particular age groups differs. A table on the Companion Website describes age-specific competencies, which are summarized here.

DENTAL HYGIENIST SPOTLIGHT:
Tammy Keller, RDH, BS

Tammy Keller, recipient of a 2008 RDH Sunstar Award of Distinction, went to dental hygiene school at North-central Technical College for her associate's degree and graduated with a bachelor of science degree from the University of Minnesota. She currently works as a dental hygienist with the Menominee Indian Reservation in northern Wisconsin. In this role, she not only provides dental care to patients but also coordinates the school-based fluoride rinse program, is the health promotion/disease prevention representative, and is a member of the Menominee County AIDS Task Force, and Diabetes Committee.

In addition to her RDH Sunstar Award, Ms. Keller has received an outstanding Service Award from the Menominee Tribal Clinic and an Award for Excellence in Dental Hygiene from the Indian Health Service Division of Oral Health.

Her answers to a number of career-related questions follow.

Why did you decide to go into dental hygiene?

I chose dental hygiene because I loved the health field, and I found the dental profession to be very interesting. I have always enjoyed working with and helping others.

How did you get into the dental public health? Did you need additional education?

After five years of clinical hygiene in private practice I accepted a full-time clinical hygiene position on the Menominee Indian Reservation. Realizing the oral health needs of the population, I wanted to be able to improve their oral health. I enrolled in the Community Dental Health Certificate program at Northeast Wisconsin Technical College in Green Bay. The program was phenomenal in teaching me how to develop evidence-based oral health programs and how to effectively assess the community's needs, cultural diversity, and more. I strongly recommend this program.

What are your current positions?

I am the school-based mouth rinse and sealant program coordinator. I serve as the oral health representative on the AIDS task force, Tobacco Coalition, Health Promotion/Disease Prevention Committee, Head Start Health Advisory Board, and the Indian Health Service Bemiji Area Dental Hygiene Mentor. I currently work three days a week doing clinical hygiene and devote two days to community oral health programs. I am part of the diabetes team, seeing patients in the medical department and offering oral health education. I work with the Women, Infants and Children (WIC) Program and Head Start programs applying fluoride varnish four times per year. I have written a maternal child health grant working with pregnant women and infants using xylitol products to reduce tooth decay.

Can you discuss any particularly interesting experiences you have had in your dental public health position?

The most interesting thing to me in public health is the significant impact that you can make on a community. Community oral health prevention programs work! The most rewarding experiences in my life are seeing the significant oral health disparities in the native population and knowing that over the past ten years, there has been a documented decrease in tooth decay in native children.

What type of advice would you give to a practicing hygienist who is thinking of doing something different?

Think outside the box. Dental hygiene is not a job; it is a passion. It is a lot of work but very rewarding. I saw the opportunity to make changes and make a difference to better oral health in the community. I created my position, and others can too.

Source: Christine Nathe writes the Public Health Column in RDH magazine published by Pennwell Publishing. For more public health spotlights please see RDH magazine online at http://www.rdhmag.com/index.html.

- **Prenatal:** Women who are pregnant present with a variety of oral health needs. They may suffer periodontal conditions exacerbated by hormonal fluctuations. Pyogenic granulomas and pregnancy-induced gingivitis occasionally occur during pregnancy. These conditions can be prevented by meticulous oral hygiene and professional dental hygiene care, information about which dental health educators provide.
- **Infancy:** Periodontal disease in the mother has been associated with preterm births and babies with low birth weights.[10] Many infants are fed milk in bed or sugary drinks from a bottle, which causes early childhood caries, sometimes referred to as *nursing (baby bottle) tooth decay.* In addition, many parents have questions about teething, the functions of the primary dentition, when to begin

regular dental hygiene visits, and home care regimens. Dental hygienists who serve as dental health educators, promoters, or clinicians can refer infants and parents to dentists as needed.

- **Preschool:** Preschoolers are interested in learning and are busy striving for independence. They are impressionable, and, therefore, their education is vital for a lifetime of good oral hygiene. Early childhood caries is a preventable disease. In particular, in this stage of development, children rapidly assume a positive dental role model and respond to education. It is important to discuss with them the role of dental hygienists and other dental care providers as well as basic dental and nutrition information. Interactive learning with coloring and other hands-on methods is effective. (See Box 10-1 ■.)

BOX 10-1   Recommendations for Providing Dental Treatment to Early Childhood Patients

- Develop rapport with children and their parents as a foundation for cooperation and trust.
- Regard parents as partners in the children's oral health care.
- Talk to children in short sentences using simple words without double meanings; do not use metaphors because children interpret language literally.
- Maintain a calm, slow, reassuring voice that does not intimidate children.
- Explain all procedures in simple, concrete terms.
- Clarify what the children's role is during treatment, and set acceptable rules for behavior.
- Demonstrate the use of equipment, and involve the children in the dental care as much as possible.
- Use substitution words (eg, refer to the *suction* as a *straw, handpiece* as a *tooth tickle,* and *x-ray procedures* as *using a camera to take pictures of the teeth*).
- Give simple instructions and directions one at a time.
- Use gestures and facial expressions.
- Use a confident manner and positive voice when inviting children to sit in the dental chair independently.
- Consider allowing children to sit on the parents' lap, depending on parental attachment.

- Allow children to explore the environment through smell, taste, touch, sight, and sound (eg, smelling the fluoride, tasting prophylactic paste, handling a mirror, seeing the mask and gloves donned, or listening to the compressed air).
- Do not lie to children about pain; describe exactly what the procedure will feel like.
- Avoid using logic because children lack reasoning skills.
- Allow children to make choices whenever possible, and give them a way to interrupt treatment, such as raising a hand to signal discomfort.
- Answer questions and encourage curiosity.
- Avoid overdirecting very cooperative children.
- Be aware that negativism (saying "no") may be the only way children know for control and that temper tantrums are a possibility.
- Teach parents and children appropriate oral hygiene care according to their specific needs.
- Offer suggestions and/or recommendations to parents concerning risk factors and ways to assist children to perform oral hygiene activities.
- Ignore inappropriate behaviors, but praise appropriate behaviors and cooperation.
- Reward good behavior with a tangible gift (eg, toothbrush, sticker, toy).

Source: Donald T. Pediatrics. In: Harris NO, Garcia-Godoy F, Nathe C. *Primary Preventive Dentistry.* 7th ed. Upper Saddle River, NJ: Pearson; 2008.

- **Elementary Age Children:** This population is interested in obtaining knowledge and continuing to strive for independence. It is important for dental hygienists to discuss a detailed concept of dental health care and using preventive interventions such as fluoride and dental sealants. Dental hygienists can easily schedule educational presentations for children through their school or their teachers. Teachers influence this age group, so dental educational materials integrated with the math, reading, and social sciences curricula are helpful for this age group. (See Box 10-2 ■.)
- **Teenagers:** This population generally strives for total independence and prefer presentations on dental health without parental supervision. Moreover, many teens are concerned with their looks or basic presentation. Discussing halitosis or tooth color may be effective for them. In addition, teens look for positive reinforcements, which can take the form of rewards such as T-shirts and hats for a job well done in oral home care. Because many teenagers are involved in athletics, a discussion of mouth guards with them is critical. (See Box 10-3 ■.)
- **Adults:** This population tends to be more cooperative in the oral health learning process if they are aware of the benefits. They focus on time constraints and want to learn only what is practical for them. Moreover, adults may have issues such as fear and anxiety concerning dental care. To treat them, dental hygienists must understand the individual's capabilities and values. Individuals who have no value for oral care will have little interest in its education. Dental hygienists must determine how to make oral health of real value to them. The presentation of information about dental care delivery in general and their children's oral health is interesting to adults.

BOX 10-2 Recommendations for Providing Dental Treatment to School-Age Children

- Develop rapport with children as a foundation for cooperation and trust.
- Talk with children about their friends, school, and outside interests.
- Direct questions to children first.
- Develop rapport with the parents, and consider them partners in children's oral health care.
- Dispel myths that children may have learned about dental visits from other children and/or adults.[6]
- Clarify what children's role is during treatment, and set acceptable rules for behavior.
- Encourage questions and give straight answers.
- Explain procedures using simple vocabulary.
- Regularly ask children to repeat (in their own words) what has just been said or explained to them to ensure that they understand.
- Describe the operation of equipment and reasons for its use.
- Give clear explanations of what children will experience in terms of pain or discomfort; do not lie to or mislead them.
- Help children retain control by including them in decision making, soliciting their help, giving them the opportunity to make choices involving their care when possible, and providing them a way to interrupt treatment, such as raising a hand to signal discomfort.
- Introduce children to routine care of their teeth and gums, including regular brushing, flossing, and reductions in sugar consumption (eg, candy, sodas).
- Teach parents to monitor their children's oral hygiene activities and offer suggestions to parents who struggle with their children regarding these issues.
- Be positive to and supportive of the children; avoid making judgments and causing embarrassment.
- Be aware that children at this age can have difficult-to-control temper tantrums and their behavior can be unpredictable, from cooperative to obstructive to withdrawn to enthusiastic.
- Distinguish between emotional crying (pain, fear) and crying used to manipulate the environment (tantrums); handle emotional crying with patience and empathy; use behavior management techniques with tantrums.
- Use praise as positive reinforcement and rewards (not necessarily tangible) for appropriate behaviors.

Source: Donald T. Pediatrics. In: Harris NO, Garcia-Godoy F, Nathe C. *Primary Preventive Dentistry.* 7th ed. Upper Saddle River, NJ: Pearson; 2008.

BOX 10-3   Recommendations for Providing Dental Treatment to Adolescents

- Develop rapport with adolescents as a foundation for cooperation and trust.
- Talk with the adolescents about friends, school, interests, and hobbies.
- Allow sufficient time for patients of this age to adjust and feel comfortable before beginning treatment, because they are at first distrustful of authority.[6]
- Reassure adolescents about confidentiality and privacy issues.
- Set reasonable limits and standards for cooperation and behavior.
- Help these patients retain control by including them in decision making, soliciting their help, giving them the opportunity to make choices involving their care when possible, and providing them a way to interrupt treatment, such as raising a hand to signal discomfort.
- Allow self-expression and avoid being judgmental.
- Listen, be attentive, and attempt to understand the adolescents while making sure to respond in consistent standard English.
- Be supportive and be a good role model and resource.
- Set goals for oral hygiene activities and future appointments.
- Appeal to the impact of their oral health on social interactions (eg, plaque and oral bacteria can cause bad breath).
- Dispel myths of idealized media images of dental health (eg, extremely white teeth).
- Understand that adolescents can exhibit arrogant and disrespectful attitudes.
- Treat all questions seriously and provide full explanations.
- Discuss oral health in terms of disease and infections; give explanations and consequences, especially physical consequences.
- Give clear explanations of what the patient will experience in terms of pain or discomfort; do not lie to or mislead the patient.
- Include dietary habits and tobacco, alcohol, and drug use in health education messages.
- Strive for a positive dental hygiene experience, allowing the adolescents to gain more self-esteem.

Source: Donald T. Pediatrics. In: Harris NO, Garcia-Godoy F, Nathe C. *Primary Preventive Dentistry.* 7th ed. Upper Saddle River, NJ: Pearson; 2008.

- **Elderly Adults:** Many elderly adults remain independent, but others may have limited independence. Understanding this group's capabilities is necessary. A number of normal but significant changes occur during aging. Fortunately, few of them cause oral diseases. Instead, the cumulative effects of both oral and systemic diseases result in the prevalence of oral disease among elderly people. Interestingly, increasing numbers of well elderly are able to retain their natural teeth and enjoy normal oral function.[11] Furthermore, this group may be entitled to government funding for dental care. Therefore, it is important for dental hygienists to serve as liaisons between elderly people and the dental care delivery system. This population may also be interested in information about dental caries, periodontal diseases, oral cancer, disease etiology and prevention, nutrition, holistic health care, and specific dental services such as tooth bleaching and cosmetic dentistry.

TARGET POPULATION PROFILES

Researching the target population is necessary for dental hygienists to determine a profile much like the initial assessment that is made during a clinical appointment. A comprehensive overview of the target population that includes specific descriptions is termed a **target population profile** or community profile.

Areas to be assessed in creating a target population profile include the population's location, available resources, and partnerships. Dental hygienists may gather this information by conducting surveys, attending community meetings, and reviewing existing data. Numerous government agencies provide baseline data that can be used to profile a target population. (See Table 10-2 ■.)

Demographic Information

Dental hygienists must include demographic information when profiling a target population. *Demographic*

Table 10-2   Government Resources for Target Population Data

Agency/Survey	Function	Web Site
Agency for Health Care Research and Quality (AHRQ)	Collects data on the utilization of health and dental care services throughout the country through the Medical Expenditure Panel Surveys (MEPS)	http://www.meps/ahrq/gov
Bureau of the Census	Conducts the US Census	http://www.census.gov
CDC, Behavioral Risk Factor Surveillance (BRFSS); CDC, Youth Risk Behavior Survey (YRBS)	Collects ongoing state-based data to measure behavioral risk factors among adults and youth	http://www.cdc.gov.brfss http://www.cdc.gov/healthyyouth/yrbs.index.htm
CDC, DATA2010	Tracks data for Healthy People 2010	http://wonder.cdc.gov/data2010
CDC, National Notifiable Diseases Surveillance System	Lists and collects national data on diseases required by law to be reported to official health authorities	http://www.cdc.gov/epo/dphsi/nndsshis.htm
CDC, National Oral Health Surveillance System (NOHSS)	Monitors dental health, disease, and use of dental services within states for a collaboration between the CDC and the Association of State and Territorial Dental Directors	http://www.cdc.gov/nohss
CDC, National Health and Nutrition Examination Survey (NHANES)	Collects data on health and nutrition	http://www.cdc.gov/nchs/nhanes.htm
CDC, Health Interview Survey (NHIS)	Uses household interviews on the health of noninstitutionalized, civilian adults in the United States	http://www.cdc.gov/nchs/nhis.htm
CDC, National Nursing Home Survey	Performs continuing series of national sample surveys of nursing home staff and residents	http://www.cdc.gov/nchs/nnhs.htm
CDC, National Vital Statistics (NVSS)	Collects data on births, deaths, fetal deaths, etc.	http://www.cdc.gov/nchs/nvss.htm
CDC, Pregnancy Risk Assessment Monitoring System (PRAMS)	Collects data on maternal attitudes and experiences	http://www.cdc.gov/reproductivehealth/srv_prams.htm
CDC, School Health Policies and Program Study (SHPPS)	Conducts national survey to assess school policies and programs	http://www.cdc.gov/HeathyYouth/shpps.index.htm
CDC, Water Fluoridation Reporting System	Monitors public water fluoridation	http://apps.nccd.cdc.gov/gisdoh
Centers for Medicare and Medicaid (CMS)	Collects data on Medicaid utilization	http://www.cms.gov/medicaid/mcaidsad.asp
Health Resources and Services Administration (HRSA)	Collects data on the dental workforce and patients with special needs	http://www.hrsa.gov/data.htim
National Institutes of Dental and Craniofacial Research (NIDCR)	Provides resources for dental diseases and oral manifestations of disease	http://drc.nidcr.nih.gov
National Cancer Institute (NCI)	Collects information on cancer rates, trends, etc, through its SEER program	http://seer.cancer.gov

information includes such factors as age, gender, and ethnicity, which are important to describe when discussing a population's dental health. Other areas to address include family lifestyles, living arrangements, cultural backgrounds, religious beliefs, social attributes, social structure, social networks, community stability, and values of dental health.

The location of the target population is of course assessed and its boundaries determined. Important factors are community size, geographic isolation, physical conditions of its neighborhoods, and community infrastructure. Organizational facilities should be described including their equipment and maintenance.

Funding opportunities such as grants or donations as well as the history of previous dental or health endeavors should be assessed. Local government structure and community organizations of the population should be described.

The ability to develop or strengthen partnerships is paramount to serving a target population. Too often dental hygienists develop programs without enough support. Community and political leaders, organizations, and other health providers are potentials partnerships with dental hygienists to improve the community.

Did You Know?

Collaborative efforts that are multidisciplinary in nature in public health initiatives tend to last longer and be more effective than stand-alone dental programs because they have more *owners* of the initiative.

FAITH-BASED INITIATIVES

Many religious groups play significant roles in health care. Religious leaders tend to have great influence on health care delivery and work diligently to help those who need it. In 2001, the federal government created the Center for Faith-Based and Community Initiatives (CFBCI), an agency that ensures collaboration between the government and religious groups to improve life for people in need. CFBCI's mission is to create an environment within the Department of Health and Human Services (HHS) that welcomes **faith-based initiatives** and the participation of community-based organizations as valued and essential partners to assist Americans in need. An example of a faith-based organization could be a local church group that fundraises for a dental clinic that provides care to the underserved populations, specifally those populations that have difficulty accessing dental care.[12]

BARRIERS TO DENTAL CARE

Many populations within a society face restrictive barriers to obtaining dental hygiene and dental care. **Barriers to care** can be defined as anything that limits an individual's ability to receive dental services. Barriers can include age, cultural variances, language difficulties, lack of information, disabilities, transportation issues, and financial limitations as well as laws preventing registered dental hygienists from providing dental hygiene care in a school setting. (See Box 10–4 ■.). Some barriers are easily

BOX 10-4 Possible Barriers to Obtaining Dental Hygiene and Dental Care

- Age
- Language
- Habit(s)
- Culture
- Financial situation
- Lack of confidence in treatment
- Education
- Lack of understanding
- Fear
- Transportation
- Values

- Safety of treatment
- Attitudes
- Denial of disease
- Unavailability of dental providers
- Sense of invulnerability
- Inconvenience
- Social issues
- Provider conflicts
- Inconvenient office hours
- Requirements for supervision of dental hygienists

overcome; for example, a state program offering rides to medical and dental appointments can address transportation problems. Addressing others, such as laws preventing practice in specific locations, are more complicated.

An individual's values may also be a barrier to care. For example, a teenage boy may believe that his teeth are invulnerable to the effects of periodontal disease. He may not understand that keeping his teeth for a lifetime takes a commitment to home as well as professional care. Consequently, he may not respond to information presented about the periodontal condition of his mouth, which could limit the services sought from a dental hygienist. Dental hygienists can alleviate this barrier by gearing the educational therapy toward the teenager's values. For example, the dental hygienist may be able to discuss the effect of periodontal disease on halitosis, which could interest him.

Barriers to care are often combinations of factors. For instance, a two-year-old child with Medicaid insurance who has severe stages of early childhood caries may receive no care if pediatric or qualified general dentists in the area are unwilling to provide treatment. The providers' reluctance could be caused by the child's age, severity of the disease, or the type of insurance to pay for the services. For this child, access may be limited by one factor or several.

Professional dental hygienists assume the responsibility for increasing access to quality dental hygiene and dental care. This responsibility requires understanding the barriers to them and working to alleviate them.

SUMMARY

For dental health initiatives to be effective, it is vital that dental hygienists learn about a target population before treating it or providing education to it. The first step in understanding what needs must be addressed is to identify a target population profile. Dental hygienists practicing in community settings must be aware of the barriers some populations face when trying to access dental hygiene care.

SELF-STUDY TEST ITEMS

1. A group from a local church youth group could be considered a
   a. Target population
   b. Target population profile
   c. Faith-based initiative
   d. Community agency

2. It is important not to frighten child patients. It is better not to tell the truth if a procedure could involve some discomfort.
   a. The first statement is true; the second statement is false.
   b. The first statement is false; the second statement is true.
   c. Both statements are true.
   d. Both statements are false.

3. Faith-based initiatives funded by the federal government do not generally include health care.
   a. The first part of the statement is true, but the second is false.
   b. The first part of the statement is false, but the second is true.
   c. Both parts of the statement are true.
   d. Both parts of the statement are false.

4. Social workers and dental hygienists can work together during programs for target populations
   a. To provide dental hygiene care
   b. To assess dental health
   c. To ensuring social services for the population
   d. To implement periodontal treatment

5. Inconvenient office hours of a dental practice can become a
   a. Target population profile technique
   b. Faith-based issue
   c. Barrier to care
   d. Long-term strategic plan

REFERENCES

1. Horn J. *Osteoporosis Prevention and Screening: Potential Role for Oral Health Professionals?* Grand Rounds in Oral-Systemic Medicine, Vol. 2, No 2. 2007.
2. *Competencies for the Advanced Dental Hygiene Practitioner (ADHP).* Chicago, IL: American Dental Hygienists' Association; 2008.
3. Zastrow C. *Introduction to Social Welfare Institutions.* 3rd ed. Chicago, IL: Dorsey Press; 1986.
4. Sanchez Dils EM. Medically Compromised Populations. In: Harris NO, Garcia-Godoy F, Nathe C. *Primary Preventive Dentistry.* 7th ed. Upper Saddle River, NJ: Pearson; 2008.
5. Sanchez Dils EM. Populations with Developmental Disabilities. In: Harris NO, Garcia-Godoy F, Nathe C. *Primary Preventive Dentistry.* 7th ed. Upper Saddle River, NJ: Pearson; 2008.

6. DeBiase CB. *Dental Health Education Theory and Practice.* Philadelphia, PA: Lea and Febiger; 1991.

7. Proctor BD, Dalaker J. *Poverty in the United States: 2001.* Washington, DC: US Government Printing Office; 2002.

8. Sawhill IV. Poverty in the United States. In: Henderson, DR. *Concise Encyclopedia of Economics.* Indianapolis, IN: Liberty Fund; 2003.

9. A Culture of Poverty Develops When the Poor Are Left Behind. http://www.poverty.smartlibrary.org/newinterface/segment.cfm?segment=1566 Accessed September 12, 2008.

10. US Department of Health and Human Services. *Oral Health in America: A Report of the Surgeon General.* Rockville, MD: US Department of Health and Human Services, National Institute of Dental and Craniofacial Research, National Institutes of Health; 2000.

11. Tatlock CD. Geriatrics. In: Harris NO, Garcia-Godoy F, Nathe C. *Primary Preventive Dentistry.* 7th ed. Upper Saddle River, NJ: Pearson; 2008.

12. Center for Faith-Based & Community Initiatives. http://www.hhs.gov/fbci/. Accessed September 12, 2008.

Multimedia Extension Activities

Use this address to access the interactive Companion Website created for this textbook. Simply select "Dental Hygiene" from the choice of disciplines. Find this book and log in using your username and password. To obtain a username and password, please register using the scratch-off access code on the inside front cover of this book.

Chapter 11

Cultural Competency

Irene Connolly, RDH, MS

OBJECTIVES

After studying this chapter, the dental hygiene student should be able to:

- Describe how cultural values regarding health care can affect oral health habits
- Identify how culture influences the way people communicate
- Define cultural competency and its significance in caring for a culturally diverse population

KEY TERMS

Acculturate

Assimilate

Complementary alternative medicine

Cultural competency

Cultural sensitivity

Ethnocentrism

Eurocentric

Sociocultural theory

Subculture

Transcultural communication skills

Zone of proximal development

COMPETENCIES

After studying this chapter and participating in the accompanying class activities, the dental hygiene student should be competent to do the following:

- Communicate effectively with individuals and groups from diverse populations both verbally and in writing
- Provide care to all clients using an individualized approach that is human, empathetic, and caring
- Respect the goals, values, beliefs, and preferences of patients/clients while promoting optimal oral and general health

"Culture is a complex and multifaceted social phenomenon that has powerful influences on all aspects of modern life."[1] Culture encompasses attitudes, values, and beliefs. On a grand scale, culture influences global business dealings, trade agreements, and negotiations. It is often the reason for continued conflict between groups of people as is evident around the world today. Most critical events facing the world today result from cultural differences. The subject of culture can include differences in ethnic background, socioeconomic standing, gender, religion, beliefs, language, and all aspects of work and family life.[2] An individual raised in one culture never completely understands another culture because the person did not internalize values and traditions of the other culture during childhood.

Traditional descriptors of a population such as *race* no longer reliably distinguish a population, since many races are mixed with populations from many different countries. For example, cultural groups such as the Irish and the Germans living within the Caucasian population may display entirely different characteristics. The Hispanic population in the United States, which constitutes 13% of total population, has many countries of origin, and recent immigrants from Mexico may communicate using a mixture of Native American and Spanish languages. Knowledge of these cultures can enhance communication efforts between health care providers and the population they serve.[3]

The 2000 US Census categorized race in five populations:

- White
- Black or African American
- American Indian and Alaska Native
- Asian
- Native Hawaiian and Other Pacific Islander

A sixth category, "Some other race," was established in 2000 for people unable to identify with any of the five races. Most who fell into this category were Hispanic. The Office of Management and Budget (OMB) defines Hispanic or Latino as "a person of Cuban, Mexican, Puerto Rican, South or Central American, or other Spanish culture or origin regardless of race."[3] In accordance with this definition, the Census Bureau provides data for the basic categories in the OMB standards: Hispanic or Latino and Not Hispanic or Latino. People who identify their origin as Spanish, Hispanic, or Latino may be of any race.[3] (See Table 11-1 ■.)

Did You Know?

In general, the Census Bureau defines ethnicity or origin as the heritage, nationality group, lineage, or country of birth of the person or the person's parents or ancestors before their arrival in the United States.

Table 11-1 Population of the United States by Race According to 2000 Census

	Number	*Percent of Total Population*
RACE: Total population	**281 421 906**	**100.0**
White	211 460 626	75.1
Black or African American	34 658 190	12.3
American Indian and Alaska Native	2 475 956	0.9
Asian	10 242 998	3.6
Native Hawaiian and Other Pacific Islander	398 835	0.1
Some other race	15 359 073	5.5

Source: US Department of Commerce, US Census Bureau. Washington, DC: US Census Bureau; 2000.

Theories of Cultural and Development of Self-Awareness

The **sociocultural theory** proposed by educational psychologist Lev Vygotsky suggests that an individual's social interaction as a child leads to continuous changes in thought and behavior that can vary greatly from culture to culture. This theory explains why, as stated earlier, fully understanding a culture that is not a person's own is difficult. Vygotsky's theory suggests that development depends on interaction with people and the tools that the culture provides to help form a view of the world. He theorized that there are three ways for cultural tools to pass from one person to another: (1) *imitative learning* by which a person tries to imitate or copy another, (2) *instructed learning,* which involves remembering the instructions of the teacher and then using these instructions to self-regulate, and (3) *passing along cultural tools* through collaborative learning, which refers to a group of peers striving to understand each other and working as a unit to learn a specific skill.[4]

Educator and researcher Barbara Rogoff elaborated on the relationship of Vygotsky's theory of zone of proximal development to culture. The **zone of proximal development** is the difference between a child's actual level of development displayed by unassisted performance, and the child's potential level as indicated by assisted performance. Rogoff suggests that children actually seek assistance of adults around them to guide them through the process of problem solving until they are experienced to do it themselves. Through this guidance, children are expected to adapt to their specific cultural surroundings, and the zone of proximal development is where culture and cognition meet.[5]

Experts agree that the first step in effectively dealing with diverse populations is for people to be aware of their own cultural habits and values.[2,4] This is not an easy task. One way to become self-aware is to read books about one's culture as viewed from the perspective of someone outside it. Another way is to ask a colleague or friend from another culture to frankly describe the person's culture.

Culture-general training, which seeks to enhance receptiveness and sensitivity to cultural differences, is another venue for learning about a culture. Culture-general training helps promote adaptation and effective functioning in any type of culture. Courses such as this can increase awareness about the limitations of one's own culture.[5]

Professional Culture

Professional groups such as dental care providers have their own culture. Dental providers share similar values regarding the importance of good oral health and its relationship to total health. It could be said that dental providers belong to a subculture based on a professional and occupational affiliation.[6] **Subculture** refers to a group of people with a culture that differentiates them from the larger culture to which they belong.

Instructors of dental hygiene students introduce a new value system regarding oral health, and over time, the student is assimilated into the culture or mores of the professional health care subculture.[1,5,6] Although dental hygienists and dentists internalize these values, many populations place little importance on them and see no connection between oral health and total health.

CULTURAL DIVERSITY IN THE UNITED STATES

The population of the United States, which was at one time composed predominately of persons of white European descent, is now truly multiracial and multicultural. The influx of immigrants has brought cultures that are vastly different from those of white European descent. Immigrants embrace different religions, diets, dress, beliefs, and values.[2]

Immigrants, such as those who came in the 1850s and the decade 1900–1910, arrived in the United States with **Eurocentric** beliefs, those reflecting a tendency to interpret the world in terms of Western and especially European or Anglo-American values and experiences. They strove to **acculturate,** or **assimilate,** or adapt to another culture by assuming its practices and beliefs to become part of the great "melting pot." However, research shows that while outward behavior might indicate acceptance of the dominant culture, these changes rarely take place in the inner self.[5] People rarely achieve complete assimilation because culture is an inseparable part of their being and is the foundation from which they form their values and beliefs.[1]

Recent immigrants to the United States are now choosing to preserve their cultural heritage and belief systems, including dress, customs, language, and religious beliefs.[1] People are less likely to aspire to completely assimilate into what is considered the "mainstream." America can now be described as a "salad bowl." Many people in the United States now embrace pluralism instead of assimilation.

Although not falling into the category of immigrants, Native American populations including American Indians, Alaska Natives, and Native Hawaiian and Pacific Islanders have cultures that differ from each other and from that of "mainstream" populations. In regions such as the Southwest, dental hygienists have many opportunities to serve this population. See Figure 11-1 ■ for locations of Native Americans in the United States. A culturally sensitive clinician taking into account the Native American's respect for tradition will garner more credibility and success with health education than one who views traditional remedies or ceremonies as being primitive or foolish. People display **cultural sensitivity** when they are aware of and understand cultural differences during interactions with people.

Did You Know?

Pluralism exists when numerous distinct ethnic, religious, or cultural groups are present and tolerated within a society.

Cross-Cultural Communication

Practice management courses identify poor communication between patients and health care providers as the leading cause of lawsuits. Clear, concise communication can be difficult to achieve between people of the same culture; imagine the difficulties practitioners without preparation for cultures vastly different from the practitioner's own experience. Communication difficulties can cause barriers to health care, including the inability to explain health problems and the failure to understand outcomes of preventive measures.

Stereotyping refers to members of one group holding a common standardized mental picture that represents an oversimplified opinion or prejudice of that group. Stereotyping a population can quickly shut down communication and understanding for its concerns. Communication is more than verbal; it encompasses gestures, eye contact, physical proximity, and formal versus informal speech. Failure to understand these nonverbal cues can impair effective communication. As an example, many people in US society consider eye contact to be important, and avoiding it could be interpreted by some groups as having something to hide or being dishonest. However, other ethnic groups view direct eye contact as being disrespectful or rude. A culturally insensitive oral health professional may view avoidance of eye contact as lack of interest when it is actually communicating a cultural sign of respect.

Effective communication is always the key to any successful transaction or interaction between people or groups of people. A diverse population urgently needs health care professionals to develop **transcultural communication skills,** or ability to interpret and transmit information to someone from a different culture. Good communication is often considered the cornerstone of effective health care practice.[7] Successful communication with other cultures requires time, patience, caring, and dropping assumptions. (See Box 11-1 ■).

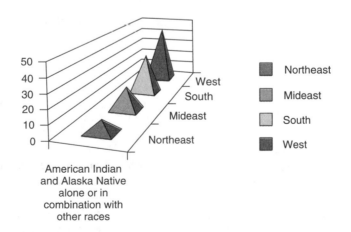

FIGURE 11-1   Geographic Location of Native Americans

Source: US Census. Census 2000 Summary File 1. http://www.bls.gov/cps/cpsaat11.pdf

---

BOX 11-1 Processes to Develop Cultural Sensitivity

- Assess one's own cultural beliefs and values.
- Recognize one's culture influences affecting communication.
- Recognize one's own cultural biases.
- Be knowledgeable of the patient's belief system.
- Be sensitive to gestures, concerns, and questions.

- Be able to collect culturally relevant data concerning the population's health background and level of understanding of the presenting problems.
- Listen and observe.
- Be aware and respectful of cultural differences.

Beware of the *cultural blind spot syndrome.* This is the belief that because a patient or population looks and behaves much like the provider, there are no cultural differences or potential barriers to care.

CULTURE ISSUES IN HEALTH CARE

The rapidly changing demographics of the United States requires the adaptation of cultural skills to communicate and interact successfully in all aspects of life, especially business, education, and health care. The constructs of culture, health, and disease are so interrelated that experts in the field maintain that lack of cultural sensitivity can lead to invalid diagnosis. Inability to recognize health care–related cultural differences can result in treatment failure, frustration for both providers and patients, and withdrawal of patients from the health care system. Health care practitioners have a major responsibility to be culturally sensitive in a society of increasingly interdependent cultures and people.[1]

> **Did You Know?**
>
> Culture plays an important role in health care because beliefs and values concerning wellness, disease, and illness are culturally determined.

Dental hygienists are not responsible for knowing all details of the values, language, character, and behavior expectations of different populations, but they must recognize how different populations perceive disease, health, and the dental hygienist as a health care provider.

Ethnocentrism

The belief that one's own culture or traditions are better than other cultures is **ethnocentrism.** Although many Americans may fail to recognize or deny their ethnocentrism, it does exist. Many health care providers practice from the point of view that their culture is the privileged culture.[2] For example, a practitioner in the United States who values traditional Western medicine may fail to recognize that many Asian cultures use acupuncture and acupressure to control pain or discomfort.[7]

The provider who is ethnocentric tends to antagonize and alienate patients from other cultures. To avoid cultural biases that distort perceptions of other people's values and behavior, which damage the ability to communicate, a person must first acknowledge that ethnocentrism exists.[1,6]

Complementary Alternative Medicine

The use of herbs, natural products, and practices such as massage or yoga is referred to as **complementary alternative medicine (CAM)** in health care. Their use often comes from cultural practices that differ from those used in Western medicine. Most people who use alternative therapies do not discuss it with health care providers, which can lead to problems.

Clinicians should always question their patients about the use of such products. People frequently use herbs as prophylactic measures to prevent disease and/or maintain good health, and dental hygienists should be aware of how their use can impact treatment options. Some supplemental herbs can be contraindicated with use of Western medicines. For instance, some in the Korean population use ginseng as a panacea, which could be contraindicated for people with high blood pressure.

Cultural Representation in Health Professions

Minority populations are still underrepresented in the health professions. In the 1960s, as a result of the Civil Rights movement, many programs were initiated to improve minority access to the health professions. More than 40 years later, however, minorities are still underrepresented in both health science programs and the workforce relative to their representation in the US population.[1] The need for culturally competent health care providers to meet the needs of the underserved, who are often culturally diverse, is tremendous.

CULTURAL COMPETENCY AND DENTAL HYGIENISTS

Dental hygienists who desire to achieve culturally sensitive attitudes while serving in community programs and public health to provide care to diverse populations must consider cultural diversity as an important factor in every encounter with every person. **Cultural competency** is defined as the awareness of and respect for an individual's or a population's cultural differences, the recognition of how these differences impact a specific group, such as health care providers, and the ability to communicate effectively and work cross-culturally.

Being culturally competent when treating patients of different cultures can help the dental hygienist deliver care and education effectively. In addition, when dental providers understand values and perspectives of different cultures, they are more likely to respond to oral health disparities in an appropriate manner.

In a very diverse society, dental hygienists must be able to disseminate oral health care information and treatment while recognizing populations' cultural differences. In collaborative practice and community-based settings, dental hygiene care must meet the needs of these populations. See Table 11-2 ■ for a guide to working with people of various cultural groups.

Table 11-2 Guide to Cultural Practices Affecting Health Care

All individuals from a given culture do not act or think in the same way. All individuals possess an inherent variability within cultural groups. The information in this table is not meant to generalize populations but to serve as a beginning guide.

Population	*Health-Related Practices and Ways to Address Them*
Native Americans/ American Indian/ Alaska Natives	• This group believes that healing results from sacred ceremonies that rely on having visions and using plants and objects that may be symbolic of the individual, the illness, or the treatment. • Traditional Navajo medicine includes chanting, praying, sand painting, dancing, and using herbs. • Many Native American tribes go to a sweat lodge to cure a variety of physical and emotional ills. • Alternative medical practitioners widely use Native American herbal medicine such as echinacea, goldenseal, and burdock.
Asian	• Chinese medicine is a complex and well-established therapeutic tradition that uses acupuncture, acupressure, and herbs, often in combination with dietary therapy, Western medicine, and supernatural healing. • Some Chinese believe that illness is a result of moral retribution by ancestors or deities because of a person's misdeeds or negligence. Rituals are performed to appease this anger. Other health beliefs include cosmic disharmony due to a poor combination of year of birth, month of birth, day of birth, and time of birth, and poor Feng Shui—improper placement of objects inside a room or orientation of the room or house itself (north, south, east, or west). • Asian mothers often prefer their children to be cared for by female providers. • Chinese and Cambodian medicine classifies food, illness, and medications according to the perceived effects of each on the body as "hot" or "cold" as does the ayurvedic system of medicine, widely used among people of Indian and Chinese descent. It identifies causes of illness as excess association of "hot" or "cold" foods, wind, and other environmental factors, emotional states, and sexual activity and may be remedied by treatment such as restoring the balance of foods in the diet. • Some Chinese and Cambodians believe in interference from malevolent spirits. Spiritual healers are sought for illnesses thought to be caused by spirits. • Some Cambodians may cup, pinch, coin, or rub an ill person's skin to treat a range of ailments.[a]

(continued)

Table 11-2   Guide to Cultural Practices Affecting Health Care

Population	Health-Related Practices and Ways to Address Them
Pacific Islanders	• Some Pacific Islanders believe that illness and other misfortune can be attributed to the loss of *mana,* defined as special power or life force. Healing requires the restoration of the imbalance of mana by analyzing damaged relationships with one's self, extended family, ancestors, environment, or spirituality. • The ideal concept of health has four components: spiritual, psychological, physical, and family relationship. All four must be incorporated into any treatment regimen. • Some Pacific Islanders believe that the traditional food called *taro* holds great mana. • Storytelling may be used as a therapeutic method of teaching and healing. • Restoring health may involve a search into the cause of the problem, open expression of feelings by all concerned, expressions of apology, and asking for forgiveness.
Eastern Europeans	• Traditional healing approaches include treatments using teas, herbs, grasses, and ointments. • Coughs and congestion are relieved by inhaling steam from chamomile tea. • Honey and pollen are consumed to ensure longevity. • Some may cup, pinch, coin, or rub an ill person's skin to treat a range of ailments.[a]
Muslim	• Muslims can be reluctant to share personal information with others. Explain the importance of disclosing such information to health care providers. • To gain a patient's trust, the provider should consider sharing a small bit of personal information with the patient. • Be aware that a family spokesman or even a community spokesman may represent the patient when dealing with health care providers. • Being frank when communicating bad news or prognosis may not be appropriate. • Muslim women prefer to be seen by a female.
Mexican American/ Hispanic	• Be aware that religion and spirituality are important parts of this culture. Allow religious items, rosary beads, etc, at the bedside if the family and patient so wishes. • Be aware that prayer is important and may take place at the bedside and include family and friends.
African American	• Address patients by their formal names, especially elderly patients. • Make direct eye contact. • Because patients may be reluctant to disclose personal information, explain why the information is needed before asking. • Be aware of historic mistrust of the health care profession by some African American people.
Russian	• In the Russian culture, bad news is not given to patients. Talk with the family first to decide whether bad news should be given directly to the patient. • Some Russian patients may overreact. Be optimistic and cautious when explaining prognosis and treatment options. • Some may distrust doctors and health care professionals, resulting in poor adherence to treatments, medicines, and appointments. • Homeopathics and natural remedies are important in the Russian culture. Encourage discussion of such practices with health care providers before starting alternatives and homeopathics.

[a]It is important that these techniques not automatically be labeled as abuse without further culturally sensitive investigation.

Sources: Management Sciences for Health (MSH), US Department of Health and Human Services, Health Resources and Services Administration and the Bureau of Primary Health Care. The provider's guide to quality and culture. http://erc.msh.org. Accessed March 13, 2009. University of Michigan Health System. Program for multicultural health. http://www.med.umich.edu/Multicultural. Accessed March 13, 2009.

Professional Policies

The American Dental Hygienists' Association (ADHA) has responded to the disparities identified in the Surgeon General's 2000 document *Oral Health in America: A Report of the Surgeon General* by encouraging and funding dental hygiene research pertaining to the influence of cultural values on oral health.[8,9] The timeliness and importance of this issue is reflected in the ADHA's recently revised National Dental Hygiene Research Agenda. This document, generated by the ADHA Council of Research, identifies areas of research needed in dental hygiene. Threaded throughout this document are references to cultural diversity specifically when related to health promotion and disease prevention in diverse populations. (See Box 11-2 ■.)

The 84th Annual Session of the ADHA emphasized the need for cultural competency in the field of dental hygiene.[10] Its House of Delegates adopted the following definitions pertaining to cultural and linguistic competencies:

Cultural competence

Awareness of cultural differences among all populations, respect of those differences and application of the knowledge to professional practice.

Linguistic competence

The ability to communicate effectively and respond appropriately to the health literacy needs of all populations.

The generation and adoption of these definitions clearly recognize and emphasize the need for dental hygienists to be aware of individual or population cultural differences, have respect for these differences, and understand how these cultural differences impact oral health. The ADHA encourages hygienists to expand their knowledge of diverse populations so they have the ability to communicate and work effectively in cross-cultural situations. Additional policy adopted by the 2007 House of Delegates stated, "The American Dental Hygienists' Association advocates cultural and linguistic competence for health professionals."

Educational Challenges

Health care educators have a major responsibility to prepare culturally sensitive health care practitioners for a world of increasingly interdependent cultures and people. Student dental hygienists should be prepared to serve all clients without discrimination and to appreciate the diversity of the populations they care for. When addressing cultural competency, the American Dental Association's Commission on Dental Accreditation called for all graduates to be competent in interpersonal and communication skills to effectively interact with diverse population groups.[11]

To meet this challenge, educational institutions often require students to treat a specific number of culturally diverse individuals in the clinical environment. However, community health courses afford students the best opportunities to be involved with diverse populations. The ability of the educational institution to make these opportunities available to the students depends largely on the cultural makeup of the community in which the school is located.[12]

Barriers to Oral Health Care

The values of a population or an individual can be a barrier to care.

National Issues

Barriers to oral health care for diverse populations exist in the United States, a fact that the 2000 document *Oral Health in America: A Report of the Surgeon General*

BOX 11-2   Health Promotion/Disease Prevention for Diverse Populations

- Validate and test assessment instruments/strategies/mechanisms that increase health promotion and disease prevention among diverse populations.
- Investigate how diversity among populations impacts the promotion of oral health and preventive behaviors.
- Investigate the effectiveness of oral self-care behaviors that prevent or reduce oral diseases among all age, social, and cultural groups.
- Investigate how environmental factors (culture, socioeconomic status, education) influence oral health behaviors.

emphasized. The first of its kind, this national report on oral health revealed that members of ethnic minority groups experienced a disproportional amount of oral health problems. The following are excerpts from the report's Executive Summary.[8]

What Is the Status of Oral Health in America?

Despite improvements in oral health status, profound disparities remain in some population groups as classified by sex, income, age, and race/ethnicity. For some diseases and conditions, the magnitude of the differences in oral health status among populations groups is striking.

What Is the Relationship Between Oral Health and General Health and Well-being?

Cultural values influence oral and craniofacial health and well-being and can play an important role in care utilization practices and in perpetuating acceptable oral health and facial norms.

As the Surgeon General's report emphasized, obvious disparities in access to oral health care for certain ethnic populations exist.[8] These barriers can include financial limitations, language differences, perceptions of good oral health, and, foremost, lack of access to professionals qualified to provide oral health care services. Although interest in public health programs has increased in recent years, recruiting dental professionals willing to work with the underserved remains a constant challenge.[12]

A language barrier may also deter people from seeking care or reduce the effectiveness of care that they receive. Use of family members to interpret is not recommended because of privacy concerns and emotional involvement. Utilizing a trained interpreter may prove helpful, but establishing rapport with the clients in this situation is difficult. The use of visual aids, repetition, clarification, open-ended questions rather than questions calling for yes or no answers is a practical technique to overcome the language barrier.[7] Learning all languages and customs is not feasible, but dental hygienists should strive to learn as much as they can to communicate with, educate, and motivate populations they serve to achieve good oral health.

When working with diverse cultures, the dental hygienist should realize that the tradition of some cultures do not emphasize dental. Members of these cultures may fail to understand the financial impact of poor oral health care and may not realize how disruptive and costly missed appointments are.

The fact that only a small number of minorities working in the oral health care professions may be considered a barrier to oral health care. A study of the racial and ethnic composition of the health care workforce reveals that the dental workforce is the least diverse of all the health professions.[12] Further investigation reveals that of all those included in the dental health care providers category—dentists, dental hygienists, dental assistants, and dental laboratory technicians—the dental hygiene profession is the least culturally diverse.[7] (See Figure 11-2 ■.)

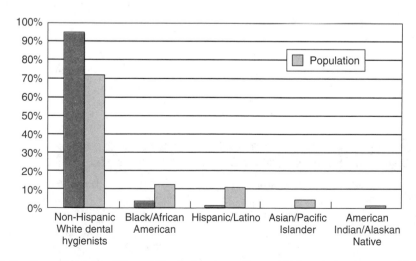

FIGURE 11-2 Race/Ethnicity of Dental Hygienists According to US Population Percent, 1999

Note: The most recent year for which data on dental hygienists in Illinois were available is 1997.

Source: Bureau of Labor Statistics, American Dental Association, Bureau of the Census. http://www.bls.gov/cps/cpsaat11.pdf

Table 11-3 Guidelines for Delivering Oral Health Care to Diverse Populations

To Develop Cultural Awareness	*To Deliver Culturally Competent Care*
• Recognize how your culture influences your values, behavior, beliefs, and decision making. • Become a lifelong learner of diverse cultures, particularly those whose population you serve. • Know about your population's cultural background. • Assess your population's values, beliefs, and knowledge of oral and total health. • Consider the effects of religious beliefs on oral and total health. • Investigate cultural dietary practices and how they affect total health.	• Incorporate cultural practices into education and treatment when appropriate, but sensitively discourage harmful practices. • Incorporate culturally competent communication into oral health education. • Deliver dental hygiene services in a culturally sensitive manner and environment. • Develop relationships with health professionals from other ethnic and minority groups to promote a collaborative effort to improve the groups' oral health.

Value of Dental Hygiene

People from other cultures do not always share the American belief that present action can change future events. Americans tend to measure the success or failure of prevention by the statistical rate of disease occurrences over time, and they generally believe that improvements in public health result from prevention. However, many people from other cultures do not see the value of prevention if no disease is evident. If there is no pain or discomfort, why be subjected to periodontal scaling? Why fluoridate the water when caries may not occur? How could dietary changes affect already formed and erupted teeth? Concerns such as these must be acknowledged before public health dental hygienists can educate a culturally diverse population.

Cross-cultural dental hygiene is the effective integration of a patient's or population's socioethnocultural background into the dental hygiene process of care. See Table 11-3 ■ for basic guidelines for delivering oral health education and care to diverse populations.

DENTAL HYGIENIST SPOTLIGHT: Meg Zayan, RDH, MPH, EdD

Meg Horst Zayan, RDH, MPH, EdD, is the current dean of Fones School of Dental Hygiene in Bridgeport, Connecticut, the original dental hygiene school. Fones recently added a graduate degree in dental hygiene and opened a remodeled state-of-the-art dental hygiene clinic.

In addition to her teaching and management experience, Dr. Zayan has worked for the US State Department in Niger, Africa, as a volunteer to help in the treatment of dental disease, and as a dental hygienist in the Colorado migrant health program. She continues to teach students about the integral relationship between dental public health and dental hygiene. Not surprisingly, she has received numerous honors including membership in Sigma Phi Alpha, the national dental hygiene honor society, and Phi Kappa Phi, the nation's oldest, largest, and most selective all-discipline honor society. Dr. Zayan has been awarded the Outstanding Teacher Award at Fones School of Dental Hygiene.

I recently asked her some questions about her career.

Why did you decide to go into dental hygiene?

As a child, I frequently visited the dentist and dental hygienist for routine appointments and restorations. I also experienced extractions of four primary and four permanent noncarious teeth to prevent crowding and the need for orthodontia.

These experiences allowed me to understand the dental office personnel and the advantages of serving the public and providing education. As I was in the decision-making process to choose a college major, it seemed beneficial to combine health care with education, and I chose dental hygiene. My grandfather always remarked that "a trade and an education will get you far and allow you to be financially stable." His words helped direct me into the dental hygiene profession.

How did you get into dental public health? Did you need additional education?

After graduating with a BS degree in dental hygiene education, I taught for one year. During that year, I realized the need for an advanced degree if I wanted to pursue a career in academia. I thought of various options that would allow me to obtain a dental hygiene "specialty" and expand my job opportunities in venues other than academia.

I was not particularly fond of dental public health as a dental hygiene student, but as I became aware of the many opportunities a degree in public health created, I began to read more and ask questions, and my interest flourished. As a clinician, I understood what it meant to serve the private sector. I wanted to learn more about serving the public sector.

I was fortunate to have received a scholarship the first year I applied for a master's degree in public health. The curriculum I chose required eighteen months of education to earn an MPH. For my minor, I chose health care administration. In retrospect, going into public health was one of the best decisions I made in regard to my education.

What are your current positions?

My current position is dean of Fones School of Dental Hygiene, Bridgeport, Connecticut. I also hold the positions of director of graduate studies and associate professor there.

Can you discuss any particularly interesting experiences you have had in your dental public health positions?

Two experiences come to mind.

First, I had the opportunity to work a summer in the Colorado migrant health program. This gave me insight to the benefits of a state-run oral health care initiative.

Dental hygienists, dentists, nurses, doctors, and nutritionists collaborated to provide education and health services to the migrant farmers and their children. We were dispersed by team throughout the state of Colorado based on need and access. During the summers, these elementary school-aged children attend school while older siblings and parents farm. Our responsibility as dental hygienists was to provide classroom education, screenings, oral prophylaxes, fluoride treatments, and sealants to the children in the schools. If dental work was indicated, we scheduled transportation to local dental offices. During the evenings, we worked in dental offices providing services to the older children and the adults. We all worked together to improve health care, and the rewards were outstanding.

The second experience was living in Niger, West Africa, for two years. My husband, as a public health physician, was hired to work in Niger to help in the program to prevent blindness and eye diseases. I came on board as a volunteer to help in the treatment of dental disease. Due to the lack of integration of preventive dental hygiene in Niger, my role was small. However, I worked with dentists, assisting them in providing treatment and at times used my own dental hygiene instruments to remove calculus. Because Niger is a French-speaking country, I was forced to improve my French so that communication when providing education was positive. This experience instilled a long-term interest in international dental hygiene in me.

What type of advice would you give to a practicing hygienist thinking of doing something different?

I would encourage everyone to always consider the various job opportunities we have in the dental hygiene profession. We have chosen a career for which there will always have be a public need in the foreseeable future. I foresee the job opportunities for dental hygienists to increase in number and type. Clinical dental hygiene is the core of who we are. Anyone considering other opportunities will continually utilize their clinical knowledge to maintain and improve oral health care. I encourage dental hygienists to periodically search the various career options available to them. It is not so much that we need to change, but that if we want to change, we can. A dental hygienist who knows the options will have a better chance of job satisfaction with the choice made.

Source: Christine Nathe writes the Public Health Column in RDH magazine published by Pennwell Publishing. For more public health spotlights please see RDH magazine online at http://www.rdhmag.com/index.html.

SUMMARY

Dental hygienists have been challenged to respond to current and projected demographic changes in the United States. Cultural competency in health care refers to the ability to provide care to populations that have beliefs, values, and behaviors that differ from those of the provider. Consideration must be given to the health beliefs and values as well as disease prevalence and incidence in each particular group. Although dental hygienists are educated to treat people equally, it is important to recognize that people do have differences and to respect them.

SELF-STUDY TEST ITEMS

1. The fact that only a small number of minorities work in the oral health care professions may be considered a barrier to oral health care. A study of the racial and ethnic composition of the health care workforce reveals that the dental workforce is the least diverse of all the health professions.
   a. The first statement is true; the second statement is false.
   b. The first statement is false; the second statement is true.
   c. Both statements are true.
   d. Both statements are false.

2. Which of the following could prevent a patient from seeking care or reduce effectiveness of care?
   a. Unhealthy behaviors
   b. Severe pain
   c. Language barrier
   d. None of the above

3. A country in which people strive to acculturate into a new society and make valiant attempts to change their cultural patterns to those of their host society is colloquially called
   a. A melting pot
   b. A Salad bowl
   c. Jello
   d. Amalgam

4. Which of the following is or are guidelines to effective communication?
   a. Assess one's own cultural beliefs and values
   b. Recognize those culture influences that affect communication
   c. Understand a patient's belief system
   d. All of the above

5. Cross-cultural dental hygiene is the effective integration of a population's socioethnocultural background into the process of care. Recognizing how your culture influences your values, behaviors, beliefs, and decision making is part of cross-cultural dental hygiene.
   a. The first statement is true; the second statement is false.
   b. The first statement is false; the second statement is true.
   c. Both statements are true.
   d. Both statements are false.

REFERENCES

1. Kreps GL, Kunimoto, EN. *Effective Communication in Multicultural Health Care Settings.* Thousand Oaks, CA: Sage Publications; 1994.
2. Connolly IM, Darby ML, Tolle-Watts L, Thomson-Lakey E. Cultural adaptability of health science faculty. *J Dent Hyg.* 2000;74(II), 102–109.
3. US Department of Commerce, Economic and Statistics Administration, US Census Bureau. 2000.
4. Gallagher C. *Lev Semyonovich Vygotsky.* http://www.muskingum.edu. Accessed June 19, 2009.
5. Rogoff B. *The Cultural Nature of Human Development.* New York, NY: Oxford University Press; 2003.
6. Stewart EC, Bennett MJ. *American Cultural Patterns: A Cross-Cultural Perspective.* Boston, MA: Intercultural Press; 1991.
7. Darby, ML, Walsh MM. *Dental Hygiene Theory and Practice.* 2nd ed. St. Louis, MO: Elsevier; 2003.
8. US Department of Health and Human Services. *Oral Health in America: A Report of the Surgeon General—Executive Summary.* Rockville, MD: US Department of Health and Human Services, National Institute of Dental and Craniofacial Research, National Institutes of Health, 2000.

9. American Dental Hygienists' Association. *National Dental Hygiene Research Agenda.* http://www.adha.org/research/index.html. Accessed June 19, 2009.

10. American Dental Hygienists' Association, 84th Annual Session, New Orleans, LA, 2007.

11. *Accreditation Standards for Dental Hygiene Education Programs.* Chicago, IL: Commission on Dental Accreditation, American Dental Association; 2008.

12. Mertz E, O'Neil E. The growing challenge of providing oral health care services to all Americans. *Health Affairs.* 2002;21(5):65–77.

PEARSON

Multimedia Extension Activities

Use this address to access the interactive Companion Website created for this textbook. Simply select "Dental Hygiene" from the choice of disciplines. Find this book and log in using your username and password. To obtain a username and password, please register using the scratch-off access code on the inside front cover of this book.

Chapter 12

Program Planning

After studying this chapter, the dental hygiene student should be able to:

- Define the dental hygiene process of care program planning paradigm
- Describe the various program planning paradigms
- Describe various dental public health programs
- Develop a dental public health program plan

KEY TERMS

Dental hygiene process of care
Paradigm
Prevention program
Program planning

COMPETENCIES

After studying this chapter and participating in accompanying course activities, the dental hygiene student should be competent to do the following:

- Promote the values of oral and general health and wellness to the public and organizations within and outside the profession
- Assess a community's oral health needs and the quality and availability of resources and services to address those needs
- Provide screening, referral, and education to bring consumers into the health care delivery system
- Provide community oral health services in a variety of settings
- Facilitate client access to oral health services by influencing individuals and/or organizations to support the provision of oral health care
- Evaluate the outcomes of community-based program and plan future ones

Dental hygienists frequently provide dental health presentations to target populations. Before planning for a dental health program can begin, the dental hygienist must review past programs and identify a **paradigm,** an outstandingly clear or typical example or framework that explains or illustrates a concept or theory. Although many different paradigms are available, all possess common threads necessary in developing programs of all types. These common threads are described later in the section on dental hygiene program planning paradigm.

Program planning encompasses the assessment, diagnosis, implementation, and evaluation stages of a dental public health program. This chapter discusses paradigms and the process of plannning a new dental hygiene program following a paradigm.

Did You Know?

A *paradigm* is a model of a specific concept such as the development and operation of a public health program.

COMMON DENTAL HEALTH PROGRAM PLANNING PARADIGMS

One of the reasons that dental public health may be difficult for students to grasp is that so many paradigms exist for developing public health programs.

Dr. A.C. Fones developed the first program planning paradigm or model in 1927 (see the Companion Website for a figure describing this paradigm). It reflected the efforts at that time to prevent and cure disease. He was a staunch believer in prevention and, when presenting this model, emphasized the fact that very few elementary schools had a well-defined health program.[1] Everything in the paradigm above a horizontal line represented efforts to prevent disease. He used the top of a tube to represent the ways that those who became ill, chiefly from preventable disease, convalesced, and then emerged in a healthy status. Everything below the line represented mortality.

DeBiase suggests that planning a dental health educational program includes identifying the target population, conducting a needs assessment, designing the program, and then implementing and evaluating it.[2] Although this model uses the same language dental hygienists use for lesson planning, its purpose is to develop an educational program rather than a dental treatment program.

Another model, the *planning and implementation strategy flowchart,* emphasizes the necessity for making ongoing needs assessments and revisions as well as the importance of assessment and planning. The emphasis on having an ongoing needs assessment and implementing revisions as needed are important functions in public health program operation. The Association of State Territorial Dental directors proposed a seven-step model for assessing oral health needs and developing community plans. (See Figure 12-1 ■.) The comprehensive plan addresses existing state infrastructure and policies and emphasizes quality assurance.[3]

Core Program Planning Functions for Government Agencies

The Institute of Medicine (IOM) in Washington, D.C., has identified core functions to be conducted by government public health agencies: assessment, policy development, and assurance to ensure effective dental care delivery. These core functions can be critical to program planning and evaluation. *Assessment* involves monitoring communities and populations at risk to identify their health needs and to set priorities for meeting them. It includes monitoring public health, collecting and interpreting data, examining case findings, and evaluating outcomes of programs and policies. *Policy development* is the process by which society makes decisions about problems, chooses goals and strategies to reach them, and allocates resources. Public policy formulation usually occurs through collaboration between the community, private sector, and government. *Assurance* involves making certain that all populations have access to appropriate and cost-effective services to reach agreed upon public health goals. In addition to treatment services for individuals, assurance activities include promoting health promotion and disease prevention. *Serving all functions* describes the research for new insights and innovative solutions to health problems.[4]

DENTAL HYGIENE PUBLIC HEALTH PROGRAMS

Program planning and implementation are quite possibly the most exciting areas of public health. Studying a population's needs and creating dental programs to meet them are motivating and intriguing. This first part of this section discusses generic program types, and final section describes specific private and publicly funded programs.

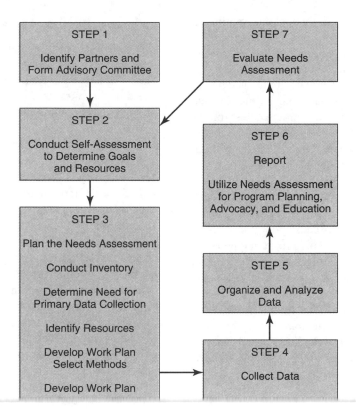

FIGURE 12-1   Assessing Oral Health Needs and Developing Community Needs

Source: Seven-Step Model for Assessing Oral Health Needs and Developing Community Plans.
Guidelines for State and Territorial Oral Health Programs. July 1997.

General Prevention Programs

A health **prevention program** is designed to prevent disease in a target population. Prevention programs can occur in a wide range of settings, including communities, schools, long-term care facilities, health care support groups, and day care facilities. Dental health educational programs seek to provide preventive dental health tools to large populations. Many are instituted in schools, such as a program consisting of a dental hygienist visiting a third grade class to present twenty minutes of dental health education are often sporadic and have no measurable outcome assessment.

A widely recognized and successful prevention program supports the use of fluoride to prevent caries. Historically, localities fluoridated their school water supplies, but now many local areas across the country implement a school fluoride mouth rinse program instead. In this program, students take time out to "swish and spit," as it is sometimes called. Dental hygienists coordinate the program and instruct the teachers in administering it.

Did You Know?

School fluoride mouth rinse programs represent a great preventive alternative for areas that have no public water supplies, such as those using well water.

Dental sealant programs are also common in schools. Dental hygienists and, when required, dentists travel to schools placing sealants on children's teeth and providing them oral hygiene instruction. This type of program enables students who may not visit the dental office to have the preventive benefits of dental interventions. It is an inexpensive program to prevent dental caries, especially for the 50% of the population who do not receive dental care via private dental offices.

Programs to promote dental health include having dental hygienists develop and implement a dental hygiene association–sponsored poster-designing contest for students during dental health month. The introduction of public health interdisciplinary programs is vital to the success and effectiveness of dental programs.

Through another program, dental hygienists in a school fabricate athletic mouth guards for all sports teams. Programs of this type are designed to prevent oral trauma and concussions because young athletes are often prone to dental trauma. This program type is frequently offered in middle and high schools because the number of school-sponsored athletics in the upper grades is high.

In a nonschool setting, long-term care facilities, commonly referred to as *nursing homes,* often hire dental hygienists to coordinate and provide a dental care program as a cost-effective way for their residents to obtain oral care. Such programs provide preventive services on a routine basis to help residents maintain their quality of life and dignity. Dentists are unable to visit long-term care facilities as frequently as dental hygienists and are therefore limited to providing urgent or restorative dental services. Facilities benefit from the resulting family satisfaction and enhanced reputation for providing total care to residents.

Collaborative dental programs are generally the most effective ones. For example, the collaborative relationship between dentist and dental hygienist long-term care facility programs benefits dental hygienists by providing a career option beyond private practice, and it allows dentists working in private practice to increase job satisfaction and care for the people who are underserved. Collaboration between teachers, social workers, case managers, and other health care providers in the operation of dental programs helps to integrate oral health into general health and promotes oral health as a valued service.

Did You Know?

Oral health screenings are mandated in all nursing facilities that receive Medicare or Medicaid funding, but many nursing facilities do not hire dental hygienists or dentists.

Existing Public Health Programs

One of the first practice settings for dental hygienists was in the Bridgeport, Connecticut, public school system. Since then, numerous organizations have offered preventive dental clinics and/or mobile dental practices that serve various populations.

University of New Mexico School-Based Dental Hygiene Clinics

The University of New Mexico (UNM) initiated the first school-based permanent dental clinic. Its Division of Dental Hygiene, Delta Dental of New Mexico, and the Albuquerque public schools have collaborated to develop school-based dental hygiene clinics.[5,6] Cooperative endeavors such as this one showcase the advantages of having the public sector and the private sector work together to create a program to improve public health.

These clinics provide restorative as well as preventive services in a coordinated effort with the nearby UNM Southeast Heights Dental Clinic. They offer UNM dental hygiene students the opportunity to work in a school-based environement. The dental clinic provides dental cleanings, fluoride treatments, sealants, individualized and classroom oral health education, dental exams, and referrals for needed treatment. The dental hygienist works with parents, teachers, and dentists to ensure optimal dental health for all students.

The University of New Mexico School-Based Health Center in cooperation with the Division of Dental Hygiene maintains a coordinated group of licensed dental providers to ensure access to quality oral health care to students attending Van Buren Middle School. Its goal is to improve the overall health of Van Buren Middle School students by striving to meet established program goals. (See Box 12-1 ▪)

Did You Know?

Many states have mobile prevention programs that travel to schools providing dental hygiene services to increase access for all children.

Collaborative Oral Prevention Program at Sandoval County, New Mexico, Health Commons

The New Mexico Department of Health, Sandoval County Government, Women with Infants and Children (WIC), and the UNM Division of Dental Hygiene

BOX 12-1 Program Goals, University of New Mexico School-Based Dental Clinic

1. **Patient Care.** Provide comprehensive dental hygiene assessment, treatment, and subsequent referrals that are in the best interest of the patient.
2. **Education.** Inform students of the significance of high-quality personal oral hygiene, proper diet and nutrition, diagnoses and maintenance of systemic diseases, and avoidance of addiction-forming substances in order to maintain a state of health.
3. **Oral Hygiene Instruction.** Evaluation of student's initial oral hygiene level and subsequent verbal and mechanical demonstration of oral hygiene measures including, but not limited to, tooth brushing, flossing, and pertinent oral hygiene adjuncts based on individual patient needs.
4. **Increase Access to Dental Care.** Raise the overall number of students that seek and receive preventive dental hygiene care by providing an environment that is readily available on site within the school setting.
5. **Non-traditional Practice Setting.** Generate a group of qualified oral health care practitioners who will provide oral health care in a non-traditional practice setting.
6. **Promote Oral Health Needs of Children.** Create a network of participating oral health care practitioners, school administrators and educators, and allied health care professionals that will serve as advocates for the oral health needs of school aged children.

UNM School-Based Dental Clinic Goals. Albuquerque: University of New Mexico, Division of Dental Hygiene. June 19, 2009.

DENTAL HYGIENIST SPOTLIGHT:
Tammi Byrd, RDH

Tammi Byrd is a wonderful inspiration for showing how many lives a dental hygienist can touch by reaching out! She is an excellent example of public health dental hygienists reaching out to the dentally underserved population—and she is an entrepreneur! She started the successful school-based dental program Health Promotion Specialists, which treats thousands of children every year in South Carolina. Many of these children would not be treated without her tireless efforts to operate the program. Ms. Byrd also teaches at Midland Technical College in South Carolina and has held numerous officer and council positions with the American Dental Hygienists' Association, including her tenure as president of the ADHA. She is the recipient of the ADHA Distinguished Service Award, the South Carolina Dental Hygienist of the Year Award (twice), and the South Carolina American Association of University Women/Women of Distinction Award.

I asked some questions about her career.

Why did you decide to pursue a dental hygiene degree?

A very close family friend who was a grandfather figure to me inspired me to want to serve others in the health care field. He was a physician, a family practitioner, who was always on the cutting edge. He designed the first neck brace, invented numerous "burn" creams and ointments used to this day, and dabbled in acupuncture yet always had time to attend medical association meetings, paint, travel, and spend time with his family. I knew I didn't want to work hospital hours; dental hygiene intrigued me, and my dental visits had always been pleasant.

How did you get into dental public health?

That's a good question. If you had asked me ten years ago if I'd be working in public health, I would've said no. I loved private practice periodontics and was a good clinician. But since my graduation, I've always been very active legislatively. When I graduated, dental hygienists in South Carolina were not able to work in schools and provide the same services my current program offers. Organized dentistry strongly opposed the original program, which allowed dental hygienists to work in schools, to the point that our state oral health division was shut down. I had seen the benefits of having dental hygienists provide preventive care in schools and become involved in the lobbying efforts to allow dental hygiene services to be delivered again with or without the division. To make a long story short, twenty years later, passage of new statutes to allow dental hygienists to deliver services without an exam by a dentist was imminent. Dental hygienists would again be able to work in school settings. I met with the policy adviser for the South Carolina Department of Health to discuss restarting our state public health dental hygiene division, but I was told that the state was not interested in being involved with the delivery of services. I asked how the law could be implemented without such a program.

The Department of Health understood the need for the program but did not know how it would come about. I left there feeling bewildered. After much soul searching and prayer, I knew it had to be done and that I, with God's help and the support of my husband, would make it happen.

Did you need additional education?

I had researched the supporting evidence for public health programs and saw how they operated when preparing to provide testimony to the legislature. Hindsight tells me that having a better understanding of business prior to starting one would have been beneficial. However, with the wealth of friends and colleagues that I have developed throughout my membership in ADHA, I had wonderful mentors I could count on for advice.

Can you discuss any particularly interesting experiences you have had in your dental public health position?

The entire experience has been interesting. I'm still amazed that even after seven years, a ruling by the South Carolina administrative law judge in our favor, a civil suit settlement with the South Carolina Dental Association, and an FTC ruling against the South Carolina Board of Dentistry, I'm still having to defend the merits of dental sealants to school board members, principals, and school nurses because the "local" dentists have told them that dental hygienists are sealing in cavities and the children will end up with "blown-up" teeth. It can be frustrating. But, one by one and group by group, we are educating the masses about the benefits of prevention.

When I see the smiles of the children we treat and hear the school nurses say there are fewer dental problems now, I know we're making a difference. We now have some dentists calling and asking our school-based program to add them to our referrals list.

What type of advice would you give us?

Understand cash flow, that being a boss can ruin friendships, that you must have the passion to stick with it, and you must have the desire to continue climbing the ladder of lifelong learning. Dental hygienists are in the best position ever to make a difference in the oral health of this nation. Consumers are going to demand increased access to services. We need to be prepared to deliver.

Source: Christine Nathe writes the Public Health Column in RDH magazine published by Pennwell Publishing. For more public health spotlights please see RDH magazine online at http://www.rdhmag.com/index.html.

are collaborating on a program at the Sandoval County Health Commons that provides an innovative dental hygiene clinical management program targeting pregnant women and their children. Oral health teams from UNM composed of a dental hygienist, dentist, and dental assistant focus on preventive dental hygiene services to pregnant women and children. They provide local oral health care management assessment, preventive service and practice as outreach workers, and serve as a referral resource for the WIC program and county health department for restorative dental care for patients in need. Sandoval County Health Commons provides UNM dental hygiene students "real-life" dental practice experience in an interdisciplinary setting.[7]

Matthew 25 Dental Clinics

More than thirty years ago, a dream of helping those in need became a reality for a group of parishioners from St. Mary's Catholic Church in Indiana who wanted to exemplify the verses from Matthew 25, a biblical call to care for the poor[8] (personal communication, Matthew 25, October 1999). The program Matthew 25 is a faith-based initiative. Its goals are to provide direct health care to those in need and promote health through education and screenings. It opened a medical clinic in 1976 and a dental clinic two years later. Matthew 25 provides dental care for individuals with low income who are not eligible for Medicaid. Its services include dental exams, cleanings, simple extractions, and restorations, and it provides dentures made by Indiana University dental lab students in the clinic's lab. Matthew 25, which does not rely on government grants for funding, continues to grow.

Operation Smile's International Dental Health Educational Program

Operation Smile (OS) is a private nonprofit, volunteer medical service organization that provides free dental work, reconstructive surgery, and related health care to indigent children and adults in the United States and developing countries. Dr. William Magee, a plastic surgeon and dentist, and his wife Kathy, a nurse and clinical social worker, founded OS in 1982.[9,10] The Magees traveled to the Philippines with a group of American physicians and nurses in 1981, where they provided surgery to children with cleft lip and palate deformities. Their frustration on realizing that more children needed treatment than could be seen during one visit led to the founding of OS. (See Box 12–2 ■.)

OS volunteer health care teams travel to various locations to provide surgeries for disfigurements such as cleft lip and palate deformities, tumors, orthopedic problem cancrum oris, and burn scars. Cancrum oris or noma, a commonly seen disease, is an acute, necrotizing process involving the mucous membrane of the mouth. It is characterized by rapidly spreading and painless destruction of bone and soft tissues. The condition is most commonly seen in children with poor oral hygiene,

malnutrition, and debilitating disease. Healing frequently occurs but often with disfiguring effects, and OS physicians perform reconstructive surgeries on patients affected by cancrum oris. Dental hygienists have an important role in preventing and controlling this disease.

Operation Smile provides education and training to achieve a long-term self-sufficiency dental hygiene program. It focuses on training teachers and health care workers to prevent and control oral disease and to promote dental health though an organized effort.

Dental hygienists are crucial in facilitating dental care in the countries OS serves. They implement the program in conjunction with a dental counterpart from the host country and secure funding for the program's dental care and educational supplies. Their primary role, however, is to plan and implement two-week training programs to educate teachers and health care providers on dental hygiene fundamentals. The training program presents basic lectures on oral anatomy, oral pathology, oral hygiene techniques, fluoridation, nutrition, dental screenings, dental emergencies, and teaching strategies. At the end of the didactic portion of the program, the participants present an oral health lesson to local schoolchildren and provide oral screenings under the supervision of OS dental hygienists. More important, these individuals serve the community as dental hygiene consultants when dental health concerns arise.

Many developing countries often place a low priority on dental conditions because they experience tremendous health issues. One way to improve the quality of life and challenge the exhausting health issues is through prevention. For this reason, dental hygiene plays a critical role in these countries.

BOX 12-2 Operation Smile

Operation Smile (OS), headquartered in Norfolk, Virginia, is a worldwide children's medical charity. It currently supports international and local, in-country medical missions to 25 countries.

Operation Smile partner countries include: Bolivia, Brazil, Cambodia, China, Colombia, Ecuador, Egypt, Ethiopia, Gaza Strip/West Bank, Honduras, India, Jordan, Kenya, Mexico, Morocco, Nicaragua, Panama, Paraguay, Peru, Philippines, Russia, South Africa, Thailand, Venezuela, and Vietnam.

Since 1982, more than 100,000 children and young adults have been treated by thousands of volunteers worldwide and thousands of healthcare professionals have been trained globally.

Operation Smile. Norfolk, VA. http://www.operationsmile.org. Accessed June 19, 2009.

DENTAL HYGIENE PUBLIC HEALTH PROGRAM PLANNING PARADIGM

The dental hygiene program planning paradigm in Box 12-3 ■ uses the steps of the dental hygiene process of care model in program planning. *Assessment, dental hygiene diagnosis, planning, implementation,* and *evaluation* are its basic elements. Refer to Chapter 9 for a detailed discussion of these steps.

Assessment

During the assessment phase, the dental hygienist assesses the population's needs, facility needs, resources, and funding. Population needs can be assessed by administering surveys or performing dental screenings using specific dental indexes that provide objective information, which often can be found in documentation from the facility, community, or existing grant applications. Surveys or personal

---

BOX 12-3 Dental Hygiene Program Planning Paradigm

Assessment

Assess via surveys, existing data, or dental screenings
Population's dental needs
Population's demographics
Facility availability and state
Workforce needed and available
Existing resources
Funding needed

↓

Dental Hygiene Diagnosis

Prioritize needs
Diagnose to provide goals and objectives for blueprint

↓

Planning

Develop blueprint
Identify methods to measure goals
Address constraints and possible alternatives

↓

Implementation

Begin program operation
Revise and make changes identified
Identify workforce and operation management

↓

Evaluation

Measure to determine success in meeting goals via surveys and dental indexes
Make qualitative and quantitative evaluation
Make ongoing revisions as needed

interviews aid in gathering information about demand, perceived needs, the population's approximate knowledge level, and existing problems and issues.

The assessment phase should identify facilities (public school, nursing home, or other organization) involved, specifically regarding available space, equipment, and dental and educational materials as well as workforce needs, sometimes referred to as *labor force planning*. In regard to this, it is essential to determine whether dental hygienists are allowed to work without supervision of dentists, which would decrease personnel needs. Dental coordination should be addressed for a program combined with a larger one.

> **Did You Know?**
>
> Ensuring an interdisciplinary approach to care using nurses, teachers, social workers, and other health care providers in addition to dental health providers enhances a program's value to the public.

Dental Hygiene Diagnosis

A dental hygiene diagnosis basically identifies needs, which is the natural conclusion to the assessment phase. Dental hygienists must prioritize these diagnoses in order of severity and offer care following that order.[11] An example of a dental hygiene diagnosis based on an assessment follows. The majority of prison inmates diagnosed using two dental indexes had moderate to advance periodontal diseases and heavy calculus. While analyzing this information, the dental public health planner noted that most inmates had not had their teeth cleaned for more than fifteen years and then made the dental hygiene diagnosis of periodontal disease associated with no regular dental hygiene care.

Planning

Planning involves reviewing the target population assessment that was used in making the diagnosis. This information provides the basis for formulating program operations. The first step is to draw a dental program blueprint identifying the goals, objectives, and methods to measure the program's effectiveness; activities planned; possible constraints and detailed strategies to address them; and funding for the program. A program's effectiveness can be measured both quantitatively by using pretest/posttest exams and dental indexes and qualitatively by conducting surveys and interviews and obtaining personal statements from those who participated.

Implementation

The dental hygiene program actually begins to operate at the implementation stage. It can be revised as necessary during this stage. Most programs require revisions as a result of unforeseen difficulties or needs not originally assessed.

> **Did You Know?**
>
> Implementation includes managing the program and the people working in the program. Effective communication results in a more effective team.

Evaluation

The program must be evaluated to determine its success and to ensure that it functions at the optimum level. The methods used to evaluate the program are determined in the planning phase. Program evaluation is discussed in more detail in Chapter 13.

SUMMARY

Dental hygienists working in public health typically develop dental programs for target populations. These programs assess a population's needs and then plan an appropriate intervention directed at the needs identified. During the need assessment, evaluative mechanisms should be identified.

Effectively planning and implementing a dental public health program can be challenging and exhausting. It is important to remember the dental hygiene process of care at each stage.

SELF-STUDY TEST ITEMS

1. Which of the following is part of the planning phase of program development?
   a. Identify methods to measure goals
   b. Assess the population's dental needs
   c. Begin program operation
   d. Revise program as needed

2. Dr. Fones's original paradigm for the school dental hygienist program focused on
   a. Restoration
   b. Utilization of a case manager
   c. Prevention of disease
   d. All of the above

3. Which school program is particularly advantageous for middle school athletes?
   a. Sealant program
   b. School fluoridation
   c. Case management
   d. Athletic mouth guard program

4. During which stage of the program paradigm planning should the target population's needs be identified?
   a. Assessment
   b. Dental hygiene diagnosis
   c. Planning
   d. Evaluation

5. A dental hygienist employed in a nursing home could provide routine preventive care. In addition, the dental hygienist could have a collaborative relationship with a dentist so that restorative and urgent care is provided as needed.
   a. The first statement is true; the second statement is false.
   b. The first statement is false; the second statement is true.
   c. Both statements are true.
   d. Both statements are false.

REFERENCES

1. Fones AC. *Mouth Hygiene*. 3rd ed. Philadelphia, PA: Lea and Febiger; 1927.

2. DeBiase CB. *Dental Health Education Theory and Practice*. Philadelphia, PA: Lea & Febiger; 1991.

3. *Seven-Step Model for Assessing Oral Health Needs and Developing Community Plans*. Guidelines for State and Territorial Oral Health Programs. July 1997. http://www.astdd.org/docs/Introduction.pdf. Accessed June 19, 2009.

4. Institute of Medicine. The Future of the Public's Health in the 21st century. Washington, DC: National Academy Press; 2003.

5. Nathe CN. Back to school. *RDH*. July 2008.

6. Nathe CN. School-based dental clinics: Collaboration and partners. *RDH*. April 2008.

7. Nathe CN. UNM Clinical Programs. *Educ Update*. January 2008.

8. Matthew 25 Health/Dental Clinic. http://www.matthew25online.org/services.html. Accessed September 8, 2008.

9. Nathe C. Operation Smile: Dental hygiene program. *Den Hyg News*.1994;7:9–10.

10. Operation smile: About us. http://www.operationsmile.org/aboutus/history/. Accessed September 9, 2008.

11. Darby ML. The dental hygiene process. *Dent Hyg*. 1981;55:6,10.

PEARSON

myhealthprofessionskit™

Multimedia Extension Activities

Use this address to access the interactive Companion Website created for this textbook. Simply select "Dental Hygiene" from the choice of disciplines. Find this book and log in using your username and password. To obtain a username and password, please register using the scratch-off access code on the inside front cover of this book.

Chapter 13

Program Evaluation

With contributions from

Elaine Sanchez-Dils, RDH, MA

OBJECTIVES

After studying this chapter, the dental hygiene student should be able to:

- Describe the mechanisms of program evaluation
- Compare qualitative and quantitative evaluation
- Identify various dental indexes and define their purposes

KEY TERMS

Clinical evaluation
Dental index
Formative evaluation
Measurement
Nonclinical evaluation
Summative evaluation

COMPETENCIES

After studying this chapter and participating in accompanying course activities, the dental hygiene student should be competent to do the following:

- Assess the oral health needs of the community and the quality and availability of resources and services
- Provide screening, referral, and education to bring individuals into the health care delivery system
- Evaluate the outcomes of community-based programs and plan future activities

During a dental public health program and at its completion, the program planner must use scientific techniques to ascertain its effectiveness. Without evaluations, dental health programs cannot be promoted as effective tools in preventing and/or treating dental diseases.

When planning a program, including those addressing the health needs of a target population and to formulate meaningful content, planners identify the methods that will measure how well goals are being met. Planners also identify the strengths and weaknesses of the program's workforce, strategies, and organization. Evaluations of the perceptions and attitudes of the target population should serve as guidelines for discussion and recommendations related to specific problems and their solutions. Formal and informal results of the evaluation, which is ongoing during all program phases and activities, are regularly reported. The process involves obtaining and interpreting baseline data. Baseline data are the data that are collected during the assessment phase, before a program has been started and can be used to identify needs and subsequently evaluate a program.

Qualitative and quantitative documentation of the program must be reported to its administrators, funding agency, and target population, and the general public on an ongoing basis. See Box 13-1 ■ for questions to ask when planning a program's evaluation. *Qualitative evaluation* involves non-numerical data such as perceptions and attitudes of the population from observations, survey results, and interviews to determine how well a goal is being accomplished. Although not reported numerically, a numerical coding system for qualitative data should be developed in order to summarize the results. *Quantitative evaluation* identifies measures expressed as a quantity or amount, often on a numerical scale. **Measurement** refers to the process of using a particular method to gauge or evaluate something; counts, proportions, ratios, rates, prevalence, and incidence are all quantitative measures. An evaluation enables planners to revise the program as needed to improve its outcomes.

Did You Know?

Both qualitative and quantitative measures are equally important when evaluating a program because each provides a unique perspective of it.

BOX 13-1 Questions to Ask When Planning a Program

- What should be evaluated?
- Whom should be evaluated?
- Who should administer the evaluation?
- When should the evaluation be conducted?
- How should the evaluation be conducted?

Formative evaluation is an internal examination of a program's process and is usually conducted while planning the program. **Summative evaluation** is an examination of a program's merit after it has been implemented. *Performance management* refers to the systematic process by which an organization involves its employees as individuals and members of a group in improving program effectiveness in accomplishing its mission.

EVALUATION TECHNIQUES

Many methods are available to evaluate a dental public health program's effectiveness. They are grouped into two areas: nonclinical and clinical. (See Table 13-1 ■.) **Nonclinical evaluations** are studies or appraisals employing questionnaires, individual or group interviews, telephone interviews, focus groups, direct observations, document analysis, and surveys. **Clinical evaluations**

Table 13-1 Methods Used to Evaluate the Effectiveness of Dental Public Health Programs

Nonclinical Methods	Clinical Methods
Face-to-face personal interviews	Basic screenings
	Epidemiological examinations
Telephone interviews	
Surveys	
Document analysis	
Focus groups	
Observation	

are studies or appraisals supported by clinical data such as basic screenings and epidemiological examinations that utilize dental indices. *Basic screenings* can be performed quickly using a tongue blade and dental mirror. In contrast, *epidemiological examinations* consist of detailed visual-tactile assessment of the oral cavity with dental instruments, a dental mirror, and a dental light. When conducting an oral health survey, the public health practitioner must communicate the limitations of the examination using either type of method to the population. When disease is identified during an oral health survey, the practitioner has a responsibility to provide a referral for treatment. Refer to Box 13-2 ■ for different areas of dentistry to be evaluated. These areas can be indicators such as disease status of a population, modalities used to prevent disease, or use of dental care by a population.

Did You Know?

Oral health screenings provided during health fairs are least likely to yield usable data, especially when they are performed without adequate illumination.

Dental caries examinations are classified according to the comprehensiveness of the examination; Type 1 is the most comprehensive and Type 4 is the basic, or least comprehensive; an epidemiologic examination is

---

BOX 13-2 Dental Indicators to Evaluate

- Access to care
- Dental caries
- Dental care delivery
- Dental hygiene treatment
- Dental fluorosis
- Dental treatment needed
- Dental sealants
- Occlusion
- Oral cancer
- Oral and craniofacial diseases and conditions
- Oral disease disparities
- Oral health and quality of life
- Oral trauma
- Periodontal diseases
- Social impact of oral health
- Tooth loss
- Water fluoridation

Type 3. (See Box 13-3 ■.) Because neither basic nor epidemiologic examinations constitute a thorough dental examination for diagnostic and treatment purposes, a Type 1 or Type 2 examination must be performed when treatment is planned. However, if treatment will not be provided by a dental program, the comprehensiveness of Type 1 and Type 2 examinations is unnecessary, costly, and unethical due to the radiographic exposure.

BOX 13-3 Classification of Dental Caries Examinations

Type 1—Complete Examination

Comprehensive including all tests, it is the least commonly used in public health and is not required for epidemiologic studies.

Type 2—Limited Examination

Performed with a mouth mirror, explorer, and adequate illumination and exposed posterior bite-wing radiographs and selected periapicals, this is useful for a public health treatment program but is not required for oral health surveys.

Type 3—Inspection

The most common type used in public health programs employs a mouth mirror, explorer, and adequate illumination.

Type 4—Screening

The least valid type uses a tongue depressor and available illumination and produces the largest number of false negatives.

DENTAL INDEXES

A **dental index** is a standardized quantitative method for measuring, scoring, and analyzing oral conditions in individuals and groups. During a program's planning stage, the planner identifies the index to be used in the implementation phase. A dental index score is used to educate, motivate, and evaluate a patient and can serve as a legal record. A comparison of index scores from an initial exam during a follow-up exam can indicate the effects of personal daily care and/or a program or specific treatment. Characteristics of a dental index include clarity, simplicity, objectivity, validity, reliability, that it is relatively easy and quantifiable. See Table 13-2 ■ for a definition of these desirable characteristics.

> **Did You Know?**
>
> A dental index used during program evaluation or research can be compared to a dental examination of a patient, which is then evaluated at subsequent appointments.

Indexes can be described as simple, cumulative, irreversible, and reversible. A *simple* index measures the presence or absence of a condition; a *cumulative index*

Table 13-2 Desirable Characteristics of a Dental Index

Characteristic	Definition
Clarity	Criteria are understandable
Simplicity	Results are easily measured
Objectivity	Results are not subject to individual interpretation
Validity	Index measures what is intended
Reliability	Examiner consistency and calibration are reproducible
Quantifiability	Statistics can be applied
Sensitivity	Small degrees of difference can be detected
Acceptability	Subjects experience no pain and index expense is minimal

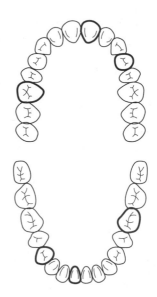

FIGURE 13-1 Ramjford Teeth

measures all past and present evidence of a condition. An *irreversible index* measures conditions that will not change, such as dental caries, whereas a *reversible index* measures those that can be changed, such as the presence of plaque.

Many index types screen only a few teeth or tooth surfaces. Usually these teeth are the six teeth numbered 3, 9, 12, 19, 25, and 28 as shown in Figure 13-1 ■, referred to as *Ramjford teeth*. The Ramjford teeth are six teeth that are representative of all the teeth, in other words, these teeth can be generalized to the entire dentition. See the interactive Companion Website created specifically to accompany this textbook for more information on the labeling of tooth surfaces and teeth numbers. A few frequently used indexes are described next.

Common Dental Indexes for Plaque, Debris, and/or Calculus

Patient Hygiene Performance (PHP) and Patient Hygiene Performance Modified (PHP-M) (Table 13-3 ■)

Purpose: Assesses extent of plaque and debris over facial surfaces of incisors and maxillary molars and ingual surface of mandibular molars; PHP-M used for Ramjford teeth with same scoring process.[1,2]

Table 13-3 Patient Hygiene Performance (PHP) Rating Scale

Rating	Scores
Excellent	0
Good	0.1–1.7
Fair	1.8–3.4
Poor	3.5–5.0

Procedure: Divide each tooth numbered 3, 8, 14, 19, 24, 30 into five subdivisions (two in interproximal portion) and direct lingual and facial areas into thirds (cervical, middle, and coronal). After application of disclosing solution, score each area retaining plaque and/or debris up to 5 points per tooth (basically, the tooth is divided into 5 subsections). Divide total points given to all teeth by total number of teeth assessed.

Example Question Answered: Will the use of dental plaque charting during oral hygiene instruction result in adolescent motivation to improve oral hygiene as measured by this index?

Plaque Control Record (PCR)

Purpose: Records presence of bacterial plaque on individual tooth surfaces.

Procedure: After application of disclosing solution, examine gingival margins for plaque.

Scoring: Count and record number of surfaces with retained plaque; calculate the index by dividing the number of plaque-containing surfaces by the total number of available surfaces.[1,3]

Example Question Answered: Does the Plaque Control Record indicate that the use of a mouth rinse prior to toothbrushing significantly reduces in the amount of plaque?

Plaque-Free Score

Purpose: Determines the location, number, and percent of plaque-free areas of teeth.

Procedure: Record the number of surfaces of plaque marked by the applied disclosing solution.

Scoring: Multiply total number of teeth by 4 to calculate number of available surfaces; subtract number of surfaces with plaque to find number of plaque-free surfaces. To determine percentage, multiply last number by 100.[1,3]

Example Question Answered: What are the clinical effects of power toothbrushing on the presence of gingivitis and supragingival dental plaque as measured by the Plaque-Free Score?

Plaque Index (Pl I)

Purpose: Assesses thickness of plaque in gingival area in evaluating each of four tooth surfaces—distal, facial, lingual, and mesial—for plaque retention.

Procedure: Use a periodontal probe to identify the plaque level on each tooth evaluated.

Scoring: Plaque levels: free = 0, small amount = 1, moderate amount visible to the naked eye = 2, large amount in the sulcus or at the gingival margin = 3. Add scores for all teeth and divide by number of teeth assessed.[1,3]

Example Question Answered: Which is more effective in improving a patient's oral health, the recognition of gingival bleeding as infection or the use of disclosing tablets to see dental plaque?

Oral Hygiene Index (OHI) and Oral Hygiene Index Simplified (OHI–S) (Table 13-4 ■)

The OHI has two components, the debris index and the calculus index; either or both can be evaluated.

Applied to: Tooth numbers 3, 8, 14, 24; lingual surfaces of tooth numbers 19, 30 (both OHI and OHI–S).[1,3]

Purpose: Measures existing plaque and calculus as oral cleanliness indication.

Table 13-4 Oral Hygiene Index (OHI) and Oral Hygiene Index Simplified (OHI-S)

OHI and OHI-S Ratings	OHI Scores	OHI-S Scores
Excellent	0.0	0.0
Good	0.1–0.6	0.1–1.2
Fair	0.7–1.8	1.3–3.0
Poor	1.9–3.0	3.1–6.0

DENTAL HYGIENIST SPOTLIGHT:
Lynn Bethel, RDH, BSDH, MPH

Lynn Bethel, RDH, BSDH, MPH, is a dental hygienist who has a wealth of experience in public health. Currently, she serves as Interim Director of the Office of Health in Massachusetts. In addition, she is the Association of State and Territorial Dental Directors (ASTDD) liaison to the ADHA. She also mentors other dental hygienists as an adjunct faculty member at the Department of Dental Hygiene of Mount Ida College, Massachusetts. She has lectured and published articles pertaining to public health in various venues. She also has served as the program coordinator for school oral health programs in Massachusetts and has been very active in various dental organizations, including service as president of the Massachusetts Dental Hygienists' Association.

What is so amazing about Ms. Bethel is the way she became interested in dental public health—not necessarily dental hygiene. She answered questions about her story.

Why did you decide to go into dental hygiene?

During the summers of my junior and senior years in high school in the late 1970s, I worked as a teacher's assistant in a Head Start program. A woman would come in and talk to the children about their teeth, look at their teeth, and so on. I decided from that experience that I wanted a job like that. My goal for my life at that point was to drive from school to school to teach toothbrushing and check teeth. It wasn't until my senior year of high school that I learned that the woman who visited the Head Start programs was a dental hygienist; so I then decided I was going to be a dental hygienist. The funny thing was that I had no idea that the "red-haired lady" who cleaned my teeth every six months was also a dental hygienist. It wasn't until the first week of hygiene school when the mirrors and explorers are passed out that I had any knowledge that dental hygienists worked in dental offices. A dental office was not where I wanted to work; I wanted to work in schools, but I stuck it out for the next eighteen months to get to the fourth semester when community dental health was in the curriculum.

How did you get into dental public health?

I don't think I got into dental public health. I think dental public health was always in me, and dental hygiene was the path I took to express it.

Did you need additional education?

After graduating from hygiene school with my associate's degree in 1983, I transferred to Old Dominion University in Norfolk, Virginia, for my bachelor's degree. I received a bachelor's degree in dental hygiene with a minor in sociology in 1984. While I was there, I volunteered to spend some of my summer on the Delmarva Peninsula providing dental treatment to the migrant workers on the Eastern Shore. During the day, I would go into the schools and provide oral health education to the children, and at night I would work on a mobile dental van where the workers who had come directly from the fields would receive both preventive and restorative treatment. I always knew I wanted a master's degree in public health (MPH), so in 1991, I began working toward that part-time by attending the Boston University School of Public Health. I was the only person with a dental background. The other students worked in medicine or law, for large companies, nonprofits, and so on, which made it a great educational experience. I wasn't learning about dental public health, but public health and, in that, I learned how to apply the principles of public health to my interests in dental hygiene. I graduated in 1995 with my MPH.

What are your current positions?

I am the Interim Director in the Office of Oral Health, a consultant for the Massachusetts Department of Public Health, and I serve on the Massachusetts Coalition for Oral Health. In addition, I am a clinical dental hygienist (part-time) in the same pediatric practice I have worked in since 1987. I teach dental hygiene as a faculty member at Mount Ida College. I also serve as editor of *Prevention Matters.*

Do you have any exciting experiences to share?

Every day is a learning experience for me both professionally and personally. I have learned so much (and am still learning) about fluoride and fluoridation issues. One day, I might be consulting with local water operators, a dental professional, or listening to a resident of the state who has a question or concern about fluoridation. Another day, I could be meeting with partners on a program we are developing, writing a grant, or working with dental hygiene students on a school-based sealant program. I can tell you honestly that I have never left work wishing I wasn't doing what I was doing or wishing that I wasn't a dental hygienist.

What advice would you give to a practicing hygienist who is thinking about doing something different?

These are my five recommendations in order:

1. Stop thinking and do!
2. Go back to school! If you have an associate's degree, go get a bachelor's degree. If you have a BS, go get

a master's degree. Education opens not only doors but also your mind. From one degree to the next, you learn so much beyond your normal scope of thinking, and you experience yourself in different situations. Education is invaluable.

3. Consider every opportunity offered to you. It may be to join an oral health coalition or assist with a fluoridation campaign or a sealant program. But with each opportunity, you'll network with other professionals in public health and gain a lot of knowledge and experience.

4. Don't let money be your guide. I noticed a few years ago that I always have just what I need. It may not be everything that I think I want, but it has always been what I have needed.

5. Remember that dental hygiene isn't just about scaling.

Source: Christine Nathe writes the Public Health Column in RDH magazine published by Pennwell Publishing. For more public health spotlights please see RDH magazine online at http://www.rdhmag.com/index.html.

Procedure: Select one tooth with most debris or calculus from each sextant; use periodontal probe or explorer to estimate amount of its debris or calculus and assign a score.

Scoring: Add all scores for all sextants, and divide by number of sextants evaluated.

Example Question Answered: What is the state of oral cleanliness of school children at age 10 as measured by the Oral Hygiene Index?

Common Dental Indexes for Gingival Bleeding

Gingival Bleeding Index (GBI)

Purpose: Records presence or absence of gingival inflammation as determined by bleeding from interproximal gingival sulci.

Procedure: Pass unwaxed dental floss interproximately into the gingival sulcus on both sides of the interdental papillae alternately using new length of clean floss for each interproximal unit. Then evaluate floss and site for bleeding and reevaluate nonbleeding sites after 30 seconds for delayed bleeding.

Scoring: Add number of all bleeding points.[1,4]

Example Question Answered: Does use of a power flosser positively enhance oral hygiene status?

Sulcular Bleeding Index (SBI) (Table 13-5 ■)

Purpose: Locates areas of gingival sulcus bleeding upon gentle probing.

Procedure: Evaluate four gingival areas (marginal from the facial and lingual aspects, mesial and distal papillary) per tooth for bleeding. After probing, wait 30 seconds before scoring.

Table 13-5   Sulcular Bleeding Index (SBI) Scoring Criteria

Score	Criteria
0	Healthy appearance of gingiva, no bleeding upon probing
1	Healthy appearance of gingiva, no change in color, no swelling or bleeding upon probing
2	Bleeding upon probing, change of color, no swelling
3	Bleeding upon probing, change of color, slight swelling
4	Bleeding upon probing, change of color, obvious swelling
5	Bleeding upon probing, spontaneous bleeding, change of color, marked swelling

Scoring: Divide sum of all surfaces scored by 4.[1,4]

Example Question Answered: Is there a significant reduction in the amount of bleeding when a chlorhexidine rinse is used as an adjunct to normal oral hygiene practices?

Eastman Interdental Bleeding Index (EIBI)

Purpose: Measures papillary bleeding after interproximal stimulation as indicator of inflammation in papillary gingiva.

Procedure: Depress the papilla with wooden interdental cleaner inserted horizontally between the teeth from the facial aspect 1–2 mm and then remove cleaner; repeat four times. Record presence or absence of bleeding within 15 seconds.

Scoring: Divide sum of the interdental spaces that bled by total number of spaces evaluated.[1,5,6]

Example Question Answered: Does the addition of a flossing aid to a toothbrushing regime decrease interproximal bleeding as measured by the Eastman Interdental Bleeding Index?

Common Dental Indexes for Gingival Changes

Gingival Index (GI) (Table 13-6 ■)

Purpose: Assesses severity of gingivitis of facial, lingual, mesial, and distal aspects of each tooth based on color, consistency, and bleeding when probed.

Procedure: To evaluate one tooth or more or all teeth, insert probe into sulcus 1–2 mm, gently press against gingiva to determine firmness, and move probe circumferentially in horizontal stroke along soft tissue side of the pocket.

Scoring: Give each tooth assessed a score of 0–3 and divide score for each tooth by 4. For multiple teeth, total all scores and divide by total number of teeth.[1,7,8,9]

Example Question Answered: Is brushing with a hydrogen peroxide-sodium bicarbonate paste as effective as brushing with fluoridated toothpaste in reducing gingival inflammation and bleeding in patients with periodontitis?

Common Dental Indexes for Periodontal Diseases

Periodontal Index (PI) (Table 13-7 ■)

Purpose: Measures periodontal disease in populations based on the clinical exam alone or combined with radiographic evaluation.

Procedure: Perform a clinical examination with periodontal probe and diagnostic radiographs.

Scoring: Give each tooth assessed score of 0–8 and then average scores to determine index (for a population, average all individual scores). The higher the score, the higher is incidence of periodontal disease.[3,10]

Example Question Answered: What are the effects of having lifelong access to free dental care on the periodontal disease status of adults?

Gingival Periodontal Index (GPI)

Purpose: Combination of Gingival Index and Periodontal Index discussed previously to assess gingivitis and pocket depth in dentition. This index

Table 13-6 Gingival Index Criteria for Scoring Facial, Lingual, Mesial, and Distal Aspects of Each Tooth Assessed

Points	Appearance	Sulcular Bleeding	Inflammation
0	Normal	None	None
1	Slight color change, mild edema, slight texture change	None	Mild
2	Redness, hypertrophy, edema, glazing	Bleeding on probing	Moderate
3	Marked redness, hypertrophy, edema, ulceration	Spontaneous bleeding	Severe

Table 13-7   Criteria for Scoring Periodontal Index

Score	Criteria for Field Study	Additional Radiograph Criteria
0	Negative	Normal appearance
1	Mild gingivitis	None
2	Gingivitis	None
4	Not used in field study	Early resorption of the alveolar crest
6	Gingivitis with pocket formation	Horizontal bone loss involving the entire alveolar crest and up to half of the length of the root
8	Advanced destruction of bone	Advanced bone loss involving more than half of the length of the root

can be used to provide detail regarding both gingivitis and periodontitis.

Periodontal Disease Index (PDI) (Table 13-8 ■)
It is a modified version of the Periodontal Index (PI) for Ramjford's teeth.

Purpose: Assesses prevalence and severity of gingivitis and periodontitis and shows the periodontal status of an individual or a group.

Procedure: Perform a clinical examination of the tissues, including use of the periodontal probe.

Scoring: Give each Ramjford's tooth assessed a score of 0–6 and average them (for a population, average all individual scores).[3,10] Tissue is graded based on inflammation, redness, bleeding, ulceration, and loss of attachment.

Example Question Answered: Is prevalence of periodontal diseases greater in elderly patients as opposed to the general population as measured by the Periodontal Disease Index?

Community Periodontal Index of Treatment Needs (CPITN) and Periodontal Screening and Recording (PSR) (Tables 13-9 ■ and 13-10 ■)

Purpose: CPITN classifies individual or group periodontal treatment needs quickly and efficiently. Gingival recession does not result in a higher score.

Table 13-8   Criteria for Scoring Periodontal Disease Index

Score	Appearance
0	Absence of inflammation
1	Mild to moderate inflammatory gingival changes not extending completely around tooth
2	Mild to moderately severe gingivitis extending completely around tooth
3	Severe gingivitis, characterized by marked redness, tendency to bleed, and ulceration
4	Periodontal loss of attachment on any portion of tooth extending no more than 3 mm
5	Periodontal loss of attachment on any portion of tooth extending 3–6 mm
6	Periodontal loss of attachment on any portion of tooth extending more than 6 mm

Table 13-9 Criteria for Scoring Community Periodontal Index of Treatment Needs (CPITN) and Periodontal Screening and Recording (PSR)

CPITN Status	Score	PSR Status
Healthy periodontal tissues	0	Colored area of probe completely visible
Bleeding after probing	1	Colored area of probe completely visible with bleeding after probing
Supra- or subgingival calculus present, or a defective margin found on a restoration	2	Colored area of probe completely visible with supra- or subgingival calculus present, or a defective margin found on a restoration
4–5 mm pocket	3	Colored area of probe partially visible
6 mm or deeper pocket	4	Colored area of probe not visible
Not used	*	Furcation involvement, mobility, a mucogingival problem or recession

Table 13-10 Criteria for Classifying Community Periodontal Index of Treatment Needs (CPITN)

Classification	Criteria
0	No need for treatment
I	Oral hygiene instruction given
II	Oral hygiene instruction with scaling and root planing and removal of defective margins
III	I+II and any recommended complex periodontal therapy such as surgery

Procedure: Probe each sextant to determine deepest pocket depth using specially designed probe for CPITN and PSR.

Scoring: Use classification from 0–III (for a population, average all individual scores or compile frequency data).[1,11,12]

Example Question Answered: Are marked periodontal probe depth changes found when comparing advanced periodontal patients on three-month recalls with those on six-month recalls following scaling and root planing?

Common Dental Indexes for Dental Caries

Decayed, Missing, or Filled Permanent Teeth or Surfaces (DMFT or S) (Table 13-11 ■)

Purpose: Determines status of dental caries activity of decayed, missing, or filled teeth or surfaces of permanent dentition.

Procedure: Evaluate twenty-eight teeth, excluding third molars, by clinically examining five surfaces of each posterior tooth (occlusal, lingual, facial, mesial, and distal) and four surfaces of each anterior tooth (facial, lingual, mesial, and distal) and record using stated criteria.[1,3,13] DMFT stands for total number of teeth, whereas DMFS stands for total number of surfaces and can only be completed with the use of radiographs. Because DMFS accounts for all surfaces it is much more detailed. The totals are calculated per each indicator including decayed, missing and filled (D, M, or F).

Scoring: Sum totals within each category scored D, M, or F.

Example Question Answered: What effects does exposure to a dental health fair have on the total caries rate of attendees as measured with the DMFT preattendance and three-year postattendance?

Table 13-11 Criteria for Recording a Decayed, Missing, or Filled Permanent Teeth or Surfaces (DMFT or S) Score

Score	Criteria
D	Dental carious lesion is present
	Dental caries and a restoration are present
	A tooth is broken because of caries
	Third molars with dental carious lesions are not counted
	Supernumerary teeth with dental carious lesions are not counted
	Teeth restored for reasons other than dental carious lesions such as esthetics purposes or use as an abutment tooth are not counted
M	Tooth has been extracted or is not restorable and indicated for extraction
	Teeth that have been extracted for orthodontic purposes or impactions are not counted as missing
	Third molars that have been extracted are not counted as missing
	Unerupted teeth are not counted as missing
	Congenitally missing are not counted
F	Permanent or temporary restoration is present
	Third molars with restorations are not counted
	Supernumerary teeth with restorations are not counted

Decayed, Extracted, Filled Primary Teeth or Surfaces (DEFT or S)

This index is always written in lowercase letters as opposed to uppercase DMFT because it is used for the primary dentition.

Purpose: Determines status of decay, extractions, and filled primary teeth or tooth surfaces

Procedure: Evaluates twenty primary teeth using same procedure as DMFT or S index.[1,3]

Scoring: Use same scores as DMFT or S index.

Example Question Answered: Is there increased risk of developing nursing bottle caries in children in day care facilities?

Root Caries Index (RCI)

Purpose: Calculates ratio of teeth with carious lesions of the root and/or restorations of the root to teeth with exposed root surfaces.

Procedure: A clinical examination is conducted by counting the number of root caries in the dentition.

Scoring: Add numbers of caries and root restoration together, divide sum by total number of teeth showing gingival recession, and multiply this number by 100. 0 = minimum score; 100 = maximum score; the higher the score, the more diffuse is the caries.[11]

Example Question Answered: What are the effects of fluoride varnish on root caries development?

Common Dental Index for Malocclusion

Treatment Priority Index (Table 13-12 ■)

Purpose: Measures malocclusions according to the Malocclusion Severity Estimate (MSE) and records results; mesio-, nuetro-, and disto-occlusion measured keeping nuetro-occlusion constant.

Procedure: Perform a clinical examination of the occlusions, measuring occlusal defects.

Rating: Maloclussion is assessed according to the rating of the scale shown in Table 13-12: 0 to >10.[14,15]

Table 13-12 Ratings for the Treatment Priority Index

Rating	Description
0	Virtually classic normal occlusion
1–3	Minor manifestations of malocclusion and treatment
4–6	Definite malocclusion, but treatment is elective
7–9	Severe handicap, treatment highly desirable
>10	Very severe handicap, treatment mandatory

Example Question Answered: What are the types of malocclusions found in a group of Argentinean primary school children and what is the need for orthodontic treatment in relation to age by using the Treatment Priority Index?

Common Dental Indexes for Dental Fluorosis

Developmental Defects of Dental Enamel (DDE)

Purpose: Scores enamel opacities regardless of origin of opacities to avoid any bias.

Procedure: Examine entire mouth for any enamel mottling and select two worst teeth for evaluation. If two teeth have unequal amounts of mottling, chose the one less affected. Dry tooth for 2 minutes and then score it.

Scoring: 0 = no fluorosis present, 1–2 = mild fluorosis, 3–9 = advanced changes to enamel.[16,17]

Example Question Answered: What is the prevalence of caries and developmental defects of enamel in nine- to ten-year-old children living in areas in Mexico with different water fluoride amounts?

Dean's Index of Fluorosis (Table 13-13 ■)

Purpose: Rates fluorosis within a population; is sensitive to mild through severe cases.

Procedure: Same as for DDE index.

Criteria: Normal to severe.[10,18]

Example Question Answered: What is the estimated prevalence and level of fluorosis attributable to fluoridation using Dean's Index of Fluorosis?

Table 13-13 Criteria for Classifying Dean's Index of Fluorosis

Classification	Description
Normal	Smooth, glossy, pale creamy-white translucent surface
Questionable	Few white flecks or white spots
Very mild	Small opaque, paper white areas covering less than 25% of tooth surface
Mild	Opaque white areas covering less than 50% of tooth surface
Moderate	All tooth surfaces affected; marked wear on biting surfaces; brown stain may be present
Severe	All tooth surfaces affected; discrete or confluent pitting; brown stain present

Fluorosis Risk Index

Purpose: Assesses fluorosis, particularly the specific time of enamel formation.

Procedure: Divide enamel surfaces of permanent dentition into two developmentally related surface zones: classification I for enamel formation begun during first year of life, and classification II for enamel formation begun in years 3–6.

Scoring: Give each zone a negative for fluorosis or positive for mild to moderate fluorosis. Zone with more than 50% display of pitting, staining, or deformities indicates severe fluorosis.[19]

Example Question Answered: Is there an association between enamel fluorosis and infants given formula?

Tooth Surface Index of Fluorosis (TSIF) (Table 13-14 ■)

Purpose: Rates fluorosis within a population more sensitively than Dean's Index.

Procedure:

Scoring: Give separate score 0–7 (0 = no fluorosis evidence, 7 = missing enamel surface large areas of enamel with altered tooth anatomy, dark

Table 13-14   Criteria for Scoring Tooth Surface Index of Fluorosis (TSIF)

Score	Description
0	No evidence of fluorosis appears
1	Parchment white fluorosis involves < 33% of visible tooth surface
2	Parchment white fluorosis involves ≥ 33% but < 66% of visible tooth surface
3	Parchment white fluorosis involves ≥ 66% of the visible tooth surface
4	Enamel staining occurs in conjunction with any of preceding findings
5	Discrete pitting of enamel surface occurs without staining of intact enamel
6	Discrete pitting of enamel surface and staining of intact enamel occur
7	Enamel surface shows confluent pitting, large areas of enamel may be missing with altered tooth anatomy, and dark brown stain is usually present

brown stain) to each facial and lingual surface of anterior teeth and buccal, occlusal, and lingual surface of posterior teeth.[11]

Example Question Answered: What fluorosis effects are seen in people living in a community with four times the optimal concentration of fluoride?

Other Common Dental Indexes

Several other indexes are calculated as rates or proportions that describe a portion of a whole that possesses a particular characteristic. Two of the most commonly used are incidence and prevalence rates, which typically refer to the occurrence of an attribute, for example a disease, in a population. *Incidence rates* refer to how many new cases are seen, and *prevalence rates* refer to the total number of cases at a given time. Some examples of dental conditions that may use rates for description are cleft lip or palate cases and oral cancer. An example question might be this: What is the prevalence rate of oral cancer diagnoses in Turkey?

GOVERNMENTAL EVALUATION OF ORAL HEALTH

The oral health goal of *Healthy People 2010* is to prevent and control oral and craniofacial diseases, conditions,

and injuries and to improve access to related services.[20] All oral health objectives in *Healthy People 2010,* managed by the Office of Disease Prevention and Health Promotion of the US Department of Health and Human Services, include a way to measure each objective. See Table 13-15 ■ for specific objectives and evaluation mechanisms.

The National Oral Health Surveillance System (NOHSS), a collaborative effort between the Centers for Disease Control and Prevention and The Association of State and Territorial Dental Directors, is based on a set of oral health indicators from *Healthy People 2010*.[21] NOHSS is designed to aid public health programs in monitoring the prevalence of oral diseases, the dental care delivery system, and the use of fluoridation. (See Box 13-4 ■.) The oral health indicators include the list in Box 13-5 ■.

Did You Know?

The specific oral health disease patterns or dental rates for each state can be found at http://www.cdc.gov/nohss/.

Table 13-15 Healthy People 2010: Oral Health Objectives and Evaluation Mechanism

Objectives	Evaluation Mechanism
Decrease deaths from oral and pharyngeal cancer	Number of oral cancer deaths per 100,000 population
Increase early detection of oral and pharyngeal cancer	Percentage of individuals with recent oral and pharyngeal examination within the past year
Increase annual examinations for oral and pharyngeal cancer	Percentage of persons with recent oral and pharyngeal cancer diagnosed at earliest stage
Decrease dental caries experience	Percentage of persons with > 1 dft or DMFT
Decrease untreated dental decay	Percentage of persons with > 1 dt or DT
Decrease permanent tooth loss	Percentage of persons with 28 teeth, no teeth extracted
Decrease complete tooth loss	Percentage of persons with all teeth extracted, edentulous
Reduce periodontal diseases	Percentage of persons with > 1 bleeding site
	Percentage of persons with > 4 mm Loss Of Attachment (LOA) in at least one site
Increase use of dental sealants	Percentage of persons with > 1 sealant on permanent molars
Increase community water fluoridation	Percentage of people served by community water systems with optimal fluoride levels
Increase use of oral health care system	Percentage of individuals with annual dental visits
Increase use of oral health care system by residents using long-term care facilities	Percentage of nursing home residents with dental service within last year
Increase dental services for low-income children	Percentage of low-income children and adolescents with preventive dental service within last year
Increase school-based health centers with oral health component	Percentage of school-based health centers with an oral health component
Increase health centers with oral health component	Percentage of local health departments and community-based health centers with oral health component
Increase referral for cleft lip or palate	Percentage of states with system for recording and referring orofacial clefts

Source: http://www.healthypeople.gov. Accessed September 14, 2009.

BOX 13-4 National Oral Health Surveillance System

Analytic Considerations of Behavioral Risk Factor Surveillance System (BRFSS), National Health and Nutrition Examination Survey (NHANES), National Health Interview Survey (NHIS), and Youth Risk Behavior Surveillance System (YRBSS)

Estimates for certain population subgroups based on small numbers may be subject to relatively large sampling error. When both the number of events and their probability are small, considerable caution must be observed in interpreting the conditions (cell size < 50). Data from multiple years may be pooled to obtain adequate sample size.

Behavioral Risk Factor Surveillance System

BRFSS is a state-based, ongoing data collection program that measures behavioral risk factors in the noninstitutionalized population eighteen years of age or older. Each state selects a random sample of adults monthly to participate in a telephone interview. This selection process results in a representative sample for the state so that statistical inferences can be made from the information collected.

Basic Screening Survey (BSS)

BSS is a standardized set of cross-sectional and descriptive surveys that collect information on the observed oral health of participants; self-reported or observed information on age, gender, and race and Hispanic ethnicity; and self-reported information on access to care for preschool, school-age, and adult populations. Dentists, dental hygienists, and other appropriate health care workers observe gross dental or oral lesions in accordance with state law. The health care worker or dental provider records the presence of (1) untreated cavities and urgency of need for treatment for all age groups, (2) early childhood caries and caries experience for preschool children, (3) sealants on permanent molars and caries experience for school-age children, and (4) edentulism (no natural teeth) for adults. States may use one or more of the surveys in the BSS in screenings to obtain oral health status and data related to dental care access at a level consistent with monitoring *Healthy People 2010* objectives. Training materials are provided with the surveys and technical assistance on sampling and analysis is available to states taking these surveys using standard protocol. BSS was developed by the Association of State and Territorial Dental Directors with technical assistance from the Division of Oral Health, National Center for Chronic Disease Prevention and Health Promotion, Centers for Disease Control and Prevention.

1992 Fluoridation Census

The 1992 Fluoridation Census is a record of the fluoridation status for each state. It identifies each state's fluoridated water system and the communities each system served; the status—adjusted, consecutive, or natural—of fluoridation; the system from which water was purchased, if consecutive; the population receiving fluoridated water; the date on which fluoridation started; and the chemical used for fluoridation, if adjusted. Adjusted means that fluoride is added or removed, whereas natural means that the fluoride was naturally present.

2000 Water Fluoridation Reporting System

Populations Receiving Optimally Fluoridated Public Drinking Water—United States, 2000* provides the most recent information on the status of water fluoridation by state.

National Health and Nutrition Examination Survey

NHANES I, NHANES III, and NHANES IV collected oral health data. Conducted between 1971 and 1975, NHANES I was based on a national sample of about 28,000 persons between the ages of one to seventy-four (but not persons of Hispanic/Latin origin according to survey design). Extensive data on health and nutrition were collected by interview, physical examination, and laboratory analyses.

NHANES III, conducted between 1988 and 1994, included about 40,000 people selected from households in eighty-one counties across the

United States. To obtain reliable estimates, infants and young children (one to five years), older persons (sixty years and older), Black Americans, and Mexican Americans were sampled at a higher rate. NHANES IV, a continuous survey visiting fifteen US locations per year, began in April 1999. Approximately 5000 people will be surveyed annually. Oral health data from the completed NHANES IV will be added to NOHSS.

National Health Interview Survey

The NHIS is a cross-sectional household interview survey on the health of the civilian noninstitutionalized population of the United States. The plan follows a multistage area probability design that permits the representative sampling of households. NHIS data are collected annually from approximately 43,000 households including about 106,000 persons.

Pregnancy Risk Assessment Monitoring System (PRAMS)

PRAMS collects state-specific, population-based data on maternal attitudes and experiences prior to, during, and immediately following pregnancy. It provides data for state health officials to use to improve the health of mothers and infants. Each participating state annually samples between 1300 and 3400 women who have had a recent live birth. The sample participants are taken from the state's birth certificate file. Women from some groups are sampled at a higher rate to ensure that adequate data are available in smaller but higher risk populations. Selected women are first contacted by mail but if they do not respond to repeated mailings, they are contacted and interviewed by telephone. Data collection procedures and instruments are standardized to allow comparisons between states. PRAMS enables the Centers for Disease Control and Prevention (CDC) and the states to monitor changes in maternal and infant health indicators (eg, unintended pregnancy, prenatal care, breast-feeding, smoking, alcohol use).

Synopses of State Dental Public Health Programs

The Synopses of State Dental Public Health Programs is a collection of oral health program information provided to the Association of State and Territorial Dental Directors (ASTDD) annually by each state's dental director or oral health program manager. ASTDD, in conjunction with CDC's Division of Oral Health, includes that information with data from standard sources (US Census, Department of Education, Bureau of Labor Statistics, etc) on the State Synopses Web site. Each state's synopsis contains information specific to it on demographics and oral health infrastructure, program administration, and activities. An interactive national trend table aggregates that information to track changes over time. Maps indicate which states conduct each of twelve types of oral health activities and which have full-time dental directors.

Youth Risk Behavior Surveillance System

A school-based survey conducted biennially to assess the prevalence of health risk behaviors among high school students, YRBSS includes national, state, territorial, and local school-based surveys. The surveys employed a cluster sample design to produce a representative sample of students in grades 9–12 and to protect the students' privacy by allowing for anonymous and voluntary participation.

*MMWR. 2002;51(7):144–147.

Source: http://www.cdc.gov/nohss/DSMain.htm.

BOX 13-5 Specific National Oral Health Surveillance System Indicators

• Caries experience
• Complete tooth loss
• Dental sealants
• Dental visits
• Fluoridation status
• Oral and pharyngeal cancer
• Teeth cleaning
• Untreated caries

SUMMARY

Evaluation is a mandatory phase of any type of dental hygiene program. A variety of evaluation mechanisms can be utilized during all phases of program planning. Dental indexes are frequently used to determine effectiveness of program planning.

SELF-STUDY TEST ITEMS

1. Program goals should be evaluated based on
   a. Measurement tools
   b. Baseline data
   c. National guidelines
   d. State surveillance records

2. During which phase of program planning should evaluation be started?
   a. Assessment
   b. Dental hygiene diagnosis
   c. Planning
   d. Evaluation

3. Which type of evaluation refers to the internal evaluation of a program?
   a. Formative
   b. Summative
   c. Quantitative
   d. Qualitative

4. Which type of evaluation is a basic screening?
   a. Nonclinical
   b. Clinical
   c. Provider driven
   d. Educational

5. An index that measures a condition that will not change, such as dental caries, is termed a(n)
   a. Clinical index
   b. Nonclinical index
   c. Irreversible index
   d. Reversible index

REFERENCES

1. Wilkins E. *Clinical Practice of the Dental Hygienist.* 10th ed. Philadelphia, PA: Lippincott, Williams and Wilkins; 2009.
2. Darby M. *Mosby's Comprehensive Review of Dental Hygiene.* 6th ed. St. Louis, MO: Elsevier; 2006.
3. Darby M, Walsh M. *Dental Hygiene Theory and Practice.* 2nd ed. St. Louis, MO: Saunders; 2003.
4. Tomko P. *Kaplan National Dental Hygienist Licensure Exam.* New York, NY: Simon and Schuster; 2005.
5. Caton J, Polson A. The interdental bleeding index: A simplified procedure for monitoring gingival health. *Compendium Continuing Educ Dent.* 1985;6:88–92.
6. Caton J, Polson A, Bouwsma O, Blieden T, Frantz B, Espeland M. Associations between bleeding and visual signs of interdental gingival inflammation. *J Perodont.* 1988;59:722–727.
7. Bollmer BW, Sturzenberger OP, et al. A comparison of 3 clinical indices for measuring gingivitits. *J Clin Periodont.* 1986;13:392–395.
8. Loe, H. The Gingival Index, the Plaque Index, and the Retention Index. *J Periodont.* 1967;38:610–616.
9. Marks RG, Magnusson I, et al. Evaluation of reliability and reproductivity of dental indices. *J Clin Periodont.* 1993;20:54–58.
10. Dentistry and Oral Medicine. *The Medical Algorithms Project.* Houston, TX: Institute for Algorithmic Medicine; 2006–2007.
11. Ainamo J, et al. Development of the World Health Organization (WHO) Community Periodontal Index of Treatment Needs (CPITN). *Int Dent J.* 1982;32:281–291.
12. Periodontal Screening and Recording (PSR) Index: Precursors, utility and limitations in a clinical setting. *J Lebanese Dent Assoc.* 2002;40(2):81–87.
13. Caries Prevalence: DMFT and DMFS from the World Health Organization: Switzerland. www.whocollab.od.mah.se/expl/orhdmft.html. Accessed June 17, 2009.
14. Ugur T, Ciger S, Aksoy A, Telli A. An epidemiological survey using the Treatment Priority Index (TPI). *Eur J Orthod.* 1998;20:189–193.
15. Ununcu N, Ertugay E. The use of the Index of Orthodontic Treatment Need (IOTN) in a school population and referred population. *J Orthod.* 2001;28:45–52.

16. Wozniak K. Changes in developmental defects of dental enamel with in the space of centuries. *Durham Anthropol J.* 2005;12(2–3).

17. Clarkson J. Review of terminology, classifications, and indices of developmental defects of enamel. *Adv Dent Res.* 1989;3(2):104–109.

18. Pereira A, Moreira B. Analysis of three dental fluorosis indexes used in epidemiological trials. *J Dent Braz.* 1999;10:1–60.

19. Pendrys DG. The Fluorosis Risk Index: A method for investigating risk factors. *J Public Health Dent.* 1990;50:291–298.

20. US Department of Health and Human Services. *Healthy People 2010: Understanding and Improving Health.* 2nd ed. Washington, DC: US Government Printing Office; 2000.

21. National Oral Health Surveillance System. CDC: Atlanta. http://www.cdc.gov/nohss. Accessed June 17, 2009.

PEARSON
myhealthprofessionskit™

Multimedia Extension Activities

Use this address to access the interactive Companion Website created for this textbook. Simply select "Dental Hygiene" from the choice of disciplines. Find this book and log in using your username and password. To obtain a username and password, please register using the scratch-off access code on the inside front cover of this book.

Unit III

Dental Hygiene Research

Dental hygiene practice is based on published research, meaning that practitioners derive decisions from documented evidence rather than anecdotal tradition. This is commonly referred to as *evidence-based practice*. Moreover, dental hygienists share the responsibility not only to practice science-based modalities but also to increase the scientific body of knowledge that encompasses the dental hygiene sciences.

Although many dental hygienists choose to practice in the clinical field, those working in other settings also incorporate research into their daily practice. It is imperative for the practitioner to fully understand basic research principles. Additionally, dental hygienists must be able to critically evaluate scientific literature and dental care products and modalities and subsequently communicate accurate information to the public whom they serve.

Chapter 14

Research in Dental Hygiene

Beth E. McKinney, RDH, MS

OBJECTIVES

After studying this chapter, the dental hygiene student should be able to:

- Explain the purpose of dental hygiene research
- Discuss the use of evidenced-based practice in dental hygiene
- Describe the role of ethics in research
- Identify the role of government and private entities in research
- Explain the connection between research and private practice

KEY TERMS

bioethics
hypothesis
informed consent
institutional review board (IRB)
literature review
null hypothesis
research proposal
research (positive) hypothesis
sampling techniques
scientific method

COMPETENCIES

After studying this chapter and participating in accompanying course activities, the dental hygiene student should be competent to do the following:

- Use evidence-based decision making to evaluate and incorporate emerging treatment modalities
- Assume responsibility for dental hygiene actions and care based on accepted scientific theories and research as well as the accepted standard of care

Dental public health seeks to prevent disease and control it when it does occur in populations through evidence-based programs that are cost-effective to administer. Conducting research is necessary to develop new programs that meet these criteria and to ensure that entrenched programs have not become obsolete. To accurately interpret research, dental hygienists must understand basic research principles.

Much of dental hygiene practice exists within the confines of a private clinical setting in which the practitioner is concerned with a single patient at any given time. Dental hygienists' ability to assess an individual's condition, plan and carry out an intervention, and expect predictable results from treatment is predicated on a much larger sphere in which the study of dental disease and the creation of dental practices originate: the world of public health research.

The number of dental professionals who practice research full-time is small, yet the volume of information generated by medical, dental, and pharmaceutical researchers is more that the average practitioner has time to review thoroughly. Conducting research often can seem distant and unrelated to a practitioner's daily concerns; however, practice is based on this same research. The encounter of a dental hygienist with a single patient bears many commonalities to the structure of research methodology. (See Table 14-1 ■.)

Table 14-1 Analogy between Private Practice and Research Methodology

Private Practice Methodology	Research Methodology
Identifies chief complaint	Takes survey or makes observations about a population
Takes health history	Conducts literature review
Makes diagnosis	Develops research question or hypothesis
Determines treatment plan	Writes research proposal
Obtains informed consent for treatment	Obtains informed consent
	Obtains research funding
Imitates treatment intervention	Conducts research
Recalls or reevaluates patient	Analyzes and publishes research results

RESEARCH AND DENTAL PUBLIC HEALTH

Throughout history, astute practitioners have made many observations about the occurrence of disease in specific populations. Some illnesses seem to run in families. Others seem confined to specific ethnic groups, and other diseases are rarely seen in certain populations. The study of disease in populations is accomplished by conducting research using the **scientific method,** which is a body of techniques using observation, reason, and experimentation to gather evidence that is empirical and measurable. (See Box 14-1 ■.) The accuracy of the research determines the usefulness of the information obtained and the conclusions that can be drawn. Good research is the foundation for understanding why disease occurs and how to prevent and control it.

Evidence-Based Practice

If dental hygiene advice and treatment are to be based on known methods with predictable results rather than anecdotes, scientific research is crucial. The requirement for using evidence-based dental hygiene means that students be taught the practice of dental hygiene based on independent research done by practitioners and scientists as reported in peer-reviewed medical and dental hygiene journals. For example, the standard treatment modality for a patient with incipient periodontal disease might be quadrant scaling. A return to health and normal probing depths would be expected in a reliable percentage of cases treated in this fashion. Evidenced-based practice also considers patient preferences. (See Figure 14-1 ■.) That would include what treatment option the patient is interested in receiving as well as patient compliance. Dental hygienists who graduated from school several decades ago were more likely to base their practices on what their instructors had learned from trial and error and anecdotal reports from other hygienists, the proverbial "what worked

BOX 14-1 Steps of the Scientific Method

1. Name the problem or question.
2. Form an educated guess (hypothesis) of the cause of the problem and make predictions based on the hypothesis.
3. Test hypothesis by doing an experiment or study (with proper controls).
4. Check and interpret results.
5. Report results to the scientific community.

DENTAL HYGIENIST SPOTLIGHT:
Gayle McCombs, RDH, MS

Gayle McCombs, RDH, MS, is a dedicated researcher with a public health agenda who helps broaden the science on which dental hygiene practice is built. She currently is an associate professor and the director of the Old Dominion University Dental Hygiene Research Center. She is the author of several published research papers and has spoken on numerous topics. Professor McCombs has also won numerous research awards. She exemplifies a dental hygiene scholar with a focus on building the knowledge base of the profession and practice.

She answered the following questions about her career.

How did you decide to pursue dental hygiene as a career?

After working as a dental assistant for many years and observing the dental hygienist in the office, I decided that I wanted to advance my career. While in dental hygiene school, one of my instructors was very instrumental in formulating my life's goals. Unfortunately, after graduation, she became very ill with cancer. One day while I was visiting her in hospice, she made me promise that I would continue my education and become a teacher.

For the next ten years, while working in private practice, I pursued my bachelor's degree, and I ended up teaching in the Florida and South Carolina community college systems. As time went by, I wanted to broaden my professional options. I decided to press on for a master's degree at the University of North Carolina-Chapel Hill. It was during graduate school that I was introduced to clinical research. Throughout the program, the mentorship and support I received from professors Rebecca Wilder and Steven Offenbacher, in addition to the experience I gained, shaped my career.

Did you need additional education or credentials for dental hygiene research?

I acquired my research foundation in graduate school; however, most of my practical experience is a result of working as a research faculty member at UNC-CH. Learning how to manage and coordinate clinical trials involves a great deal of organizational skill. In addition to sponsor and governmental regulations, there are professional and ethical responsibilities that must be adhered to.

Agencies such as the National Institutes of Health (NIH), the Food and Drug Administration (FDA), the pharmaceutical industry, local universities, and private clinical research training organizations such as the Society of Clinical Research Associates (SoCRA) offer numerous continuing education courses and workshops in clinical trial management. There are also various online training opportunities to become certified or obtain specialty training in topics such as monitoring, regulatory affairs, and clinical trial design and management.

What is the most valuable piece of advice you can give?

Be adaptable, self-motivated, and have the capability to be a leader, as well as a team player.

What do you think the future holds for this field?

I believe it is wide open for those individuals who are interested in research. When our graduate students complete the program, they have no problem finding employment. I think one of the most rewarding aspects of my job is getting students energized about research. I mentor students who are fearful of the process and then watch as they become excited about research once they realize they can be successful.

Do you have any suggestions for others who may be considering research as a career?

My suggestion to those who would like to follow this path would be start out simple. Volunteer for a study, take a course, shadow someone in research, search the Internet, and read your professional journals. Seek out someone who is involved in clinical research and observe for a day or two to see whether this is something that sparks your interest.

Source: Christine Nathe writes the Public Health Column in RDH magazine published by Pennwell Publishing. For more public health spotlights please see RDH magazine online at http://www.rdhmag.com/index.html.

FIGURE 14-1 *Evidence-Based Practice*

for them." Although this anecdotal approach has frequently been the basis for treatment, it is not the most scientific or reliable method. Clinicians are not the only people who are frequently swayed by anecdotal tales. Dental hygienists encounter patients daily who have selected an oral care product because of an advertisement or because the product worked for a friend.

Dental hygiene practice has changed as the result of research. For many years, instructors taught that fluoride treatments should be given only after scaling and polishing. Likewise, patients were instructed to brush and floss at home prior to rinsing with fluoride. The prevailing argument was that the plaque needed to be removed for the fluoride to be effective. These practices remained the standard of care for many years until one day a researcher questioned them and, discovering a lack of evidence to support them, conducted a research study to test their effectiveness. The research study revealed that fluoride can indeed penetrate plaque.[1,2] Dental hygiene practice based on documented evidence from critically reviewed research is referred to as *evidence-based practice*.[3] However, many dental hygienists continue to remove all plaque with prophy paste prior to applying fluoride. In this case, the anecdotal method and the method based on scientific research differ widely.

The importance of conducting dental hygiene research is to establish a scientifically based standard of care for the practice of dental hygiene. Understanding something about research methods benefits any dental hygienist whether directly involved in conducting research or only occasionally reading about it to be able to critically decide whether the research has scientific merit and should be applied in daily practice.

Because of what is now known about the multifactorial nature of disease, which will be discussed in more detail in Chapter 16, using the same anecdotal treatment that met with success on patient A does not guarantee that patient B will obtain the same results.

THE COMPONENTS OF A RESEARCH STUDY

Research always begins with a question. Someone wonders why something is so. Why do 25% of the children in the US have 80% of the caries? Why is the survival rate for oral cancer low? Why are communities becoming more resistant to water fluoridation? If milk were fluoridated, would it work as well as water to prevent caries? Does having soda in school vending machines affect caries rates?

The Research Question or Hypothesis

The first step when planning a research project is the development of a **hypothesis,** which is a question to be answered by a study. Hypotheses are the result of asking a question *that can be researched.*

After answering the research question, a hypothesis can be stated in terms of a positive outcome, (a **research** or **positive hypothesis**) or in terms of a negative outcome, as a **null hypothesis** (a statistical hypothesis to be tested and accepted or rejected in favor of an alternative).

Question: Which instrumentation use is superior in periodontal debridement?

Research (Positive) Hypothesis: Ultrasonic instrumentation is significantly more effective than hand scaling during periodontal debridement.

Null Hypothesis: Ultrasonic instrumentation is not significantly more effective than hand scaling during periodontal debridement.

BOX 14-2 Research Hypothesis Characteristics

A researchable hypothesis must be:

- Ethical to all participating subjects
- Necessary research, that has the possibility to
  - Improve clinical practice
  - Improve health policy
  - Confirm or change previous theories
  - Recommend future research directions
- Fundable research that
  - Includes adequate number of subjects
  - Is cost effective
  - Is manageable in terms of the project scope
  - Involves professional expertise

Question: Does brand X toothpaste really whiten teeth?

Research (Positive) Hypothesis: Brand X significantly whitens teeth.

Null Hypothesis: No statistically significant difference exists between brand X and a placebo when comparing the ability to whiten teeth.

Questions or hypotheses often arise from researcher observations and experienced occurrences. They may also come from questions arising out of previous research projects and from colleagues' experiences. For a hypothesis to be considered researchable, it must possess all the characteristics listed in Box 14-2 ■. Hypotheses are usually stated in the null form. If the researcher finds that a significant difference does exist, the null hypothesis is rejected, thereby stating that a difference does exist.[4]

Basics of Research

When a valid hypothesis has been stated, the researcher must write a detailed plan for the study called a **research proposal** or protocol. The proposal is often used not only to validate the significance of the research but also to secure funding. Funding for major research studies is highly competitive and awards are based in part on how well the proposal is written. Funding can come from private industry or the governmental sector as discussed in Chapters 3 and 4. Small studies not involving the manipulation of human subjects may be funded by grass roots organizations or local health care coalitions.

After formulating a workable hypothesis, the second step is to conduct a **literature review,** which is an examination of all pertinent reports and studies to determine what is currently known about the issue. The researcher may find that the question has already been answered or that little information on the subject is available. Literature reviews should include all issues associated with the research topic.

Reviewing the literature once required many hours of library time looking through card catalogs and journal indexes. Thanks to the technological advances of computers and the Internet, literature reviews can now be conducted online. Any clinician can conduct a literature review to find the most current information about a disease or a treatment. The largest volume of online literature in the United States is at the National Library of Medicine.[5,6] Begun in the 1800s, it now contains more than 17 million citations online going back as far as the 1950s. New journal references are added monthly. Searching for information on a subject in the Internet is now remarkably easy and will bring up a plethora of information on almost any subject. However, the quality of information on Web sites are not regulated, so researchers should carefully and critically view scientific information that does not come from legitimate and trusted sources.

The third step in writing a proposal is to design the research project. See Box 14-3 ■ for some questions to

BOX 14-3 Questions to Ask When Writing a Research Proposal

- How will the research question be answered?
- What method will be used to gather data?
- Will human subjects be needed?
- Will the project require any manipulation of subjects?
- Will collaborators be needed to conduct the research?
- How will the examiners be calibrated (standardized)?
- Will funds and/or supplies be needed?
- How will funds and/or supplies be purchased?
- Will human subjects be compensated?
- Are previously used data collection instruments valid?
- Can the resulting data be statistically analyzed?
- What statistical methods will be used?
- How many subjects are needed?
- Will a control group be used?
- How will the sample groups be selected?
- Does a pilot study need to be conducted first?
- Who will fund the research?
- How much money will be needed?

ask when deciding on the research design. All of those questions and likely others need to be carefully thought out and addressed before the researcher recruits the first subject or sends out the first questionnaire. For this reason, research is often time consuming and requires months or years to conduct. (Teaching actual methodology of research is beyond the scope of this textbook; for more detailed information, the reader is referred to specific textbooks on research and/or a separate class on the subject.)

Developing a study's methods depends on the research approach chosen. If a *descriptive approach* is chosen, for example, the researcher likely develops a survey. Designing historical approaches and retrospective studies should be done at the same time the statistical method for analyzing the data is chosen. Experimental approaches are frequently clinical, laboratory, or epidemiological in nature and tend to employ specific, well-validated designs. These approaches are discussed in detail in Chapter 15.

These three main components—the research question, the literature review, and the research study design make up the research proposal.

Until this point, the research project may have been conducted entirely by one researcher called the *principal investigator.* At the point of the study's implementation, research most often takes on a team approach. It generally takes a group of people working in concert to successfully conduct a research project.

Sampling Techniques

Researchers generally cannot study an entire population that may be affected by a particular disease. The logistics and cost of such research would be prohibitive. Therefore, researchers select a sample population to study. To generalize research results to the whole population, the researcher must be sure that the sample is a representative subset. Different techniques can be used to select a sample from a population to study. These **sampling techniques** vary in how well they represent the population and in how easy they are to employ. Random, stratified, systematic, convenience, judgmental or purposive, and cluster are all sampling techniques.

The best way to ensure adequate representation is to take a *random sample* in which every possible subject is selected independently and has an equal chance of

being selected for the project. Selection may be done by lottery for a small sample or by computer for a large sample. Ensuring that no hidden patterns exist that could threaten randomness is important.

Did You Know?

Stratifying a sample provides additional data from studies by breaking the sample into populations.

Systematic technique samples every *nth* subject, which can be determined by dividing the total population size by the desired sampling size. Every third subject could be chosen for a study or a researcher studying all 8000 residents in state nursing homes could choose a sample of 800 residents. The nth term would then be computed by diving 8000 by 800, which equals 10.

Types of Samples

A sample can be large or small depending on the type of research. A large sample is the most accurate representation of the population. This is especially important for descriptive studies for which a large sample is more likely to produce valid results. It is easier to demonstrate statistical significance of differences when large sample sizes are used in experimental studies.

Individuals have the right to participate or not in a study. This volunteer participation can result in loss of subjects from longitudinal studies. A longitudinal study involves repeated observations of the same items over long periods of time. Attrition must be planned by selecting an initial sample size adequate to accommodate the loss of study participants. Otherwise, resulting group sizes will be too small to produce valid results.

Several terms describe a group selected for evidence-based research. A *convenience sample* is composed of individuals who are most readily available to be selected for the study.[7] A researcher who wants to study the prevalence of oral cancer at a nursing home may be able to study the "whole" population there. However, the results could not be applied to other nursing homes because for the study to be generalized, a sample of residents in multiple facilities is needed.

An intact group is a *convenient* group of subjects that is already together, such as children in a classroom, an orphanage, or a head start program. This group's advantage is the convenience of the subjects, especially for certain types of research. Intact groups and volunteers are used because of the impracticality of using random or other samples. The problem with the use of intact groups, however, is that they do not represent the population in many ways; therefore, their use introduces bias.

Bias is introduced into an experiment by the method used to select the subjects who are to participate in it. For example, a clinician who understands a study's purpose and uses personal judgment to select patients to represent typical patients creates *selection bias.*[7] Although not appropriate for experimental research studies, *judgmental samples* are effective for action research, which in relation to health care involve the reflective evaluation of current community programs designed to improve health practices and behaviors by changing them.

Research should ideally represent a cross-section of the population with regard to gender, age, race, and ethnicity. Much research has been criticized recently because certain groups were not well represented in study populations. The omission of these groups can make a difference when trying to apply study information to other groups. For example, if a drug is tested only on men, does similar dosing apply to women and children? If a drug for hypertension is tested only in males, will it work the same way in females? Research often is not feasible for some populations—for example, pregnant women are not typically considered as good candidates for drug studies.

On the one hand, public health is ideal for recruiting subjects who provide an adequate cross-section of the population because public health tends to serve a wide variety of target populations. On the other hand, public health serves people who are typically socioeconomically disadvantaged and should not be targeted as research subjects. Death rates from oral cancer are higher for African Americans than for other races, even when adjusting for later diagnosis, which makes this population much more at risk and in need of research support to decrease these death rates.[8] Suppose a researcher wished to study a new treatment for oral cancer. A good way to recruit patients might be through a state-sponsored program that conducts community oral cancer screenings funded by tobacco restitution money. Patients who qualified for and enrolled in the study would receive free treatment. Would those candidates be more likely to participate in the research study because it is the only way they can afford to obtain treatment?

In summary, random samples result in the most representative samples. Judgmental and convenience samples can result in selection bias. Even when samples are large and selected randomly, results of research using such samples can never predict the effects on the whole population with complete accuracy. This is seen most frequently with new drugs that are taken off the market when serious side effects occur in widespread use that did not appear in the testing phases.

Data Analysis and Interpretation

When a study has been completed or at prescribed intervals in a long one, the data are collected for statistical analysis, the method of which is decided selected prior to the study's inception. Often not all data collected are useful for analysis. For example, subjects withdraw or are lost from studies for many reasons. Unless the researcher is experienced in statistical analysis, a biostatistician is often asked to do the mathematics, and now several computer programs available fortunately make this task simpler. Chapter 18 provides more detail on data analysis and interpretation. For an amusing look at how statistics can be misinterpreted and misused, read Mark Clifton's "The Dread Tomato Affliction" (Box 14-4 ■).

Research Conclusions and Publication

No single research study can prove a hypothesis. Hence, most research articles end with the caveat that more research in the area is warranted. No single research study can be applied beyond the population that was studied. Each bit of information gathered from a well-designed research study contributes to the overall body of knowledge and suggests additional questions for study.

For research to make the leap from the scientist's bench to evidence-based practice, it must be published. Peer-reviewed journals allow a panel of professionals from the same (or similar) discipline to assess the merits of the research and access the largest volume of readers. Without the distribution of this information, dental hygienists in private practice will not be able to incorporate new knowledge and techniques into daily practice that will benefit both clinicians and patients. Oral health and dental hygienists' occupational health can and do suffer as a result. Through professional journals, the science of the laboratories becomes the art of patient care.

BOX 14-4 The Dread Tomato Addiction by Mark Clifton

- 92.4% of juvenile delinquents have eaten tomatoes.
- 87.1% of the adult criminals in penitentiaries throughout the United States have eaten tomatoes.
- Informers reliably inform that of all known American communists, 92.3% have eaten tomatoes.
- 84% of all people killed in automobile accidents during the year 2000 had eaten tomatoes.
- Those who object to singling out specific groups for statistical proofs require measurements within a total. Of those people born before the year 1850, regardless of race, color, creed or caste, and known to have eaten tomatoes, there has been 100% mortality!
- In spite of their dread addiction, a few tomato eaters born between 1850 and 1900 still manage to survive, but the clinical picture is poor—their bones are brittle, their movements feeble, their skin seamed and wrinkled, their eyesight failing, hair falling, and frequently they have lost all their teeth.
- Those born between 1900 and 1950 number somewhat more survivors, but the overt signs of the addiction's dread effects differ not in kind but only in degree of deterioration. Prognostication is not hopeful.

- Exhaustive experiment shows that when tomatoes are withheld from an addict, invariably his cravings will cause him to turn to substitutes—such as oranges, or steak and potatoes. If both tomatoes and all substitutes are persistently withheld—death invariably results within a short time!
- The skeptic of apocryphal statistics, or the stubborn nonconformist who will not accept the clearly proved conclusions of others, may conduct his own experiment. Obtain two dozen tomatoes—they may actually be purchased within a block of some high schools, or discovered growing in a respected neighbor's back yard!—crush them to a pulp in exactly the state they would have been in if introduced into the stomach, pour the vile juice and pulp into a bowl, and place a goldfish therein. Within minutes the goldfish will be dead!
- Those who argue that what affects a goldfish might not apply to a human being may, at their own choice, wish to conduct a direct experiment by fully immersing a live human head into the mixture for a full 5 minutes.

Source: Clifton M. The dread tomato addiction *Astounding.* February 1958.

ETHICAL CONSIDERATIONS IN RESEARCH

Bioethics, an important aspect of conducting research, refers to the inherent role of ethics in health care and the established norms of conduct in performing research that distinguish between morally acceptable and unacceptable behavior. The field of ethics has its origins with the father of modern medicine, Hippocrates, who developed an oath of medical ethics in 400 BC. Since then, the deliniation of what constitutes ethical research has continued to evolve. After World War II, the Nuremberg War Crimes trials brought to light examples of medical research that had clearly exploited human beings. The United States had its own sad chapter in unethical research practices from 1932–1972 in the Tuskegee study of syphillis. As a result of these expolitations, medical research became a slow, laborious process with many checks and balances to protect human subjects. In the

1990s, activists for persons with AIDS complained to Congress about the long time required to obtain approval for new treatments and drugs. People with AIDS were willing to take some personal risk to get treatments on the market faster. As a result of their lobbying efforts, some of the protections in human research were changed to permit the Food and Drug Administration (FDA) to implement a fast-track approval process for drug companies.

Ethics in medical research goes beyond what the law requires. A course of action may be legal but not ethical. Large institutions including the FDA, Environmental Protection Agency, National Institutes of Health, and all major universities have their own code of ethics. Institutions that conduct medical research usually have an entity known as the **institutional review board (IRB)** charged with reviewing the ethical implications of every research study. The IRB has two responsibilities. First, it must ensure that the rights and safety of the research subjects are respected and protected. Second, it must protect the institution and the researchers against lawsuits and help to ensure that the research results will not be flawed because the study was ethically unsound. The IRB holds the researchers accountable to the public. A research proposal may have to pass the scrutiny of more than one IRB. The institution funding the research and the institution where it is actually conducted may each have its own board.

A number of ethical considerations involved in doing research are common to all institutions. The first is research misconduct. This includes plagiarism, copyright or patent infringement, falsifying or fabricating data, misrepresenting data, and conflict of interest. Like malpractice, research misconduct must be intentional. Bias, unintentional negligance, or disagreement about the meaning of the results does not constitute misconduct. Animal research has its own set of ethical guidelines that usually include such things as making sure the animals do not suffer needlessly, prohibiting frivolous research, and requiring proper care for the animals during the course of the studies. (See Box 14-5 ■.)

BOX 14-5 Radium Girls: Another Public Health Disaster

In the early 1900s, [a] US Radium Corporation['s] factory in New Jersey that made timepieces for the military, employed young women to paint the faces of the watch dials with luminescent paint made from radium, a radioactive substance. The work was too delicate to be done by machine. The girls used very fine sable brushes to trace the numbers on the dial, which they often moistened with their tongues. In addition they often used the glow-in-the-dark substance for more fun endeavors such as painting their fingernails. Radium was invisible, odorless, tasteless, and—according to the employer—completely harmless.

It wasn't long before a number of girls fell ill with bone pain, loose teeth, anemia, jaw tumors, and necrosis of the jaw. Joseph Knef, a dentist who treated several of the girls, suspected the radium exposure as a cause of their illness. He devised an ingenious method to ascertain a crude measurement of the radioactivity by wrapping extracted teeth and pieces of jaw in dental x-ray film for several days, and then developing the film. It is likely that the medical and dental x-rays of the time exposed the women to significant additional radiation exposure.

One woman, Grace Fryer, decided to sue. It took several years to find a lawyer but her case was finally taken up by the Consumer League of New Jersey, and she was joined in the lawsuit by four other women who also worked at the factory.

The company denied accusations that radium was to blame for the women's illness. Company doctors who knew of the dangers and monitored the women produced advertisements of the time indicating radium was a curative for cancer, and suppressed the women's company medical files. Doctors insisted the women were in perfect health. Company owners attempted to smear the women's reputation by insisting their illnesses were the result of syphilis or diptheria. The company refused to pay for the women's medical expenses. Company lawyers used delaying tactics to avoid a trial until the women were dead or too sick to assist in the prosecution. Marie Curie was even called in to give an expert deposition.

As the women began to die, an out-of-court settlement was reached. The company agreed to pay the women's medical expenses and each woman was awarded $10,000 in damages.

The first article on the association of radium and jaw necrosis was published in the *Journal of the American Dental Association* in 1924. By the mid-1930s all five of the women were dead. The total number of women affected by the radium is unknown but the plant employed thousands of workers in plants throughout the country. Additional lawsuits followed in Illinois and other states. As a result of this case, new legislation was enacted which improved industrial safety standards and gave workers the right to sue for damages. The cleanup of the factory sites, local water, soil, and subsequent buildings erected on the sites have cost the Environmental Protection Agency millions of dollars. Some towns still have radium "hotspots" to this day.

Source: Clark C. *Radium Girls: Women and Industrial Health Reform, 1910–1935.*
Chapel Hill: University of North Carolina Press; 1997.

Informed consent, another ethical consideration, requires educating a subject in a research study about the study's purpose, duration, experimental procedures, alternatives, risks, and benefits. Informed consent requires information to be presented so that prospective research subjects can voluntarily decide whether or not to participate; it is a fundamental mechanism to ensure respect for persons by having them give thoughtful consent for a voluntary act. Human study participation must always be voluntary. In the past, research projects conducted at closed institutions, such as prisons, were often coercive recruiting subjects. Participants must be free to participate or not and to withdraw at any time for any reason.

The procedures used in obtaining informed consent should be designed to educate the subject population in terms that they can understand. Therefore, informed consent language and its documentation must be written in "lay language" (ie, understandable to the people being asked to participate). The written presentation of information is used to document the basis for consent and for the subjects' future reference. The consent document should be revised when deficiencies are noted or when additional information would improve the consent process.[9] Informed consent for research involves presenting the research information orally and obtaining written consent prior to a subject's entering into a study and documenting the consent process in the subject's medical record or research file.

When research involves human subjects, an informed consent must be obtained except in one circumstance: If the research uses survey methodology, such as a questionnaire or an interview, the subjects' willing participation in answering the questions is their informed consent. They can decline to participate or can refuse to answer specific questions. However, if the study participant is a minor, a non-English-speaking person, or someone not competent to give consent (such as a person with Alzheimer's disease), a valid informed consent becomes an extremely important ethical piece of the research.

Federally established guidelines regulate research conducted on people. An outline for an informed consent and a sample document are presented on the interactive Companion Website created specifically to accompany this textbook. Other ethical considerations in human research involve confidentiality. Research subjects are never identified when research is published. However, the researcher may ask for a subject's consent to use photographs in an article. In clinical research, dental hygienists–investigators often stand in dual roles to the subject:

as a practicing dental hygienist and as a researcher. For the practicing dental hygienist, the responsibility of confidentiality has long been established under well-known legal and ethical standards. The Health Information Portability and Accountability Act (HIPAA) adds to these standards in practice and research. When a covered entity conducts clinical research involving protected health information (PHI), dental hygienists–investigators must understand the HIPAA privacy rule's restrictions on the use and disclosure of patient's PHI, such as information from a patient's medical chart or test results, as well as an individual's billing information for medical services rendered, when that information is held or transmitted by an entity. PHI also includes identifiable health information about subjects of clinical research gathered by a researcher who is a health care provider.

Another issue related to human research is the participant's right to receive treatment, as was the case with research into new AIDS treatments in the 1990s. Many prospective research studies rely on a control group who does not receive treatment to prove efficacy. Studies now offer most control groups access to the experimental treatment at the end of the study if they so chose. In contrast, participants need to be protected from experimental treatments or tests that might cause harm. A recent series of studies at the National Institues of Health on hormone replacement therapy was stopped early because the treatment was shown to be harmful and continuing the study could not be ethically justified.

Without a doubt, the worse ethical chapter in US research history is the aforementioned Tuskegee study. In 1932, the Public Health Service recruited 400 African American men from Alabama to do a historical study on syphilis to document its progression and its presentation at autopsy. At the time, there was no cure for the disease. The men were given free medical care for their participation and additional monetary benefits, which was adequate incentive because the men were poor farmers. In the late 1940s, penicillin was discovered and became the standard treatment for syphilis, but the men were never told about this cure. As the study continued into the 1970s, the men began dying. Some of them had passed syphilis to their wives and children. The ethical misconduct of the research was leaked to the media. A class action lawsuit awarded the surviving men, wives, and children free medical care for life in addition to a large cash settlement. In 1997, President Bill Clinton formally apologized to the men on behalf of the government. (See Box 14-6 ■.)

RESEARCH ROLES OF GOVERNMENT AND PRIVATE ENTITIES

The federal government has always been at the center of medical research. It has a dual role of promoting research while protecting the public. The government primarily is involved in setting standards for conducting research and ethics. Government entities such as the FDA review research conducted in the private sector. This government oversight provides strict controls on what treatments, medicines, and medical devices can be sold and on what health claims these products may make. Government oversight also prevents the intrusion of less standardized research from other countries. The government often provides funding for research; in theory, it is an ideal mechanism through which to provide grants because it neither manufacturers nor profits from the development of new products. The federal government also conducts research, mostly at the National Institutes of Health through the Public Health Service and the military.

Local governments, such as public health departments, may serve as research centers for studies and may be able to tap a minority population of interest to the research, for example, people with type 2 diabetes. In addition, local governments may benefit from grant money or medical equipment resulting from the research study. Local governments also provide tax incentives to attract private research companies to their work in their area.

Private institutions design and carry out the bulk of medical research in the United States. They can do so more quickly and cost effectively than other entities. Their funding for research may come from federal government grants, from the institution itself, from private companies, or through philanthropy. Competition for grant money is usually great, which theoretically should stimulate better research ideas. Large institutions can contribute multiple perspectives on a single topic. For example, two dental schools in different areas of the country might conduct the same study using two different populations.

Research conducted by private companies also has a negative side. Some researchers, in an effort to conduct studies more quickly and less expensively, have turned to developing countries to find participants. These researchers may pay a private institutional review board to approve the study although ethical controls over it can be poor and the research results of questionable quality.

SUMMARY

Public health has been an important component in the creation of a body of research that impacts dental hygiene practice. Every dental hygienist, whether or not directly involved in research, should be familiar with basic research design, including hypotheses, various types and merit of study designs, and the uses and limits of statistics. Each individual clinician supports a scientific discipline by incorporating evidence-based knowledge and techniques into his or her practice. To be effective in initiating, conducting, and applying research, the dental hygienist must be able to critically analyze the existing body of literature. This crucial link allows scientific study to become the standard of care in the profession.

SELF-STUDY TEST ITEMS

1. Evidence-based decisions come from research, practice, and
   a. Science
   b. Patient preferences
   c. Disciplines
   d. None of the above

2. Informed consent is an ongoing process that is initially obtained at the first step of the research process. It should be discussed in a group setting.
   a. The first statement is true; the second statement is false.
   b. The first statement is false; the second statement is true.
   c. Both statements are true.
   d. Both statements are false.

3. Which type of sample involves choosing every subject independently and all subjects have an equal chance of being selected?
   a. Systematic
   b. Random
   c. Convenience
   d. Judgmental

4. "No statistically significant difference exists between Brand X and Brand Y toothpaste in the reduction of tooth decay" is an example of a
   a. Research question.
   b. Research hypothesis.
   c. Null hypothesis.
   d. Positive hypothesis.

5. Data analysis involves
   a. Assessing the research question
   b. Developing the hypothesis
   c. Analyzing the data
   d. Performing statistical regression techniques

REFERENCES

1. Ripa LW. Open questions and form. In: Wei S, ed. *Clinical Uses of Fluoride*. Philadelphia, PA: Lea and Febiger; 1985.
2. ADHA position paper on polishing procedures. http://www.adha.org/profissues/prophylaxis.htm. Accessed June 22, 2009.
3. Fourth national research conference agenda. Chicago, IL: American Dental Hygienists' Association; 1999.
4. Burns N, Grove S. *The Practice of Nursing Research*. 2nd ed. Philadelphia, PA: W. B. Saunders; 1993.
5. US National Library of Medicine. http://www.nlm.nih.gov/. Accessed June 22, 2009.
6. PubMed. http://www.ncbi.nlm.nih.gov/pubmed. Accessed June 22, 2009.
7. Darby M, Bowen D. *Research Methods for Oral Health Professionals: An Introduction*. St. Louis, MO: C.V. Mosby; 1980.
8. Shiboski CH, Schmidt BL, Jordan RC. Racial disparity in stage at diagnosis and survival among adults with oral cancer in the US. *Comm Dent Oral Epid*. 2007;35(3):233–240.
9. Office for Protection from Research Risks. Tips on Informed Consent. http://www.hhs.gov/ohrp/humansubjects/guidance/ictips.htm. Accessed September 16, 2008.

PEARSON
myhealthprofessionskit™

Multimedia Extension Activities

Use this address to access the interactive Companion Website created for this textbook. Simply select "Dental Hygiene" from the choice of disciplines. Find this book and log in using your username and password. To obtain a username and password, please register using the scratch-off access code on the inside front cover of this book.

Chapter 15

Research Approaches and Designs

With contributions from

Beth E. McKinney, RDH, MS

Christine French Beatty, RDH, PhD

OBJECTIVES

After studying this chapter, the dental hygiene student should be able to:

- Describe and compare various research approaches
- Describe various research designs used in oral epidemiology
- Describe methods used to conduct research studies
- List the parts of a research design

KEY TERMS

Data
Descriptive approach
Double-blind study
Experimental approach
Historical approach
Pilot study
Placebo
Quasi-experimental approach
Research approach
Research design
Retrospective (ex post facto) approach
Variable
Washout period

COMPETENCIES

After studying this chapter and participating in accompanying course activities, the dental hygiene student should be competent to do the following:

- Use evidence-based decision making to evaluate and incorporate emerging treatment modalities
- Assume responsibility for dental hygiene actions and care based on accepted scientific theories and research as well as the accepted standard of care

Dental hygiene research can be conducted using a variety of approaches. It also can focus on a variety of topics: One study might focus on dental hygiene providers' comparative status of educational level versus annual salary; another might focus on patients' compliance with daily flossing regimens.

Because understanding research-related terminology is crucial, we define some of the most important ones before our discussion begins. To gather **data,** or information collected, a researcher may use various *methods:* from questionnaires to clinical testing. Some research makes no *intervention,* or experimental manipulation, of a variable in a study. A **variable** is a treatment, a drug, or an educational component whose value may change over the course of a research study.

Before the research process begins, a **pilot study,** which is a version of a proposed study, is conducted on a small, sometimes intentionally chosen sample. It is a trial run to work out unforeseen errors in the overall plan for a study, which is called the **research design.** In addition, the pilot study conserves valuable and limited research funding for the actual study. After conducting a pilot study, revisions may be made in the research design to obtain results with a higher degree of accuracy.

Did You Know?

Many times, pilot studies must be conducted before research funding can be obtained for complete studies.

Various research approaches may be utilized for dental hygiene research. A **research approach** is the type of research used to obtain information. All approaches observe, describe, measure, analyze, and interpret occurring phenomena. Research approaches may be classified as historical, descriptive, experimental (prospective), quasi-experimental, and retrospective (ex post facto). (See Table 15-1 ■ for examples.)

Dental hygiene research can be categorized in numerous ways and with a plethora of titles. This chapter discusses the wide array of research approaches and designs used in dental hygiene to enable the dental hygienist to understand scientific studies and research reports.

Research may be descriptive or analytic in nature. *Descriptive research* is characterized as the attempt to identify and describe the topic being researched whereas *analytic research* attempts to establish why something is the way it is and how it came to be that way.[1] For example, descriptive research may identify the magnitude or distribution of a disease. Analytical research may test a hypothesis about the relationship of an exposure to a disease.[2]

HISTORICAL APPROACH

The purpose of studies using the **historical approach** is to determine the meaning of past events by reviewing records and literature and conducting interviews. It is one of the approaches that does not study interventions. Historical studies help to establish the incidence and prevalence of a disease in a population over time.

DESCRIPTIVE APPROACH

The **descriptive approach** uses a variety of methods, including surveys, case studies, developmental studies, document or content analysis, trend studies, and correlational studies. Descriptive studies use the survey method to measure and describe the presence and distribution of a disease or health condition in a population or sample[2] at one point in time.

Did You Know?

Descriptive studies can be used to determine the prevalence of disease within the population. Repeating studies can be used to determine which population(s) a disease most affects.

Descriptive Approach Types

A *survey* is a type of descriptive approach that involves collecting data using written or oral questionnaires or dental indices but does not perform interventions. The larger the representative sample for a survey, the more valid are

Table 15-1 Research Approaches

Approach and Subtype	Definition/Purpose	Methods	Limitations	Application Examples
Historical	To determine the meaning of past events	Records review Interviews Literature reviews	Location of accurate data Gaps in knowledge No ability to replicate Biased reports Distortion of events	Development of ADHA water fluoridation program 1945–2005
Descriptive	To describe and indentify current events or situations			
Survey To gather broad information about status quo; usually involves large sample size		Questionnaires Opinionnaires Interviews Indices	Lack of depth	Use of pit and fissure sealants by dental hygienists Caries experience of high school sophomores
Case Study To conduct in-depth report on a single person, group, event, or situation		Interviews Observation Testing Records review	Uniqueness Replication not possible Subject to bias	Orthodontic case report Water fluoridation in Albuquerque, NM
Developmental To study growth, development, maturation, or change over period of time			Obtaining representative population	Primary teeth exfoliation patterns
Cross-Sectional To study cross section of population in limited period of time				
Cohort or Longitudinal To study same population over extended period of time			Time-consuming process Extended financial commitment Loss of subjects	Changes in the periodontium over time
Document or Content Analysis To analyze documents themselves		Examination of records or documents for specific information or presentation style	Subjectivity in evaluation	Evaluation of dental journals for types of articles printed Gender biases in dental hygiene textbooks
Trend Combines descriptive and historical research to establish patterns from the past and present in order to predict future occurrences		Records review Review of the literature Interviews Observation Surveys	Long-range prediction less valid and reliable than short-range prediction	ADHA actions 1968–2008 regarding expanding scope of dental hygienists Use of sugar substitutes in carbonated beverages

(continued)

213

Table 15-1 Research Approaches (continued)

Approach and Subtype	Definition/Purpose	Methods	Limitations	Application Examples
	Correlational Measure the relationship between variables	Comparison of two sets of data	No indication correlation indicates cause-effect relationship between variables Plausible rival hypotheses	Frequency of flossing and periodontal disease Predental hygiene grades and clinical dental hygiene grades
	Retrospective (causal-comparative or ex post facto) To investigate existing differences to determine possible causes. (Reverse of experimental approach)	Reverse of experimental approach Independent variable is not manipulated	Cannot determine causal relationship Can only determine functional relationship Independent variable cannot be manipulated	Periodontal Disease (study adults over 40 with periodontal disease and adults over 40 without periodontal disease) Oral cancer (similar methodology)
Experimental (prospective)	To investigate cause-and-effect relationships Involves manipulation of variables	Manipulation of one or more independent variables Control of extraneous variables Measurement of dependent variable(s) Use of a control group	Artificiality due to amount of control Decreased external validity	Effect of intraoral sodium bicarbonate rinses on the periodontal ligament of laboratory rats. Life expectancy of dental restorative materials in vitro.
Quasi-Experimental	Approximates true experimental approach but lacks control of true experimentation	Same as experimental except lacks the control of a true experimental design	Decreased internal validity Lack of control of extraneous variables	Effect of intraoral sodium bicarbonate rinses on the periodontal ligament of dental patients. Life expectancy of dental restorative materials in vivo

Source: Darby M, Bowen D. *Research Methods for Oral Health Professionals: An Introduction.* St. Louis, MO: C.V. Mosby; 1980.

the results. Descriptive surveys can be used to measure knowledge, attitudes, and values related to disease and health conditions, all of which can be used to determine needs for public health programs. For example, knowledge of the effectiveness of fluoride can be measured in a sample of the patient population of a community children's clinic to determine whether further fluoride education is needed. This information can be obtained by surveying parents and children by having them complete questionnaires when they come to the clinic.

A *case study* is research about a specific incidence of a disease in one person. It is an excellent way to discover possible treatment options for a variety of conditions or diseases. A case study entails assessing or diagnosing a specific patient or community population and planning, implementing and evaluating treatment. A famous case study mentioned in a previous chapter involved Dr. Jenner's patient explaining her fortune of contracting cowpox as a way to protect her against smallpox. The incentives and rewards for conducting clinical research from a simple case study were never more apparent.[3] This example clearly demonstrates an effective, practical treatment that began as a case study.

A *case series* reports on a small group of people but cannot be generalized to the overall population; however, it often is interesting to read and frequently contributes to practical ideas for clinical practice.

A *developmental study,* sometimes called an *observational study,* simply looks at events as they exist but performs no intervention. Like a natural history study, a developmental study attempts to describe a condition or situation comprehensively. It observes growth, development, maturation, or change over a period of time. Many developmental studies are classified as *cross-sectional* or *cohort.*

A *cross-sectional study* measures the outcome and the exposure at the same time to determine the association between the two.[4] By measuring outcomes and exposures at the same time, a correlation or noncorrelation between the outcome and exposures could be identified. Such a study would be conducted on a sample across the population as its name indicates. The sample is measured only once. A descriptive survey can be expanded into a cross-sectional study by going beyond simply measuring the presence of a condition. For example, a cross-sectional study could identify the characteristics of parents' return of consent forms for their children to participate in a school-based dental sealant program. A sample of the school population is studied to measures parents' socioeconomic status, dental knowledge, dental history, and other traits. Parents' attributes (suspected characteristics) and compliance (condition) are measured only one time in only one group for associations.

A *cohort (group) study* examines one population group or subset with a common characteristic (for example, age, gender, special needs classification) over a specified time period to measure the change or progress of a disease or condition.[5] The study starts with a group of individuals who do not have the disease or condition but are at risk for it and then collects information regarding exposure to that risk. The group is observed to identify members who do or do not eventually develop the disease or condition. This requires at least two measurements on the same group of people at different times.

A cohort study can be described as a *longitudinal study* (measured over time).[5] The most well-known and comprehensive longitudinal study could be the Harvard Nurses' Health Study.[6] Begun in 1976 to determine any relationship between the use of oral contraceptives and smoking, the study has followed 100,000 nurses over the three decades and has resulted in more than 400 publications on numerous health topics. Another longitudinal cohort study has tracked the use of tobacco products in the US population for more than a century to determine prevalence of smoking, incidence of new smokers each year, characteristics of the population that use tobacco, and events related to increases and decreases in use, such as the free distribution of cigarettes to US troops in World War I and the more recent policy to control the sale of cigarettes.[5]

A *document* or *content analysis* study analyzes documents to understand phenomena. One example of a document analysis is a detailed review of the content of a college course, such as reviewing all topics that have been covered. Another example is the review of dental records of a dental practice to determine its payer mix.

A *trend study* combines descriptive and historical research to establish patterns or phenomena from the past and in the present to predict future occurrences. Reviewing the consumption of sports drink over the past two decades to predict their future use is an example of a trend study. Cross-sectional studies are often compared over time to determine trends, such as oral health surveys conducted as part of an oral health surveillance system.

A *correlational study* is exploratory in nature and attempts to establish a link between two variables or conditions but does not provide evidence for a cause-and-effect relationship between them. It can consider a population's past, present, and future as well as study specific occurrences of a disease. It is followed by an experimental study to determine whether a cause-and-effect relationship actually exists. This research approach may use indices, survey methodology, ands clinical testing.

In recent years, a large number of correlation studies have linked oral health with overall systemic health. They have linked periodontal disease with heart disease, osteoporosis, obesity, Alzheimer's disease, pancreatic cancer, and preterm births.[7] This research approach is often misinterpreted to infer that having periodontal disease *causes* heart disease or vice versa—an erroneous extrapolation. When a research study has identified a possible relationship, additional prospective controlled cohort or experimental studies may be needed to determine cause and effect. Identifying causality requires repeating several such studies over several different populations that obtain the same results.

RETROSPECTIVE (EX POST FACTO) APPROACH

A **retrospective study** looks backward (**ex post facto,** or after the fact) to investigate a group of people with a particular disease, usually via medical records. For example, one retrospective study examined the impact of dental interventions before organ transplants. Persons undergoing bone marrow transplants to treat advanced cancer often receive preoperative dental evaluation and periodontal therapy as a standard of care to reduce the chance of septicemia after the transplant. For example, a retrospective study in a public health hospital with a dental clinic examined medical records to compare patients who did and did not have dental intervention prior to transplant. Contrary to expected results, no septicemia was observed for either group.[8]

One type of retrospective study is a *case–control study;* its purpose is to compare two groups to identify factors in the history of the group associated with a specific disease or condition. One group has a disease or condition (called a *case*) but the second group does not. Cases are compared to controls, hence its name.[4] Case–control studies investigate the outcome (presence or absence of a disease) and then probe for information about exposure to factors that could be associated with it.[9] The computation of risk from a case–control study is called *odds ratio.*[10] Case–control studies are sometimes referred to as *case history* or *ex post facto studies.*[11] The relationships they establish are called *functional relationships.*[11]

During the early stages of research on fluorosis, researchers conducted a case–control study by comparing two naturally occurring groups, one of people with severe fluorosis and the other without fluorosis. The researchers measured each group only once to identify the common exposure or factor(s) related to the condition's presence and then attempted to relate common exposure(s) to the presence of fluorosis (outcome). In this case, their drinking water was the common factor.[12]

An *ecologic study* also attempts to relate outcome with exposure to a suspected risk factor but does so using existing data for the population to identify any correlations rather than measuring the exposure and the outcome in the same group.[4,5] The ecologic study forms no groups and does not measure variables but uses data that had previously been recorded for another purpose. Ecologic studies, which can be useful in establishing associations, have the advantages of being low cost and quick to conduct because they do not require data collection. Their weakness is the use of existing data. Because the data are collected at different times for different purposes, the groups being compared may be different. To relate exposure and outcome, they both must be measured on the same individuals. In other words, the exposure data may come from one group and the outcome data from another group, producing what is called an *ecologic fallacy.*[10] Because of the ecologic fallacy, ecologic studies are not definitive in identifying risk factors or even risk indicators. Results of ecologic studies are sometimes reported using correlations. Measures of risk that are established with cross-sectional, cohort, and case–control studies provide more information about association for comparisons than ecologic studies.[4] Health recommendations should not be based on ecologic studies alone. These studies should be followed with analytic studies to more closely examine the risk of an exposure resulting in the disease or condition.

Antifluoridationists have conducted ecologic studies to try to implicate fluoridation as a risk factor for conditions such as cancer, Down syndrome, and infant mortality. These researchers used existing data measured at different times to demonstrate invalid relationships. Closer scrutiny using well-controlled cohort and case–control studies have disproved antifluoridationists' claims.[13]

EXPERIMENTAL (PROSPECTIVE) APPROACH

The **experimental approach,** also known as a *clinical trial,* is probably most familiar to a layperson. This research studies an experimental treatment or intervention

---

BOX 15-1   Requirements for Conducting Experimental Research

- Use a control group for comparison with the experimental group.
- Control extraneous variables.
- Randomize study participants.
- Control errors in measurement.

- Directly manipulate one or more independent variables.
- Observe and measure the dependent variable.
- Ensure occurrence of independent variable before dependent variable in the design.

---

using a *dependent variable* whose value or outcome is determined by that of one or more other variables. An independent variable is the variable that is being manipulated. The dependent variable may be a new drug or surgical procedure; its effectiveness is the outcome being studied. See Box 15-1 ■ for requirements of an experimental research.

Placebo Effect

Experimental research frequently uses placebos and control groups. The control group is the group with the disease/condition being studied that does not receive experimental treatment. The **placebo** is a control. It is not the factor being studied but can be a nontreatment or sometimes a "sugar pill." It is more likely however, to be either the standard drug of choice for a disease or the standard treatment procedure against which the experimental one is being compared, called an active control. Even in carefully controlled studies with a placebo drug or treatment, a proportion of the participants, typically 15–35% receiving the placebo actually improve, a phenomenon known as the *placebo effect.* First described in detail in 1955, the placebo effect is testimony not only to the multifactorial nature of illness and healing but also to the human mind's ability to provoke physiological change.[14]

⌐ Did You Know? ⌐

Interestingly, the research that led to the description of the placebo effect was found in the 1970s to be significantly flawed by researchers doing retrospective studies.[15]

Sometimes subjects in a study are affected simply by being subjects in it. This phenomenon, known as the *Hawthorne effect,* was discovered as a result of a study

held in the late 1920s and early 1930s. Investigators at the Western Electric Company's Hawthorne plant in Chicago found that because factory workers knew they were participating in a study, anything the researchers did caused the workers' productivity to change. This theory suggests that when subjects are singled out for a study of any kind, they may improve their performance or behavior not because of any specific condition being tested but simply because of the perception of being observed.

Double-Blind Studies

Most experimental research is conducted using a **double-blind study,** that is, a research project in which neither the subjects nor the investigators know who is in the control (or placebo) group and who is in the other (independent variable) group that receives the experimental treatment. This type of study is considered to be highly reliable because it eliminates a great deal of the researcher's bias. An investigator who does not know which treatment a subject is receiving could not make any suggestive comments to the participant, and the data collection can be done without any preconceived expectations.

Suppose, for example, a dental hygienist who was providing services in a correctional facility wanted to evaluate the relative merits of rinsing with chlorhexidine over a commercially available mouth rinse. A pharmacist could dispense two rinses: both blue and mint flavored in identical unmarked bottles. The pharmacist kept a record of which subjects received which rinse, but neither the dental hygienist nor the subjects knew. Therefore, the hygienist could not inadvertently suggest to the patients that one rinse is superior, and any indices would be scored without the preconceived expectation that the subjects on chlorhexidine "should" be healthier than the control subjects. The dental hygienist could not bias the results of the study. The subjects also would be less likely to bias the results because people who know they are getting a placebo are less likely to comply with study protocol.

Independence of Researchers

Because bias may also be introduced through the funding source of a research study, it is important that clinical trials be conducted by independent researchers. If a pharmaceutical company produces mouthwash G, its efficacy should be confirmed by independent studies that are not funded by the manufacturer. In most studies, the principal investigator is usually required to disclose that there is no financial conflict of interest.

Experimental Research Designs

An experimental study can be a pretest-posttest design or a posttest only design.[16] These and other designs appear in Figure 15-1 ■. Pretest-posttest designs are a common type of repeated measures, because the same test is given at least twice, before the independent variable is introduced and after the independent variable is introduced.[17] A *pretest-posttest* study measures the dependent variable—the treatment or intervention being studied—before and after introducing the independent variable—the pla-cebo. The advantage of the pretest-posttest design is having the pretest for comparison. The pretest also is used to check for equivalent groups before introducing the intervention.

A *posttest-only* design introduces the independent variable and then measures the dependent variable. This study is conducted when administering a pretest is impractical. For example, a study could be conducted in a school-based oral screening program to compare the percentage of compliance with two referral systems. Although randomization would be possible, no pretest could be administered, so a posttest-only design would be appropriate for this experimental study.

Posttest-only designs are used also to control the effect of a pretest on the dependent variable in a study. This effect is called *pretest sensitization*.[11] For example,

One-Group Time Series Design

Repeated Pretest Measures	Independent Variable	Repeated Post-Test Measures
Y_1 Y_2 Y_3	X	Y_4 Y_5 Y_6

Control Group Time Series Design

Group	Repeated Pretest Measures	Independent Variable	Repeated Post-Test Measures
E	Y_1 Y_2 Y_3	X	Y_4 Y_5 Y_6
C	Y_1 Y_2 Y_3	—	Y_4 Y_5 Y_6

Randomized Subjects Pretest/Post-Test Design

Group	Pretest	Independent Variable	Post-Test
(R) E	Y_1	X	Y_2
(R) C	Y_1	—	Y_2

Randomized Subjects Post-Test Only Design

Group	Independent Variable	Post-Test
(R) E	X	Y_2
(R) C	—	Y_2

Randomized Matched Subjects Post-Test Only Design

Group	Independent Variable	Post-Test
(RM) E	X	Y_2
(RM) C	—	Y_2

Solomon Four-Group Design

Group	Pretest	Independent Variable	Post-Test
(R) E	Y_1	X	Y_2
(R) C_1	Y_2	—	Y_2
(R) C_2	—	X	Y_2
(R) C_3	—	—	Y_2

FIGURE 15-1 Quasi-Experimental and Experimental Study Designs

Source: Adapted from Darby, M. L., & Bowen, D. M. Research methods for oral health professionals: An introduction. St. Louis, MO: C. V. Mosby, 1980. Reprinted by J. T. K. McCann Co., Pocatello, ID, 1993.

in educational research studies, conducting an exam to measure knowledge prior to evaluating the effectiveness of various teaching methodologies could in and of itself bring about learning. A *Solomon four-group design* can be used to determine whether the pretest affects the dependent variable.[16] The Solomon design (see Figure 15-1) combines a pretest/posttest design with a posttest only design. For example, a study of four groups using the Solomon design would place two of them in an experimental and control group with a pretest-posttest design. The other two would be an experimental and control group with a posttest-only design. The change in the dependent variable is compared across groups to determine whether the control group or pretest affects the outcome. Solomon designs are infrequently used because they are difficult to implement.[16]

Using the example of educational research, four groups would be tested to determine the effectiveness of an educational method to improve fluoride knowledge of clients in a public health program. Two would be an experimental and control group with a pretest-posttest. The other two would be an experimental and control group using a posttest only. Knowledge would be measured at pretest and posttest with a questionnaire consisting of questions about fluoride. The Solomon design would be used to determine whether completing the fluoride questionnaire results in learning about fluoride. The two experimental groups would be exposed to the educational program being evaluated, but the two control groups would not be. To determine the learning in each group, the results for two pretest groups are compared with those of the posttest-only groups. If the outcome is higher in the pretest groups, some of the learning could be attributed to the pretest questionnaire rather than the educational program. A variation of this design that eliminates the control posttest-only group is used for the same purpose and is called the Solomon three-group design.[16]

Sometimes the dependent variable is measured several times over a specific period, either at pretest or posttest to determine whether the effect of the independent variable on the dependent variable holds over time. This is called *time series design*.[18] It can be applied to a one-group before-and-after trial but is most valid when applied to an experimental study. Its measurement of the dependent variable at posttest is its most valid use. Figure 15-1 represents the measurement of

the posttest three times in a randomized pretest-posttest design. The pretest-posttest study of hypersensitivity described earlier would likely be conducted as a time series study. The reduction in hypersensitivity would be measured at posttest repeatedly over several weeks or months to make sure that the hypersensitivity did not return.

A *factorial design* is used to study two or more independent variables in combination.[11] For example, this design could compare the effectiveness in removing plaque of a power toothbrush to a manual toothbrush at the same time it compares a tufted floss to a traditional floss to determine whether they interact. Two levels of two independent variables are involved, toothbrush and dental floss, referred to as a 2 × 2 factorial design. (See Table 15-2 ■.) Four groups are formed with various possible combinations of these two levels of the two independent variables. This design can be applied with more independent variables and/or more levels of each independent variable for factorial designs that are 2 × 3, 3 × 3, 3 × 4, and so on. In a factorial design, the effect of each independent variable is tested on the dependent variable, referred to as a *main effect*, and the combined effect of the independent variables is tested on the dependent variable, referred to as an *interaction effect*.[11]

Controls

Two types of studies in which participants serve as their own control are *crossover* and *split mouth*. Participants are assigned randomly to a study and a control group in a *crossover design*. After a specified length of time, participants are switched ("crossed over") to the opposite group. Then the participants in both groups experience a period of time with no treatment, called a **washout period.** In drug trials, this is the period allowed for all of any administered drug to be eliminated from the

Table 15-2 2 × 2 Factorial Design

Manual brush	Manual brush
Traditional floss	Tufted floss
Power brush	Power brush
Traditional floss	Tufted floss

body. It reduces the effect of the first treatment on the second. After the washout period, each group receives the opposite treatment it had earlier received. This crossover design is not appropriate for regimens that have a permanent effect that the washout period cannot eliminate.

The crossover design could be applied to a study of a new power toothbrush. A sample is randomly assigned to a test group that will use a new power toothbrush or to an active control group that will use the best-selling power toothbrush currently on the market. After three weeks, all study participants are told to return to using their regular manual toothbrush for three weeks, and then those participants who were in the test group for the first three weeks are now in the control group for three weeks, and vice versa. Thus, all participants use both toothbrushes for a three-week period with a three-week washout period between.

In a *split mouth design,* one side of the mouth is used for the test treatment, and the other side of the mouth is used for the control treatment.[19] This design is common in testing treatment regimens in dentistry because it is very effective to control subject-relevant variables.

A split mouth and crossover design can be combined so that the sides of the mouth are switched. In the crossover toothbrush study discussed earlier, participants could be asked to brush with the new power toothbrush on the right side of the mouth and with the standard power brush (active control) on the left side, making it a split mouth design. In this case, the brushing should be done under supervision to ensure that the correct toothbrush is used on the proper side. The participants could then return for another supervised brushing session during which they switch sides with each toothbrush. Another example of a split mouth design is related to the earlier hypersensitivity study. The new treatment could be used to treat hypersensitive teeth on one side, and the placebo used to treat hypersensitive teeth on the other side. In this example, use of a

crossover design would not be appropriate because the test treatment could have a carryover and possibly permanent effect. A final example of a split mouth design is a test of the retention rate of a new dental sealant product by using it on one side of the mouth and using the standard sealant product (active control) on the other side of the mouth. Again, a crossover design would not be suitable for this study.

An advantage of using participants to serve as their own control is that they can provide near perfect group similarity.[2] Crossover and split mouth trials control for subject-relevant variables because results are not affected by variations in response among participants. Therefore, they have increased validity. Another advantage is that they can be conducted with small samples because each study participant is a member of both the test group and the control group. Of course, having participants serve as their own control is not feasible in all studies.

QUASI-EXPERIMENTAL APPROACH

A **quasi-experimental approach** is used in an experimental study that lacks inherent control. Results may be used when planning other studies. This approach is employed because the use of a control is not practical or necessary. For instance, when studying the use of a mandibular advancing oral appliance to treat obstructive sleep apnea, a researcher could not replace the appliance with a control that did not advance the mandible, especially when the intervention is medically necessary.

Did You Know?

A quasi-experimental study could use a historical finding as a control.

DENTAL HYGIENE SPOTLIGHT:
Christine French Beatty, RDH, PhD

Christine French Beatty is a dental hygiene educator who has taught public health and research to many dental hygienists. What is so exciting about Professor Beatty is that in addition to teaching it, she is a public health hygienist and researcher. She has published numerous studies germane to dental hygiene in peer-reviewed journals and has had a multitude of experiences in public health. Professor Beatty is a member of Sigma Phi Alpha and Phi Kappa Phi and has received numerous teaching and mentoring awards, which are a testament to her teaching skills. She has been a mentor to numerous dental hygienists interested in research.

I asked Dr. Beatty a few questions about her experiences in research and public health.

dental public health and research. The first was a three-year clinical trial to test a new formula fluoride dentifrice funded by Procter & Gamble. Through this position, I learned firsthand the skills involved in research. Because of the nature of the project, I also functioned much like a dental public health hygienist, working in the parochial schools of Houston to teach oral hygiene regularly, scheduling examinations for data collection in relation to the project, and providing follow-up for the children who had active disease. The second project was a school fluoride tablet and rinse program in two school districts outside of Houston. Again, I coordinated the research side of the project and served as an educator and community dental health program administrator.

This position was such a change from clinical practice, and I loved it! It gave me a new challenge, helped me develop new skills related to management and coordination of programs, allowed me to have a more flexible work schedule, and provided employment benefits that I did not have in clinical practice. I learned many of these new skills on the job, but I also returned to school to complete my bachelor's degree, knowing that I wanted to expand my dental hygiene career opportunities beyond clinical.

What are your current positions?

I am a professor at Texas Woman's University (TWU) Dental Hygiene Program. With my background and love for dental public health and research, I was hired to teach the community and research content areas of our bachelor's degree program. This has been a great fit for me because it requires developing and coordinating community programs and research. As well as serving as community dental health coordinator for our program, I have the wonderful opportunity to develop a research program for our dental hygiene students and to serve on research committees for master's theses and professional projects for students in dental hygiene, health studies, and occupational therapy programs.

Why did you decide to go into dental hygiene?

My decision to go into dental hygiene was not all that intentional. When I was considering what to do after high school forty-six years ago, the options for females were few. Because my dad was a dentist and professor in a dental school, I was drawn to the field of dentistry. Also, I was interested in dental hygiene because the program lasted only two years. I was anxious to be able to earn a good living soon because my parents were older and my dad was close to retirement. So it was mostly a practical decision. Even so, it was a good fit for me. I loved the detail of dental hygiene, and it afforded me the opportunities that I was seeking to become independent and earn a good living.

How did you get into dental public health? Did you need additional education?

I disliked public health in school and avoided it for a few years because of my anxiety. After practicing clinical dental hygiene for approximately ten years, circumstances led me to a position as a research associate with the Dental Science Institute of the University of Texas Dental Branch in Houston. I coordinated two projects that provided me hands-on training and experience in

Can you discuss any particularly interesting experiences you've had in your dental public health positions?

I love dental public health because of the variety of activities and responsibilities. It allows us to fill all of the roles of the dental hygienist. It not only draws on my knowledge of dental hygiene clinical practice but also challenges me as an educator, researcher, administrator/manager, and change agent.

One position early in my career was as a school dental hygienist. Among other responsibilities, I followed up with Head Start children who needed dental treatment. I remember driving through town with a carload of wiggly children, transporting them to dental offices for treatment. Also, because I was part of the health care team, I was called on to participate in lice checks!

In another position, I traveled from school to school to coordinate programs and even went to the children's homes to meet with parents to supervise the children's use of test products and follow up on treatment needs. I loved the flexibility of the schedule and the opportunity to be out in the field.

Can you discuss the research you have conducted and its importance to dental hygiene and public health?

As an educator, most of my research has been related to dental hygiene education. However, my students have had varied clinical research interests that we have pursued for their research projects. I remember the first research study that I personally conducted in the 1970s. It was when I was working at the Dental Science Institute. My immediate supervisor was a dental faculty member who taught research to students in the periodontics specialty program. I got a small grant funded by the dental school for a clinical trial to compare the effectiveness of waxed and unwaxed floss. The perio students served as subjects.

One of my first publications was a description of a community dental health program that I was involved in through my local component. So many great programs go unreported, which is unfortunate for our profession. As a result, I don't think the dental profession and the public realize the impact that dental hygiene has on the oral health of the community.

Research skills are so basic to evidence-based practice that I can't imagine making decisions as a dental hygienist, no matter the role or setting, without doing research. For example, a recent research project by a senior student was to evaluate the effectiveness of our dental hygiene clinic's referral system for sealants. We wanted to verify that we were maximizing the number of sealants placed in children who came to our clinic to help meet our nation's goal of increasing the number of children with sealants. Another student implemented a fluoride varnish program under my direction, and we evaluated the program with the goal of implementing it on a larger scale in the future. Making decisions about programs and treatment has to be data driven, and that means doing research.

What advice would you give to a practicing hygienist who is thinking of doing something different?

Network, network, network! All of my opportunities to do something other than clinical dental hygiene came as a result of talking to many people, being active professionally in the local, state, and national associations, and volunteering for community service.

I can't stress enough the importance of active involvement with your dental hygiene association. I met so many people, was continually aware of trends in the profession, and gained incredible leadership skills through this participation. It is also important to maximize whatever position we are in. For example, when I was in clinical practice, I continually evaluated our procedures and treatment to stay on the cutting edge. I also took advantage of all opportunities to attend conferences, learn more, connect with new people, and be involved in the community.

What else would you like to share?

Although the vast majority of dentists and dental hygienists practice in private settings, I am convinced that the future of oral health care is in dental public health. Only about half of our population utilizes dental care on a regular basis. One has only to read reports such as the *ADHA Dental Hygiene: Focus on Advancing the Profession,* and the USDHHS *Oral Health in America: A Report of the Surgeon General* to realize that increasing dental utilization rates will require the expansion of community programs.

Source: Christine Nathe writes the Public Health Column in RDH magazine published by Pennwell Publishing. For more public health spotlights please see RDH magazine online at http://www.rdhmag.com/index.html.

SUMMARY

Dental hygienists need to understand different research approaches and designs. Research approaches are varied and are based and conducted on the specific phenomenon(a) the researcher wishes to study. Understanding this enables dental hygienists to critically review scientific literature and make evidenced-based decisions during dental hygiene treatment.

SELF-STUDY TEST ITEMS

1. Which of the following is a descriptive approach to research?
   a. Case study approach
   b. Experimental approach
   c. Retrospective approach
   d. Prospective approach

2. Which studies combine descriptive and historical research to establish patterns from the past and present to predict future occurrences?
   a. Document analysis studies
   b. Correlational studies
   c. Trend studies
   d. Prospective studies

3. In a split mouth study, one side of the mouth is used for the test treatment. The other side of the mouth is used for the control treatment.
   a. The first statement is true; the second statement is false.
   b. The first statement is false; the second statement is true.
   c. Both statements are true.
   d. Both statements are false.

4. A quasi-experimental study is designed as an experimental study but lacks inherent control. However, results from a quasi-experimental study may be used when planning further studies.
   a. The first statement is true; the second statement is false.
   b. The first statement is false; the second statement is true.
   c. Both statements are true.
   d. Both statements are false.

5. Studying the relationship between obesity and oral health is an example of which type of study?
   a. Experimental
   b. Quasi-experimental
   c. Correlational
   d. Analytic

REFERENCES

1. Ethridge DE. *Research Epidemiology in Applied Economics: Organizing, Planning, and Conducting Economic Research.* Malden, MA: Blackwell Publishing; 2004.
2. Burt BA, Eklund SA. *Dentistry, Dental Practice, and the Community.* 6th ed. St. Louis, MO: Elsevier; 2005.
3. Berg AO. Gordon MJ, Cherkin DC. *Practice-Based Research in Medicine.* Kansas City, MO: American Academy of Family Physicians; 1986.
4. Koepsell TD, Weiss NS. *Epidemiologic Methods: Studying the Occurrence of Illness.* New York, NY: Oxford University Press; 2003.
5. Friis RH, Sellers TA. *Epidemiology for Public Health Practice.* 3rd ed. Boston, MA: Jones & Bartlett; 2004.
6. Nelson NJ. Nurses health study: Nurses helping science and themselves. *J Natl Can Inst.* 2000;92(8):597–599.
7. Oral and Whole Body Health. *Sci Am.* 2006 (special publication).
8. Akintoye SO, Brennan MT, Graber CJ, McKinney BE, Rams TE, Barrett AJ, Atkinson AC. A retrospective investigation of advanced periodontal disease as a risk factor for septicemia in hematopoietic stem cell and bone marrow transplant recipients. *Oral Surg, Oral Med, Oral Path.* 2002;94(5):581–588.
9. Morabia A. Epidemiology: An epistemological perspective. In: Morabia A. *A History of Epidemiologic Methods and Concepts.* Boston, MA: Birkhauser Verlag; 2004:3–125.
10. Gerstman BB. *Epidemiology Kept Simple: An Introduction to Traditional and Modern Epidemiology.* 2nd ed. Hoboken, NJ: Wiley-Liss; 2003.
11. Darby M, Bowen D. *Research Methods for Oral Health Professionals: An Introduction.* St. Louis, MO: C.V. Mosby; 1980.
12. National Institute of Dental and Craniofacial Research, National Institutes of Health. The Story of Fluoridation. http://www.nidcr.nih.gov/HealthInformation/DiseasesAndConditions/Fluoride/StoryFluoride.htm. Accessed January 8, 2008.
13. American Dental Association. Fluoridation facts. http://www.ada.org/public/topics/fluoride/facts/. Accessed January 15, 2008.
14. Beecher HK. The powerful placebo. *JAMA.* 1955;159(17):1602–1606.

15. Kienle GS, Kiene H. The powerful placebo effect: Fact or fiction? *J Clin Epid.* 1997;50:1311–1318.

16. Cottrell RR. *Health Promotion and Education Research Methods.* Boston, MA: Jones & Bartlett; 2005.

17. Minke, A. Conducting repeated measures analyses: Experimental design considerations. Paper presented at: Southwest Educational Research Association; 1997; Austin, TX. Ericae .net Clearinghouse on Assessment and Evaluation. http://ericae.net/ft/tamu/Rm.htm. Accessed January 18, 2008.

18. Last JM. Time series. *Encyclopedia of Public Health.* http://www.Answers.Com/. Updated 2008. Accessed January 13, 2008.

19. Hackshaw A, Paul E, Davenport E. *Evidence-Based Dentistry: An Introduction.* Hoboken, NJ: John Wiley; 2007.

PEARSON

myhealthprofessionskit™

Multimedia Extension Activities

Use this address to access the interactive Companion Website created for this textbook. Simply select "Dental Hygiene" from the choice of disciplines. Find this book and log in using your username and password. To obtain a username and password, please register using the scratch-off access code on the inside front cover of this book.

Chapter 16

Oral Epidemiology

Christine French Beatty, RDH, PhD

OBJECTIVES

After studying this chapter, the dental hygiene student should be able to:

- Define oral epidemiology and describe the uses of epidemiology
- Relate epidemiology to evidence-based practice
- Define common epidemiologic terms
- Relate measurement to epidemiology
- List and describe various publications that report oral epidemiology in the United States
- Describe ways to increase validity of epidemiologic research methods

KEY TERMS

Epidemiology
Epidemiology triangle
Multifactorial
Oral epidemiology
Surveillance

COMPETENCIES

After studying this chapter and participating in accompanying course activities, the dental hygiene student should be competent to do the following:

- Use evidence-based decision making to evaluate and incorporate emerging treatment modalities
- Assume responsibility for dental hygiene actions and care based on accepted scientific theories and research as well as the accepted standard of care

As Chapter 14 discussed, evidence-based practice combines the use of the best evidence available, clinical expertise, and patient preferences.[1] This evidence-based decision-making process requires skills in critically evaluating the evidence and accepting or rejecting it as research without merit, applying that with merit to clinical practice, and evaluating the outcomes.[2] Understanding the importance of high levels of evidence in the form of meta-analyses and randomized clinical trials and the role of analytic studies in identifying risk factors is critical to being able to participate in evidence-based practice.[3,4]

An understanding of oral epidemiology and the methodology used in epidemiologic research is essential to evidence-based practice.[5] This chapter presents an overview of the principles and methods of epidemiology and oral epidemiology so that dental hygienists will be able to analyze the scientific literature to apply it to making evidence-based practice decisions.

WHAT IS EPIDEMIOLOGY?

Timmreck has defined **epidemiology** as the study of the nature, cause, control, and determinants of the frequency and distribution of disease, disability, and death in human populations.[6] The *population* can be as large as the entire globe or as small as a nursing home or elementary school. Epidemiology also includes the process of characterizing the distribution of disease and various related factors, such as age, gender, race, socioeconomic status (SES), time, place, person, and behaviors.[6] The science and tools of epidemiology are used to study disease and trends related to health care, such as needle

stick injuries among dental workers, the success of hepatitis B immunization campaigns, and suicide rates among dentists, to name a few.

Epidemiology is multidisciplinary in that it draws upon knowledge from the biological sciences, physical sciences, social sciences, behavioral sciences, and biostatistics.[7] Research methodology is integral to epidemiology.

Epidemiology is grounded in population thinking rather than thinking in terms of what will happen with the individual.[8] It can be used to form reliable predictions at the population level; these predictions can then be applied to an individual within the population in terms of risk or probabilities that a disease will occur in an individual.[8]

In general, epidemiology is used to describe the health status of populations, to identify multiple factors associated with disease and conditions to explain their etiology, to predict the occurrence of disease and conditions, and to control the distribution of diseases and conditions within the population.[7] See Box 16-1 ■ for a more detailed list of the uses of epidemiology.[4,6,7,9,10]

Epidemiology uses a specific vocabulary that must be learned in order to understand it. For example, three common terms used to describe the distribution of disease in a population are endemic, epidemic, and pandemic.[7] *Endemic* is the relatively low but constant presence of disease in a particular geographic region. *Epidemic* is the occurrence of disease in excess of normal in a specific community or region, usually occurring suddenly and spreading rapidly; it is often referred to as an "outbreak" of disease. *Pandemic* is an epidemic that crosses international borders to affect several countries or continents.

BOX 16-1 The Uses of Epidemiology

- To study the trends of disease to help plan for health services and public health programs
- To assess disease or health conditions within a community
- To identify risk factors that affect a population group to predict individuals' risks of disease
- To assess, evaluate, and research how well public health policies and activities and health services meet the priorities and needs of the population

- To identify cause-and-effect relationships of diseases and various factors to help in the diagnostic processes of disease identification
- To identify syndromes from the distribution of clinical phenomena
- To control, prevent, and eliminate causes of diseases, conditions, injury, disability, or death

Definitions of these terms and others are summarized in Table 16-1 ▪ for easy reference.

> **Did You Know?**
>
> **Oral epidemiology** simply is epidemiology in relation to oral diseases and conditions.

Without oral epidemiology, we would not be aware of the associations of diseases to each other and to risk factors such as those for periodontal diseases; the relationship of periodontal diseases to other conditions such as heart disease, diabetes, and blood dyscrasias; the bacterial origin of dental caries and its association with sugar consumption, saliva quality, and many other factors; and how to prevent and control oral diseases and conditions.

Table 16-1   Commonly Used Epidemiologic Terms

Term	Definition
Basic screening	Rapid assessment accomplished in a short time by visual detection providing information about gross dental and oral lesions; can be accomplished with a tongue blade, dental mirror, and appropriate lighting
Calibration	Standardization of examiners as they apply epidemiologic measurements
Determinants	Factors or events capable of bringing about a change in health; various factors that make up a multifactorial approach to a disease or health condition
Endemic	Usual presence of disease in a particular geographic region
Epidemic	Occurrence of an illness or condition in excess of normal expectancy in a community or region, usually occurring suddenly and spreading rapidly
Epidemiologic examination	Detailed visual-tactile assessment accomplished with dental instruments and a light source in a survey; provides more detailed information than basic screening; differs from a clinical examination in that it does not involve a clinical diagnosis and resulting treatment plan
Epidemiology	Study of the frequency and distribution of disease, disability, and death in the population, including the nature, cause, control, and determinants of health and disease as well as related factors
Eradication	Elimination of an infectious disease agent through surveillance and containment; contrasted to control, which is to keep the disease at minimum level so that it no longer poses a health problem
Incidence	Rate of new cases of a disease during or over a given time period
Interexaminer reliability	Agreement among two or more examiners as they apply an index or instrument over time
Intraexaminer reliability	Consistency of a single examiner in the application of an index or instrument over time
Morbidity	Extent of disease, injury, or disability in a defined population
Mortality	Death rate resulting from a specific disease or condition
Multifactorial	Concept that more than a single cause must be present for a disease or health condition to occur; multiple causation
Pandemic	Epidemic in which the disease may cross international borders to affect several countries or continents
Positive reversal	Change of the measurement made in error in a logical direction
Predictive value	Ability of a diagnostic test to accurately measure both the presence and absence of disease
Prevalence	Numerical expression of the number of all existing cases of a disease or health condition in a population measured at a given point or period of time

(continued)

Table 16-1 Commonly Used Epidemiologic Terms (continued)

Term	Definition
Proportion	Type of ratio that expresses the amount of disease or health condition with a fraction that presents it in relation to the size of the population; it can be expressed as a percentage
Rate	Expression of disease in a population using a standardized denominator and including a time dimension; allows for valid comparisons
Ratio	Expression of the magnitude of one occurrence of disease exposure in relation to another with a fraction; in contrast to a proportion, not necessary to have a relationship between the numerator and denominator
Reliability	Consistency or reproducibility of a measurement over time
Reversal (negative reversal)	Change of diagnosis in an illogical direction over a period of time
Sensitivity	Ability of a test to accurately identify the presence of a disease or condition when the disease is in fact present
Specificity	Ability of a test to accurately identify the absence of a disease or condition
Surveillance	Ongoing observation, persistent watching over, scrutinizing, constant monitoring, and assessing changes in populations related to disease, conditions, injuries, disabilities, or death trends
Trend	Long-term changes or movements in disease patterns and health-related conditions identified by examining surveillance data
Validity	Accuracy of a measurement; produced by measuring what is supposed to be measured

Source: Merrill RM, Timmreck TC. *An Introduction to Epidemiology.* 4th ed. Boston, MA: Jones & Bartlett; 2006. Friis RH, Sellers TA. *Epidemiology for Public Health Practice.* 3rd ed. Boston, MA: Jones & Bartlett; 2004. Gerstman BB. *Epidemiology Kept Simple: An Introduction to Traditional and Modern Epidemiology.* 2nd ed. Hoboken, NJ: Wiley-Liss; 2003. Association of State and Territorial Dental Directors (ASTDD). Basic screening surveys: An approach to monitoring community oral health. Revised September 2003. http://www.astdd.org/docs/BSS_Manual_9-25-03.pdf. Accessed January 13, 2008. US Department of Health and Human Services. *Healthy People 2010.* http://www.healthypeople.gov/. Accessed January 13, 2008.

THE MULTIFACTORIAL NATURE OF DISEASE

Epidemiology attempts to understand the cause(s) of disease and health conditions in a population. A key aspect of epidemiology is *determinant,* which is defined as a factor and event that can bring about a change in health.[7] At the turn of the nineteenth century with the discovery of bacteria, the cause of disease was generally thought of in terms of exposure to an etiologic agent. A simple cause-and-effect mechanism was understood to be at work. Today, epidemiology is based on a **multifactorial** approach, which assumes that a disease or condition has multiple causes.[7] These factors—the host, the agent, and the environment—are organized by epidemiologists as the **epidemiology triangle** to demonstrate the interaction and interrelatedness of these factors over time in bringing about the disease or condition.[6,9,11]

Agent is the biologic or mechanical cause of a disease or condition (eg, specific bacteria in relation to dental caries or brushing with a hard toothbrush in relation to abrasion). *Host* refers to an individual's genetic or social factors that contribute to the person's susceptibility or resistance, such as tooth morphology, salivary flow, salivary composition, and personal behaviors in relation

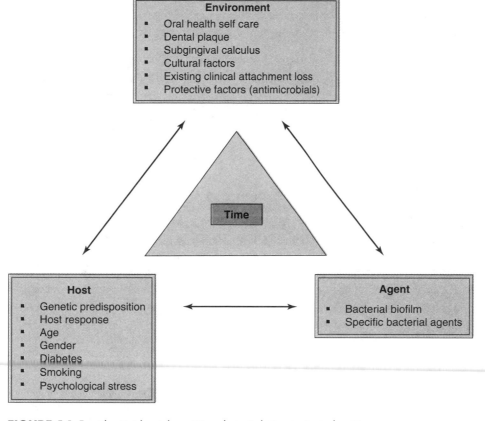

FIGURE 16-1   The Epidemiology Triangle in Relation to Periodontitis

Source: Adapted from Merrill RM, Timmreck TC. *An Introduction to Epidemiology.* 4th ed. Boston,
MA: Jones & Bartlett; 2006; Timmerman MF, van der Weijden GA. Risk factors for periodontitis.
Int J Den Hyg. 2006;4:2–7. http://www.blackwell-synergy.com/doi/pdf/10.1111/j.1601-5037.2006.00168.x.
Accessed June 7, 2008; Van Dyke TE, Dave S. Risk factors for periodontitis. *J Int Acad Periodont.*
2005;7(1):3–7. http://www.pubmedcentral.nih.gov/articlerender.fcgi?artid=1351013. Accessed June 7, 2008.

to dental caries. *Environment* refers to the physical, social, sociocultural, sociopolitical, and economic circumstances required for the disease to thrive, survive, and spread (eg, sugar in the diet and low SES in relation to dental caries as well as social norms and policies that control smoking in relation to oral cancer). Time issues include incubation periods, life expectancy, duration of the course of an illness or condition, and the severity of the illness. Approaching the diagnosis, treatment, and control of disease from a multifactorial approach requires consideration of these different factors.[11] See Figure 16-1 ■ for an example of the application of the epidemiology triangle to the multiple causation of periodontitis.

MEASUREMENT IN EPIDEMIOLOGY

Epidemiology involves the measurement of diseases, other health conditions, and death. *Morbidity* is the extent of disease, injury, or disability in a defined population, and *mortality* refers to the death rate resulting from a specific disease or condition.[6,9] The most common measures of morbidity and mortality are prevalence and incidence.[12] *Prevalence* is the numerical expression of all existing cases of a disease or health condition in a population measured at a given point or period of time.[6] This can be determined by case reports during the time period or surveying the population at a point in time. *Incidence* refers to the development of new cases of a disease or condition over a given time period or its progress over time. Determining incidence requires measuring the same people at least twice, at the beginning and at the end of the specified time period.[7] Incidence requires three important elements: a numerator (the number of new cases), a denominator (the population at risk), and a time dimension (the time period during which the new cases occurred).[6]

> ### Did You Know?
>
> A good way to remember prevalence and incidence is that *prevalence* refers to all of a disease or condition in the population at the designated time, and *incidence* refers to only new cases identified during the specific time period.

Epidemiologists also express measures using counts, proportions, ratios, rates, and indexes.[7,12,13] A *count* is the simplest form of measurement. It is simply the number of cases of the disease or condition in the population. It provides the least information because it does not communicate the size of the population.[7] An example is a statement that twenty patients presented in the community dental clinic for dental hygiene treatment with secondary oral herpetic lesions.

A count becomes a *proportion* when it is expressed relative to the size of the population. A proportion is a fraction and can be expressed as a percentage.[7] Expression of the frequency as a proportion rather than a count provides more information about the extent of the disease in the population. Using the preceding example, a proportion would be that 20 patients out of 200, or 10 percent, presented with herpetic lesions. This would be more significant than had the 20 cases been in a population size of 2000, thus representing only 1 percent. Use of a proportion versus a count communicates this information. A proportion is a type of *ratio*.[7] Prevalence is a proportion and should not be described as a rate, a commonly made mistake.[7]

A fraction is another type of ratio; it expresses the magnitude of one occurrence in relation to another.[6] We could refer to the ratio of the incidence of oral herpetic lesions in individuals who are under extreme stress in relation to individuals who are not experiencing stress. This would be expressed as a ratio, such as 5:1, but it is not a proportion because the numerator (those experiencing extreme stress) is not reflected in the denominator (those not experiencing stress); 5:1 can be translated to a relative risk of 5.0.[6,12,14]

A *rate* is the expression of disease in a population using a standardized denominator and including a time dimension.[7] The use of the common denominator allows for making valid comparisons across different populations or detecting trends within the same population. The value of the common denominator (eg, per 1000, per 100,000, or per 1,000,000) depends on the relation to the value being reported. For example, the mortality from oral cancer among African Americans in the year 2000 was 4.1 per 100,000 compared to 5.2 per 100,000 in the 1988–1992 period.[13] Expression of these rates as 0.041 per 1000 and 0.052 per 1000 would be just as correct mathematically although more difficult to interpret.[7] Incidence is a rate.[7]

An *index* reports more detailed information than a count, proportion, and rate by providing an abbreviated, standardized measurement of the amount or severity of the disease or condition in the population.[13] An index usually involves a graduated numerical scale to measure the extent of the health problem and to aid in data collection and analysis and is discussed in Chapter 13.

ORAL EPIDEMIOLOGY SURVEILLANCE AND REPORTS

Various systems of epidemiologic surveillance are used to collect data to determine the presence of disease, injury, disability, and related factors. **Surveillance,** an ongoing process, is the observation, persistent watching over, scrutiny, constant monitoring, and assessment of changes in populations related to disease, conditions, injuries, disabilities, or death trends.[6] It uses methods that are quick, simple, and practical, such as those discussed in Chapter 15, putting as little burden as possible on the health practitioners reporting the data.[11,13] Surveillance data are used to identify trends, which are the long-term changes or movements in disease patterns and health-related conditions.[6] Surveillance data are not as accurate as those collected under a strict protocol for research purposes, but this is appropriate because the purpose of identifying these trends is primarily to initiate epidemiologic investigations and to develop public health prevention and control programs.[6,11]

The primary means of surveillance in the United States is passive surveillance, which involves voluntary reporting, although this may be in response to laws that require reporting.[13] For example, some state dental boards require that HIV be reported by dental personnel who are carriers, but the authorities do not actively solicit the data. Active surveillance in which public health staff personnel go into the field to collect data is used to identify cases of disease that would be missed by passive reporting. For example, active surveillance was used when attempting to eradicate smallpox.[15]

In the United States, surveillance activities are conducted by various components of the Centers for Disease Control and Prevention (CDC) of the US Department of Health and Human Services (USDHHS). Except for oral cancer (and cleft lip and palate in some states), oral health data have not been available through these traditional surveillance systems. The Surveillance, Epidemiology, and End Results (SEER) program is a system that provides a source for data of virtually all cancer, including oral cancer, in the United States.

Surveys have been conducted to generate oral health data for other oral conditions for purposes of planning public health programs. These surveys, which are more similar to active surveillance, were originally conducted by the National Institute for Dental (and Craniofacial) Research and then by the National Center for Health Statistics, which is part of CDC.[13] The National Health and Nutrition Examination Survey (NHANES) is a national survey that has been conducted several times over the past decades. The National Health Interview Survey (NHIS) has been used to track various oral health–related conditions reflected in *Healthy People 2010* objectives. Another national survey is the Medical Expenditure Panel Survey (MEPS) conducted by the Agency for Healthcare Research and Quality of the USDHHS, which measures progress of the *Healthy People 2010* objectives related to dental events.[16]

National Oral Health Surveillance System

National surveys such as those just described provide valuable national data, but their information could not be separated into state-level data necessary for local public health program planning. In response to that limitation, the National Oral Health Surveillance System (NOHSS) was established in the mid-1990s as a joint venture of the CDC and the Association of State and Territorial Dental Directors (ASTDD). The NOHSS was designed to monitor the burden of oral disease, utilization of the oral health care delivery system, and community water fluoridation on both national and state levels. The CDC assists states in collecting their specific survey data, and the CDC then reports them in a national database. Data are collected for a set of nine oral health indicators: dental visits, (professional) teeth cleaning, complete tooth loss, loss of six or more teeth, fluoridation status, dental sealants, caries experience, untreated tooth decay, and cancer of the oral cavity and pharynx.[16]

Did You Know?

The Web site http://www.cdc.gov/nohss/ is an excellent resource for information about dental disease and dental services in your state. It can be particularly helpful for writing reports and planning and developing public health programs.

Several state-level surveys collect the surveillance data for the NOHSS. The Behavioral Risk Factor Surveillance System (BRFSS) and its companion Youth Risk Behavior Surveillance System (YRBSS) collect several indicators. Both surveys consist of core questions developed by the CDC that a state health agency can adapt to its local needs. Fluoridation status is monitored at local, state, and tribal levels for the NOHSS by using the Water Fluoridation Reporting System (WFRS), an interactive, real-time, Web-based, surveillance system developed by the CDC in collaboration with the ASTDD.

Clinical data for other indicators are collected using the Basic Screening Survey (BSS) developed by the ASTDD.[17] Its purpose is to collect valid although limited clinical data in an unobtrusive, efficient, and cost-effective manner.[13] Rather than measuring the total caries experience with a decayed, missing, filled tooth (DMFT) index, which was discussed in Chapter 13, the BSS uses the basic screening approach of oral surveying to assess the prevalence of untreated dental caries and dental caries experience on a per person basis using dichotomous (yes/no) measures. With this approach, individuals with a DMFT score of 1 or greater are classified as having caries experience; individuals with a DMFT of 0 are classified as caries free. Classification of treatment—no obvious problem, early treatment needed, or urgent treatment needed—can be utilized for referral purposes and surveillance.[17]

Morbidity and Mortality Weekly Report

The CDC publishes current, relevant epidemiologic data in the United States weekly in the *Morbidity and Mortality Weekly Report* (*MMWR*). It compiles cogent health and health-related issues currently being studied. Its primary purpose has been to report events of public health interest and importance as well as a list of nationally notifiable diseases (diseases that must be reported to the CDC) to state and local health departments as quickly as possible.[18] The CDC receives case-report surveillance data that are voluntarily contributed electronically by states and then compiles the statistics for the nationally notifiable disease list. The CDC also summarizes these case counts annually.[15] Many of these health and health-related conditions and events, such as herpes, hepatitis, asthma, autism, health behaviors, fluoridation, immunizations, and use of tobacco, are of interest to those in dental hygiene. The *MMWR* is available online free or by subscription for a paper copy.

Healthy People 2010 Objectives

Oral health surveillance in the United States has resulted in the establishment of oral health objectives for the nation for the last three decades.[19] National publications have provided a statement of these objectives designed to identify the most significant preventable threats to health and to establish national goals to reduce them. Thus, these publications have set the prevention agenda for the United States. The most recent one, *Healthy People 2010,* has two overarching goals and consists of 467 objectives organized around twenty-eight focus areas (see Table 16-2 ■).[20] Ten leading indicators have been identified to measure attainment of these objectives: physical activity, overweight and obesity, tobacco use, substance abuse, responsible sexual behavior, mental health, injury and violence, environmental quality, immunization, and access to health care.

Oral health is a specific focus area of *Healthy People 2010* and is integrated into many of the other twenty-eight focus areas (see Table 16-2). The goal for these areas is to prevent and control oral and craniofacial diseases, conditions, and injuries, and improve access to related services. The oral health objectives build on oral health initiatives over the last decades, including NOHSS surveillance data.[21] A summary of the oral health objectives is presented in Table 16-3 ■.

Table 16-2 *Healthy People 2010* Goals and Focus Areas

Goal 1: Increase Quality and Years of Healthy Life

To help individuals of all ages increase life expectancy and improve their quality of life

Goal 2: Eliminate Health Disparities

To eliminate health disparities among different segments of the population

Focus Areas

1. Access to quality health services[a]
2. Arthritis, osteoporosis, chronic back conditions[a]
3. Cancer[a]
4. Chronic kidney disease
5. Diabetes[a]
6. Disability and secondary conditions[a]
7. Educational and community-based programs[a]
8. Environmental health[a]
9. Family planning
10. Food safety
11. Health communication[a]
12. Heart disease and stroke[a]
13. Human immunodeficiency virus infection
14. Immunization and infectious diseases[a]
15. Injury and violence prevention[a]
16. Maternal, infant, and child health[a]
17. Medical product safety[a]
18. Mental health and mental disorders[a]
19. Nutrition and overweight[a]
20. Occupational safety and health[a]
21. Oral health[a]
22. Physical activity and fitness[a]
23. Public health infrastructure[a]
24. Respiratory diseases
25. Sexually transmitted diseases[a]
26. Substance abuse[a]
27. Tobacco use[a]
28. Vision and hearing

[a]Objectives related to oral health are included in these focus areas; see US Department of Health and Human Services. Oral health. *Healthy People 2010, Oral Health.* Vol. II. http://www.healthypeople.gov/document/HTML/Volume2/21Oral.htm. Accessed January 18, 2008.

Source: US Department of Health and Human Services. *Healthy People 2010.* http://www.healthypeople.gov/. Accessed January 13, 2008.

Table 16-3 Summary of Healthy People 2010 Oral Health Objectives

Oral Health (Chapter 21) Goal: To prevent and control oral and craniofacial diseases, conditions, and injuries and improve access to related services.

21-1   Decrease dental caries experience

21-2   Decrease untreated dental decay

21-3   Increase proportion with no tooth loss

21-4   Decrease edentulousness

21-5   Decrease gingivitis and destructive periodontal disease

21-6   Increase early detection of oral and pharyngeal cancer

21-7   Increase annual examinations for oral and pharyngeal cancer

21-8   Increase placement of dental sealants in permanent teeth

21-9   Increase community water fluoridation

21-10 Increase dental utilization (annual dental visits) of the general population

21-11 Increase dental utilization by nursing home residents

21-12 Increase dental services for low-income children

21-13 Increase availability of oral health in school-based health centers

21-14 Increase availability of oral health in community health centers

21-15 Increase referrals for cleft lip or palate

21-16 Increase state oral health surveillance systems

21-17 Increase availability of dental programs in tribal, state, and local health agencies

Source: US Department of Health and Human Services. Oral health. *Healthy People 2010, Oral Health.* Vol. II. http://www.healthypeople.gov/document/HTML/Volume2/21Oral.htm. Accessed January 18, 2008.

A midcourse review of progress made toward these oral health objectives was conducted and reported through January 2005.[21] Objectives that showed improvement and those that moved away from their targets are summarized in Box 16-2 ■. The other oral health objectives demonstrated no change or could not be assessed.

BOX 16-2 Summary of Progress Toward Healthy People 2010 Oral Health Objectives

Objectives That Improved

- Proportion of adolescents with untreated dental decay
- Dental caries experience and untreated dental decay in children ages 6 to 8 years
- Untreated dental decay and tooth loss among adults
- Destructive periodontal disease in adults
- Number of children who have received dental sealants on their molar teeth
- Proportion of the US population served by community water fluoridation
- Proportion of low-income persons younger than 19 who received preventive dental services in the past year
- Proportion of community health centers with an oral health component

Objectives That Moved Away from Their Targets

- Increase in the proportion of children ages 2 to 4 years with dental caries and untreated dental decay
- Decrease in the proportion of oral and pharyngeal cancers detected at an early stage
- Decrease in the number of Indian Health Service and Tribal dental programs

Surgeon General's Reports

The US Surgeon General regularly issues reports on various health conditions. *Oral Health in America: A Report of the Surgeon General,* issued in May 2000 by Surgeon General David Satcher, MD, PhD, was the first-ever comprehensive report on the status of the nation's oral health.[22] The report provided scientific information on the growth and development of oral, dental, and craniofacial tissues; described oral diseases and conditions; and underscored the critical relationship between oral health and general health throughout life. The report discussed the extensive toll resulting from the range of oral, dental, and craniofacial diseases and conditions that affect the US population. See Box 16-3 ■ for a summary of its major findings.

BOX 16-3 Major Findings from *Oral Health in America: A Report of the Surgeon General*

- Oral health is more than healthy teeth.
- Oral disease and disorders in and of themselves affect health and well-being throughout life.
- The mouth reflects general health and well-being.
- Oral diseases and conditions are associated with other health problems.
- Lifestyle behaviors that affect general health, such as tobacco use, excessive alcohol use, and poor dietary choices, affect oral and craniofacial health as well.

- Safe and effective measures exist to prevent the most common dental diseases—dental caries and periodontal diseases.
- There are profound and consequential oral health disparities within the US population.
- More information is needed to improve America's oral health and eliminate health disparities.
- Scientific research is the key to further reduction in the burden of disease and disorders that affect the face, mouth, and teeth.

Source: US Department of Health and Human Services, Public Health Service, National Institutes of Health, National Institute of Dental and Craniofacial Research. *Oral Health in America: A Report of the Surgeon General, 2000* [press release]. http://www.surgeongeneral.gov/library/oralhealth/. Accessed January 13, 2008.

The report referred to the mouth and face as a mirror of the health and disease conditions found in the rest of the body. It discussed more than twenty diseases and conditions that cause lesions of the oral mucosa. For example, the report described associations between oral infections and diabetes, heart disease/stroke, respiratory ailments, and adverse pregnancy outcomes, such as premature births and low birth-weight babies. It also addressed the effects of oral diseases on well-being and quality of life. Dental hygienists are aware of the impact of tooth pain and oral disfigurement on eating, sleeping, cultural significance, social functions, and economics.

The surgeon general's 2000 report does not mention the past or future critical role of the dental hygiene profession in preventing and treating oral diseases in the United States. However, it does highlight fluoridation, school water fluoridation, dietary fluoride supplements, fluoride mouth rinse programs, fluoride varnishes, dental sealants, and community programs as approaches to promote oral health and prevent oral disease. Water fluoridation was reported to have the single greatest impact on the prevention of oral diseases. The dental hygiene profession is an integral part of such pubic health initiatives.

The surgeon general's 2000 report discussed a framework for action including the following recommendations:

- Change perceptions regarding oral heath and ideas so that oral health becomes an accepted component of general health.

- Accelerate the building of the science and evidence base, and apply science effectively to improve oral health.
- Build an effective health infrastructure that meets the oral health needs of all Americans and integrate oral health effectively into general health.
- Remove known barriers between people and oral health services.
- Use public-private partnerships to improve the oral health of those who still suffer disproportionately from oral disease.

The Surgeon General's office released a follow-up report, *A National Call to Action to Promote Oral Health (Call to Action),* in May 2003. It describes the ongoing effort to address the country's oral health needs in the twenty-first century. Reflecting the work of a partnership of public and private organizations, the *National Call to Action* builds on *Oral Health in America: A Report of the Surgeon General* and *Healthy People 2010.*[23] It was an invitation to expand plans, activities, and programs designed to promote oral health and prevent disease, especially to reduce the health disparities that affect members of racial and ethnic groups, poor people, many who are geographically isolated, and others who are vulnerable because of special oral health care needs.[23] The report consists of five actions (see Box 16-4 ■) to which individuals from research, clinical care, and the community are

---

BOX 16-4 Five Action Recommendations in the *National Call to Action to Promote Oral Health*

1. Change perceptions of oral health so that it is viewed to be as important as and related to general health.
2. Overcome barriers to oral health by replicating effective programs and proven efforts to enhance health promotion and health literacy, improve access to care, and reduce disabilities.
3. Build the science base of oral health by enhancing oral health research and accelerating the effective transfer of science to public and private practice.
4. Increase oral health workforce diversity, capacity, and flexibility to ensure a sufficient workforce pool to meet oral health care needs.
5. Increase collaborations to enhance partnering between the private and public sectors of oral health care.

Source: Adapted from US Department of Health and Human Services, Public Health Service, Centers for Disease Control and Prevention, National Institutes of Health, National Institute of Dental and Craniofacial Research. *A National Call to Action to Promote Oral Health: A Public-Private Partnership under the Leadership of the Office of the Surgeon General.* Bethesda, MD: Author; 2003. NIH Publication No. 03-5303.

---

enlisted to work collaboratively to improve the oral health of society. It should be noted that the current emphasis on evidence-based practice in dentistry and dental hygiene is in line with the third recommended action.[23]

Global Oral Health Data Bank

The Global Oral Health Data Bank managed by the World Health Organization (WHO) contains oral epidemiologic data from around the world.[24] It uses data the WHO systematically collects from countries that use its recommended data collection methods[25] and maintains these country-specific data sets.[13] Data are provided for dental caries, periodontal diseases, tobacco use, oral cancer, and other oral conditions and programs.[24] In many cases, these data apply to large groups from the most populous parts of a country to provide an epidemiologic estimate of health conditions rather than being fully representative. Sources/references are given for every data set presented in the relevant country pages. Links to these databases are available on the Companion Website created specifically to accompany this textbook.

CONCEPTS OF EPIDEMIOLOGICAL STUDIES

Certain concepts that are germane to epipidemiological studies include risk of disease, causes of disease, and effectiveness and efficacy of treatment modalities. It is vital to understand these concepts and how they relate to and differ from each other in meaning.

Risk and Causality

To understand research, classify a study design, and be able to apply research results to dental hygiene practice, we must understand the difference between risk and causality.[14,26] *Causality,* also referred to as *cause and effect* or *causation,* means that a particular exposure results in a particular outcome.[6] This could be exposure to a causative agent that results in a specific disease, exposure to a preventive agent that results in preventing the disease, or exposure to treatment that results in resolving or controlling the disease. Causality routinely is used in dental hygiene practice to make decisions about what prevention and treatment programs to implement with individual patients or the population. Some examples are provided in Box 16-5 ■. Experimental studies are used to establish causality without question.[13] However, in many cases in oral epidemiology, causality has been accepted from analytic (observational) studies that have identified risk.

When conducting experimental studies to establish causation is not practical or ethical, observational studies may be used to infer it. For example, exposing young children to malnutrition to establish a causal link to the development of caries is not ethical, nor can a researcher ethically observe a group of malnourished

BOX 16-5 Examples of Causality in Dental Hygiene Practice

- Plaque biofilm has been shown to cause gingivitis. This was demonstrated by observing its effect on the gingiva after a week of no oral hygiene in a group of students compared to a similar group that practiced oral hygiene and did not develop gingivitis. This established causality is the reason we teach oral hygiene to our patients.
- Causation of sugar in the development of dental caries has been indicated. This was established with experimental studies that compared caries rates in children with high sugar diets with caries rates in children with low sugar diets. This causation is the reason we do diet counseling.
- The causal role of fluoridation in the prevention of caries has been demonstrated. This was done by comparing the caries rates in children in cities where fluoridation was implemented to the caries rates in children in cities where it was not. Hence, we promote water fluoridation.
- A causal relationship has been established between professional fluoride treatments and lower dental caries rates. This was accomplished by comparing caries incidence in children who received fluoride treatments to caries rates in children who did not. This causality is why we recommend fluoride treatments.
- The causality of flossing has been shown in relation to improved gingivitis healing. This was demonstrated by the reduction of interproximal bleeding when proper flossing was practiced with brushing in one group compared to continued bleeding in a comparable group that only brushed. This causation is why we recommend flossing.

children over a long period to see whether they experience more caries than a group of well-nourished children. If we were aware of their being malnourished, we would be obligated to intervene because of the other known health risks involved with malnutrition. In these cases, we must establish risk by conducting analytic studies that associate an attribute or exposure with the disease or condition. For example, the nutritional history of young children with and without dental caries can be studied to associate malnutrition with caries.

Establishing risk is not the same as establishing causality, but risk is used to infer or suggest causality. While causality means that a cause-and-effect relationship has been established, risk is the probability that a specified event will occur.[13] The purpose of analytic studies is to quantify the degree of risk in specific circumstances. Risk establishes an association or relationship between the exposure and the condition that is used to infer or suggest causality.

See Box 16-6■ for a description of the criteria that support inferring causality from observational studies. Not all of these criteria must be in place to support causality, but the more that are present, the stronger is the case for causality of a risk factor in relation to the disease or condition.[6,7,15,26] Examples of inferred causality from analytic studies in oral epidemiology are the causal relationships between malnutrition and dental caries, excess fluoride and fluorosis, tobacco use and oral cancer, and plaque biofilm bacteria and periodontal diseases. Although none of these causal relationships has been confirmed with experimental studies, causality has been accepted because of the results of observational studies that suggest it.

Some types of analytic studies establish risk more strongly than others.[13] To understand this, we must first understand the three types of attributes—risk factors, risk indicators, and risk markers, also called *risk predictors* and *demographic risk factors*—associated with diseases and conditions and how they are established.[13] Risk factors and risk indicators can refer to attributes that result in disease as well as those that control or prevent disease.

A *risk factor* is a modifiable attribute or exposure known to be associated with a health condition.[13] Increased exposure increases the risk; reduced exposure reduces the risk. Risk factors are considered important to prevent. They are identified by conducting longitudinal studies (observation over time); therefore, they are the most reliable indication of risk.

Three criteria must be met to establish an exposure as a risk factor:

- Exposure must precede the onset of disease or health condition.

BOX 16-6 Criteria for Inferring Causality from Observational Studies

- **Strength of Association.** The stronger the association between exposure and outcome, the greater is the likelihood of causation.
- **Consistency of Association.** If the association holds in a large number of studies (replication studies), it is more likely to be causal.
- **Sensitivity of Association.** If those who have the disease were exposed to the suspected causative factor, the factor is more likely to be causal.
- **Specificity of Association.** If absence of exposure is associated with absence of the disease outcome, the exposure is more likely to be causal.

- **Time Relationship.** If the exposure precedes the outcome, causality is more likely. This condition is considered to be absolute.[a]
- **Dose-Response Relationship.** If the disease outcome increases as the degree of exposure increases, causality is more likely.
- **Plausibility.** If the association is congruent with current biological, medical, epidemiologic, and scientific knowledge, causality is more likely.
- **Analogy.** If the association is similar to other associations that have been shown to be causal, the transfer of knowledge can be used to support causality.

[a]Webber R. *Communicable Disease Epidemiology and Control: A Global Perspective.* 2nd ed. Cambridge, MA: CABI; 2005.

- Exposure must covary with the frequency of the disease or health condition.
- Observed association must not be due to bias or error in sample selection, measurement, or data analysis.

These criteria can be illustrated by examining the relationship between smoking and periodontitis. Smoking precedes the development of periodontal disease, but smoking is modifiable: People can quit smoking. Multiple long-term observational studies have demonstrated that frequency of periodontal disease covaries with smoking status. In other words, we have observed smokers longitudinally to confirm that they develop periodontal disease more frequently than nonsmokers. Additionally, we have observed that smokers who have quit smoking develop periodontal disease less frequently than those who continue to smoke. These studies have been well controlled to prevent error. Although experimental studies cannot be conducted to confirm a causal relationship, we accept the causation of smoking relative to periodontitis because of the strength of these observational studies.

A *risk indicator* is a modifiable attribute that has been shown to be associated with a disease in cross-sectional and/or case–control studies. Therefore, it is assumed to have a causal role in the development of the disease.[13] Risk indicators are suspected risk factors that have not been confirmed by the necessary longitudinal studies. Note that the difference between a risk factor and a risk indicator is the type of research study used to establish the risk. Sometimes it is impractical or unethical to conduct longitudinal studies to confirm risk indicators as risk factors. For example, we would not want to expose a population to long-term malnutrition to confirm that malnutrition is a risk factor for poor oral health.

Without confirmation, there is no way to be sure that a risk indicator is truly a risk factor. Experience has shown that risk indicators can disappear when assessed in longitudinal studies.[13] Therefore, we should take care to know the difference so we do not make inappropriate recommendations to patients.

A *risk marker* is an attribute that is associated with the increased probability of disease but is not considered to have a causal role in its development. Risk markers are also established by conducting cross-sectional and case–control studies. Risk markers such as age, gender, race, ethnicity, and SES are nonmodifiable. Therefore, they are not useful when considering prevention based on controlling risk.

The significance of discriminating between these attributes relates to the way they are applied to clinical decision making about preventive recommendations in dental hygiene practice.[13] Risk factors should be considered to help patients control disease because the risks have been established such as those with tobacco, alcohol, and

Table 16-4 Summary of Risk Attributes

Attribute	Modifiability	Studies	Application to Dental Hygiene Practice
Risk factor	Yes	Longitudinal	• Established causal role • Should be an important consideration in making recommendations
Risk indicator	Yes	Cross-sectional Case–control	• Possible causal role • Should be applied with care when making recommendations
Risk marker (demographic risk factor/risk predictor)	No	Cross-sectional Case–control	• Is not important in making individual recommendations to control that factor • Indicates greater need to control modifiable risk factors and risk indicators • Should be considered to identify target populations for dental public health program

diet. Risk indicators should be applied with care in practice decisions because the risk is assumed but not confirmed as with some systemic conditions. Risk markers are not useful in controlling disease, but they point to an increased need to address modifiable known risk factors and risk indicators to reduce the risk of disease. Risk markers also have application in making decisions about what populations to target with dental public health programs. See Table 16-4 ■ for a summary of risk factors, risk indicators, and risk markers and Table 16-5 ■ for a comparison of the classifications and characteristics of nonexperimental studies.

Effectiveness Versus Efficacy Trials

Clinical trials are classified as either efficacy or effectiveness.[13] The differences relate to the trial's purpose. Understanding the difference is important to interpret the results correctly. The purpose of an *efficacy trial* is to test whether an agent or treatment regimen works. It is conducted on a population susceptible to the disease or condition being studied.[13] Susceptibility could be based on age, gender, race, SES, geographic location, or other factors identified in previous studies. Results can be generalized only to the susceptible population sampled for

Table 16-5 Comparisons of Different Types of Nonexperimental Studies

Type of Study	Number of Groups	Number of Measures	Classification	Used to Identify
Descriptive	1	1	Prevalence	Prevalence
Cohort	1	2 or more	Longitudinal Prospective Incidence	Risk factor
Case–control	2	1	Retrospective	Risk indicator Demographic risk factor
Cross-sectional	1	1	Cross-sectional	Risk indicator Demographic risk factor
Ecologic	1	2	NA	Correlation

the study. Therefore, generalizing results of efficacy trials to the population at large produces an error in interpretation. These trials are conducted under very controlled conditions. They have requirements such as the use of a control group, double-blind methods, and agent exactly as intended in terms of concentration, length and frequency of use, and application procedures as well as the random allocation to groups. The term *application procedure* refers to instructions given to study participants, application by a person who will apply it correctly (self or professional) or professional supervision if self-applied, and duplication of procedures with a control group.

An example of an efficacy trial is testing the ability of a new power toothbrush to reduce gingivitis by evaluating its use in a sample population that has high plaque, gingivitis, and bleeding scores. To ensure that it is operated correctly, the power toothbrush would be used by the study participants under close supervision after careful instruction by the researcher.

The purpose of an *effectiveness trial* is to test the way an agent or treatment regimen works in everyday conditions after its efficacy has been established.[13] This type of trial is conducted on a broad community population with varying degrees of the disease or condition under study. Results of effectiveness trials can be generalized to the population at large because they are conducted on a sample drawn from this broad population. Effectiveness trials require less control than efficacy trials because the agent is used as it normally would be

used. Professionals who apply the agent are given instructions but not supervised as they apply it. If it self-applied, participants must receive professional instructions and then take the agent home to use.

The previous example of an efficacy trial can be adapted to illustrate an effectiveness trial. The effectiveness of the same power toothbrush could be tested in a sample that represents the general population with a variety of ages, abilities, and oral health status. The toothbrush would be used at home without supervision after receiving standardized instruction from the researcher. This would be done after the efficacy trial determined that the power toothbrush reduces gingivitis under controlled conditions in a sample that exhibits gingivitis.

VALIDITY OF EPIDEMIOLOGICAL STUDIES

Chapter 13 of this textbook discussed the validity and reliability of measurements. Here validity will be discussed in relation to conducting an epidemiologic research study. *Validity* is the accuracy of a study, which is affected by procedures and controls used while conducting it.[27] The two types of validity are internal and external. Researchers are concerned with validity because they must ensure that research is meaningful. Validity is increased by controlling errors and bias when conducting a study. See Box 16-7 ■ for a summary of ways to increase validity in experimental studies.

BOX 16-7   Ways to Control Errors and Bias to Increase Validity of Experimental Research Designs

- Have a researchable hypothesis
- Base the study on valid assumptions
- Operationally define variables clearly
- Use the appropriate population for the type of study
- Use a representative sample
- Have an adequate sample size to accommodate for loss of participants
- Control extraneous variables
- Use an appropriate type of control or comparison group
- Control group differences by using randomization and stratification
- Use participants as their own control when appropriate

- Use blind and double-blind procedures
- Use a pretest for comparison
- Control for pretest sensitization
- Use valid and reliable instruments
- Control examiner error with standardization and calibration
- Carefully control and supervise procedures
- Control errors in measuring the dependent variable
- Standardize study conditions in all groups
- Use repeated measures when appropriate
- Use several measures of the dependent variable when called for
- Have a long enough trial to detect new disease or change

Internal Validity

Internal validity refers to the accuracy of a study's results.[15] Internal validity is enhanced by controlling sources of error and extraneous variables when conducting the research, increasing subject retention, achieving compliance of study participants, enhancing data quality, and applying appropriate methods for statistical data analysis. To increase an experimental study's accuracy, procedures followed during the study should be carefully controlled and supervised to standardize study conditions between the experimental and control groups.

Several procedures increase internal validity by controlling errors in the measurement of the variables.[13] For example, the validity and reliability of instruments and examiners must be ensured.[27] The measurement instrument must be valid and reliable and provide consistent, reproducible results.[15] Measuring the dependent variable with established or pretested measures and instruments that have documented reliability increases a study's internal validity.

> ### Did You Know?
>
> Double blind study designs can control the reliability of data by reducing experimenter bias and participant expectations.

The length of the study can also affect its internal validity. It must be long enough to detect new disease and extension of current disease. The ideal length varies with the disease being studied. The recommendation of the Fédération Dentaire Internationale is two to three years for caries reduction trials, eight to twenty-one days for plaque-inhibiting studies, ninety days for supragingival calculus prevention agents, longer for subgingival calculus prevention, and six months for gingivitis reduction trials.[13]

A sample's size can affect internal validity in several ways. Humans have the right to participate or not in a study. This volunteer involvement can result in the loss of participants from longitudinal studies. The sample must be large enough to compensate for this loss; otherwise, resulting group sizes can be too small to produce valid results. Even when compensating with a larger sample, the fewer participants lost, the less susceptible the study is to invalid results.[26] Loss of participants can result

in groups that are no longer equivalent, thus invalidating the study results.[26] When participants are lost from a study, it is important also to test for equivalency of the final groups and to determine whether those who dropped from the study were similar to those who completed it.[10] Research reports should include the size of the sample in terms of the number approached to participate, the number who agreed to begin the study, and the number who completed it.[13]

Finally, internal validity is affected by the validity of the statistical procedures used, which depends in part on the sample size. Group sizes must be adequate for the application of inferential statistics. The use of multiple groups as required by factorial and Solomon designs necessitates the use of a larger sample than other designs to allow for adequate group sizes. Samples also must be larger when small differences are expected in the dependent variable between the test and control group.[13] For example, early fluoride studies compared a group exposed to fluoride to a group not exposed, and large differences in caries rates were expected because other uses of fluorides were uncommon. Today, because of the prevalence of fluoride exposure in our population, we expect smaller caries differences when comparing a group exposed to fluoride to a group not exposed. Therefore, larger groups (hence, larger samples) are needed today to obtain the statistical results required to reject the null hypothesis.

External Validity

The accuracy of inferring (generalizing) the results from the sample to the population at large is referred to as *external validity*.[15] It is affected by how well the sample represents the population. If it is a good representation, we can safely generalize results to that population. If it is not representative, we cannot infer results from that single study to that population. Therefore, selection of study participants is critical. Regardless of the type of study, the sample should be similar to the population in age, gender, SES, ethnicity, other demographic factors, and variables that relate to the area of study.[25]

The type of study determines the type and sample size required to increase internal validity.[13] Use of a large, representative sample is critical for descriptive studies.[6] Distribution of several hundred questionnaires would be the goal of a survey, depending on population size.[6] Generally, at least 10 percent of the population is suggested for survey research. Also, when an interview or questionnaire is used to collect survey data, response rate must be considered to accommodate the size of the sample approached to increase external validity.

Sampling must be precise for survey research. Because the intent is to infer the results to the population, the sample must represent it. Use of a nonrepresentative sample results in a discrepancy between the sample and the population in one or more important characteristics, and the results cannot be generalized. For example, if a dental hygiene class is surveyed when studying college students, the sample clearly does not represent the population. Dental hygiene students differ from other students in the college in terms of GPA, health interest, age, and other characteristics.

Even when precise sampling methods are used, sampling error can occur.[7] Sampling error can be calculated statistically when a probability sample is used. With a probability sample, which is a method of sampling that uses some form of random selection, the chance of each person being selected in the sample is known but is not necessarily equal.[7] The degree of sampling error for a probability sample can be calculated; thus, how well the results can be inferred to the population is known. The chance of each person being selected for a nonprobability sample is not known. In this case, the sampling error cannot be calculated, and problems with interpretation of the data can arise. Many large national epidemiologic surveys, such as those described earlier in this chapter, use probability samples as a technique.[13]

A small sample can be used for a pilot study, which is a trial run in preparation for a major large research project. (See Chapter 15.) Also, nearly all randomized clinical trials are accomplished with smaller convenience samples, which are composed of subjects who are most readily available.[13] Replication studies are used to compensate for the use of unrepresentative samples in experimental research by confirming that similar results occur with different samples. Additional studies that examine the same research question using similar methods in different populations and obtaining similar results provides evidence that the observed effect is real and can be generalized to the population at large.[13]

The delimitations of the study sample to control the internal validity of efficacy trials reduce the study's legitimacy when applied to the population at large by excluding certain individuals. Also, controlling and supervising the use of a product or procedure limits the legitimacy in the uncontrolled circumstances of the real world. Thus, effectiveness trials follow efficacy trials.[13] For example, if a fluoride varnish study shows its efficacy to reduce dental caries in a Head Start program in a low SES urban population of children recently emigrated from Mediterranean and Middle Eastern countries, these results do not generalize to all children. Replication studies would be needed to test the fluoride varnish in various groups of children representing different ages, dietary practices, ethnic backgrounds, and exposure to fluoridated water. If similar results occur in these different studies, it would be possible to generalize the results to the general population.[13]

Other procedures used when conducting research also affect external validity. For example, the dependent variable measure must have reference and meaning to the real world. Also, using more than one measure of the dependent variable improves the study's external validity.[13,27] An example is the measurement of both bleeding and gingival appearance with a bleeding index and a gingival index. Pretest sensitization occurs when subjects have been pretested and as a result may act or react differently once an independent variable is studied. This can also decrease external validity but can be controlled by using posttest-only or Solomon designs. Some changes measured at posttest, such as improved plaque scores to measure success of oral health education, may not hold over time. When this is the case, measuring the dependent variable three times after introducing the independent variable is recommended.[28]

SUMMARY

Evidence-based practice requires understanding epidemiologic research methods to be able to interpret their results and apply them to dental hygiene practice. Various epidemiologic methods are used to track oral disease and related conditions in the population. Surveillance systems in place in the United States help to determine what public health programs are needed and to track trends that can be used to evaluate the success of these programs. Nonexperimental and experimental research designs are used to measure the presence and distribution of oral disease in the population, track progress of disease over time, determine population needs, and evaluate the success of programs, treatment regimens, and methods of preventing and controlling disease.

DENTAL HYGIENE SPOTLIGHT:
Missy McDougal-Plese, RDH, MS

Missy McDougal-Plese is a school dental hygienist. She graduated from the undergraduate and graduate programs at the University of New Mexico (UNM) where she now teaches and is the American Dental Hygienists' Association UNM student member advisor. Ms. McDougal-Plese has been very involved in the local and state dental hygiene associations and speaks on school-based health care initiatives to a variety of audiences.

I asked a few questions about her career.

Why did you decide to go into dental hygiene?

My first real interest in oral health developed when I was a teenager. I wore orthodontics and became obsessed with keeping my braces clean. The idea of having something stuck in my braces for everyone to see completely mortified me. So, I guess you could say my interest in dental hygiene at a personal level came from pure vanity! My personal attention to oral hygiene developed into the thought that maybe dental hygiene was a profession that I would want to pursue. My childhood dentist, realizing I was interested in the dental professions, recruited me to work in his dental office. I began working there the summer after I was graduated from high school. That same summer, he hired a newly graduated dental hygienist. Really, my dentist's encouragement and the dental hygienist's excitement and willingness to share her knowledge encouraged me to pursue dental hygiene as a career.

How did you get into dental public health? Did you need additional education?

I was introduced to dental public health while both an undergraduate and graduate student at UNM's Division of Dental Hygiene (DDH). I feel very fortunate to have been educated in a state and at a university that recognize the significance of dental public health and therefore provide a variety of opportunities to dental hygienists. As part of my graduate education, I worked in one of

UNM's school-based dental clinics. That experience really allowed me to see firsthand the benefit that public health dental hygienists can have in a community as well as the advantages of working in a nontraditional practice setting. After obtaining my MS in Dental Hygiene, I was invited to become a faculty member at UNM's DDH. The fact that I did pursue an advanced degree has been a benefit to me on many levels. The knowledge I obtained while carrying out my graduate education has definitely improved my abilities as an educator, researcher, clinician, and dental public health advocate.

What are your current positions?

I am an assistant professor at UNM, Health Sciences Center, DDH. As part of my faculty responsibilities, I coordinate and provide preventive services within our school-based dental clinics. Currently UNM has one school-based health center (SBHC) dental clinic in a public middle school, and we are working to expand our services to two additional schools.

Can you discuss any particularly interesting experiences you have had in your dental public health positions?

Everyday is a new experience with new adventures. I truly enjoy working with the students, teachers, staff, and administrators at the school. The students I treat really educate me as much as I educate them. The school in which our dental clinic is located has a large Spanish-speaking population. Although I rely heavily on the bilingual dental clinic clerical staff as well as the school staff, I have been able to improve my Spanish-speaking abilities. The students get a kick out of helping me learn new words or phrases, and I enjoy expanding my Spanish conversational skills.

I think the most notable experience I have had while working in UNM's school-based health centers is the overall demonstration of interest and support of professionals from all different disciplines once they hear that I provide dental preventive services in a school-based clinic. When people learn about school-based dental care, they have a lot of interest in how they can either get involved with or support such a program.

As we all know, access to care is an important issue within health professions, so people are looking to pursue avenues that improve access to and use of health care services. A school-based health center is a unique way to provide care to the youth of communities while addressing many of the unmet and untreated health issues that countless Americans experience. It has been exciting for me to work within an existing SBHC and participate in the expansion of school-based dental clinics within my community. It gives me personal satisfaction knowing that I am using my professional skills to help bring dental services to those children who without school-based dental clinics may otherwise not receive any dental care.

What type of advice would you give to a practicing hygienist who is thinking of doing something different?

If you are looking for a change in your work experience, I would recommend identifying what you do and don't like about your current position and seek avenues to expand on the positives of your chosen profession. Many times I hear of dental hygienists leaving our profession to pursue other careers because they are unhappy with their current work situation. I have been in that very situation of not being happy working in private practice but not really knowing what I should do about it other than considering transferring to another private dental office and running the risk that I would find myself in another position in which I felt unfilled.

By pursuing higher education in dental hygiene, other opportunities became evident to me. My increased knowledge allowed me to see that I could teach, carry out research, and serve as promoter of oral health in addition to providing clinical hygiene services. It is true that I could have done all of those things even if I had not had an advanced degree, but as I expanded my knowledge base, the more comfortable I became with pursuing other avenues within my profession. I honestly think that the more informed people become, the more likely they will be to take a risk and develop new personal and career courses that could potentially lead to a more fulfilling life. It is because of that belief that I pursued advanced education, and even though it was sometimes a difficult path to be on, I do not regret embarking on the path of higher education because as a result, I have a newly restored value of what I can accomplish as a dental hygienist.

Source: Christine Nathe writes the Public Health Column in RDH magazine published by Pennwell Publishing. For more public health spotlights please see RDH magazine online at http://www.rdhmag.com/index.html

SELF-STUDY TEST ITEMS

1. *Epidemiology* has been defined as the study of the nature, cause, control, and determinants of the frequency and distribution of
   a. Disease
   b. Disability
   c. Death
   d. All of the above

2. The agent of disease is the biologic or mechanical cause of the disease or condition. Examples of agents are the specific bacteria in relation to dental caries or brushing with a hard toothbrush in relation to abrasion.
   a. The first statement is true; the second statement is false.
   b. The first statement is false; the second statement is true.
   c. Both statements are true.
   d. Both statements are false.

3. The occurrence of an illness in excess of normal expectancy in a community or region, usually occurring suddenly and spreading rapidly, is termed a(n)
   a. Endemic
   b. Epidemic
   c. Pandemic
   d. All of the above

4. Which study attempts to relate outcome with exposure to a suspected risk factor using data that are available for the population?
   a. Case–control
   b. Case study
   c. Ecological
   d. Time series

5. What is a modifiable attribute or exposure that is known to be associated with a health condition?
   a. Risk ratio
   b. Risk factor
   c. Risk attribute
   d. Risk indicator

REFERENCES

1. Bader J, Ismail A, Clarkson J. Evidence-based dentistry and the dental research community. *J Dent Res.* 1999; 78(9):1480–1483.

2. Forrest JL, Miller S. Evidence-based decision making. *Dimens Dent Hyg.* 2005;3(9):12,14,16–17.

3. Forrest JL, Miller S. A practical guide for incorporating evidence into dental hygiene practice. *Access.* 2007; 21(10):12–18.

4. Weiss NS. Clinical Epidemiology.. In: Marmot MG, Samet JM, Savitz D, Vessey MP, eds. *Monographs in Epidemiology and Biostatistic.* 3rd ed. Vol. 36. New York, NY: Oxford University Press; 2006.

5. Hackshaw A, Paul E, Davenport E. *Evidence-Based Dentistry: An Introduction.* Hoboken, NJ: John Wiley; 2007.

6. Merrill RM, Timmreck TC. *An Introduction to Epidemiology.* 4th ed. Boston, MA: Jones & Bartlett; 2006.

7. Friis RH, Sellers TA. *Epidemiology for Public Health Practice.* 3rd ed. Boston, MA: Jones & Bartlett; 2004.

8. Morabia A. Epidemiology: An epistemological perspective. In: Morabia A. *A History of Epidemiologic Methods and Concepts.* Boston, MA: Birkhauser Verlag; 2004:3–125.

9. Gerstman BB. *Epidemiology Kept Simple: An Introduction to Traditional and Modern Epidemiology.* 2nd ed. Hoboken, NJ: Wiley-Liss; 2003.

10. Wassertheil-Smoller S. *Biostatistics and Epidemiology: A Primer for Health and Biomedical Professionals.* 3rd ed. New York, NY: Springer-Verlag; 2004.

11. Webber R. *Communicable Disease Epidemiology and Control: A Global Perspective.* 2nd ed. Cambridge, MA: CABI; 2005.

12. Hebel JR, McCarter RJ. *A Study Guide to Epidemiology and Biostatistics.* 6th ed. Boston, MA: Jones & Bartlett; 2006.

13. Burt BA, Eklund SA. *Dentistry, Dental Practice, and the Community.* 6th ed. St. Louis, MO: Elsevier; 2005.

14. Pendrys DG. Epidemiology of oral diseases. In: Gluck GM, Morganstein WM. *Jong's Community Dental Health.* 5th ed. St. Louis. MO: Mosby; 2003:173–203.

15. Koepsell TD, Weiss NS. *Epidemiologic Methods: Studying the Occurrence of Illness.* New York, NY: Oxford University Press; 2003.

16. US Department of Health and Human Services, Centers for Disease Control and Prevention, National Institutes of Health. National Center for Chronic Disease Prevention and Health Promotion, Division of Oral Health. National Oral Health Surveillance System. Published September 22, 2006. http://www.cdc.gov/nohss/. Accessed January 13, 2008.

17. Association of State and Territorial Dental Directors (ASTDD). Basic screening surveys: An approach to monitoring community oral health. Revised September 2003. http://www.astdd.org/docs/BSS_Manual_9-25-03.pdf. Accessed January 13, 2008.

18. Goodman RA, Foster KL, Gregg MB, eds. Preface. *Morbidity & Weekly Report.* 1999;48(v). http://www.cdc.gov/mmwr/preview/ind99_su.html. Accessed June 7, 2008.

19. US Department of Health and Human Services. *Healthy People 2010.* http://www.healthypeople.gov/. Accessed January 13, 2008.

20. US Department of Health and Human Services. Oral health. *Healthy People 2010, Oral Health.* Vol. II. http://www.healthypeople.gov/document/HTML/Volume2/21Oral.htm. Accessed January 18, 2008.

21. US Department of Health and Human Services. Healthy People 2010 Midcourse Review. http://www.healthypeople.gov/Data/. Accessed January 18, 2008.

22. US Department of Health and Human Services, Public Health Service, National Institutes of Health, National Institute of Dental and Craniofacial Research. *Oral Health in America: A Report of the Surgeon General, 2000* [press release]. http://www.surgeongeneral.gov/library/oralhealth/. Accessed January 13, 2008.

23. US Department of Health and Human Services, Public Health Service, Centers for Disease Control and Prevention, National Institutes of Health, National Institute of Dental and Craniofacial Research. *A National Call to Action to Promote Oral Health: A Public-Private Partnership under the Leadership of the Office of the Surgeon General.* Bethesda, MD: Author; 2003. NIH Publication No. 03-5303.

24. World Health Organization. Oral health databases. http://www.who.int/oral_health/databases/en/. Accessed January 13, 2008.

25. World Health Organization. *Oral Health Surveys: Basic Methods.* 4th ed. Geneva: WHO; 1997.

26. Savitz DA. *Interpreting Epidemiologic Evidence: Strategies for Study Design and Analysis.* New York, NY: Oxford University Press; 2003.

27. Thompson NJ, Boyer EM. Validity of oral health screening in field conditions: Pilot study. *J Dent Hyg.* 2006;80(2):1–10. www.ingenta.com. Accessed June 22, 2009.

28. Darby ML, Bowen DM. *Research Methods for Oral Health Professionals: An Introduction.* St. Louis, MO: C. V. Mosby, 1980. Reprint. Pocatello, ID: McCann; 1993.

PEARSON
myhealthprofessionskit

Multimedia Extension Activities

Use this address to access the interactive Companion Website created for this textbook. Simply select "Dental Hygiene" from the choice of disciplines. Find this book and log in using your username and password. To obtain a username and password, please register using the scratch-off access code on the inside front cover of this book.

Chapter **17**

Current Oral Epidemiological Findings

OBJECTIVES

After studying this chapter, the dental hygiene student should be able to:

- Describe the current epidemiological issues of disease
- Describe the current epidemiological issues of conditions

KEY TERMS
Incidence
Morbidity
Mortality
Prevalence

COMPETENCIES

After studying this chapter and participating in accompanying course activities, the dental hygiene student should be competent to do the following:

- Use evidence-based decision making to evaluate and incorporate emerging treatment modalities
- Assume responsibility for dental hygiene actions and care based on accepted scientific theories and research as well as the accepted standard of care

As discussed in Chapter 16, the study of disease in human populations is called *epidemiology,* but it includes more than this. The science and tools of epidemiology are used to identify health, disease, and use of dental services. Oral diseases, risks, and preventive strategies are affected by many variables including societal forces and demographics. Therefore, the epidemiology of oral diseases constantly changes, and it is important for the dental hygienist to stay informed about current epidemiological findings of diseases and conditions and the rates of dental care utilization.

THE EPIDEMIOLOGY OF ORAL DISEASES AND CONDITIONS

The range of oral, dental, and craniofacial ideas and conditions that affect the populations is extensive. Just as there is no single measure of overall health or overall disease, there is no single measure of oral health or the burden of oral diseases and conditions.[1] See Box 17-1 ■ for findings from the US Surgeon General's report on oral health.

The following sections present epidemiological data for the specific oral disease or condition named. When assessing data, it is important to understand the prevalence and incidence of diseases or conditions. For each oral disease or condition, risk factors are presented and specific preventive aspects are discussed. **Prevalence** is the number of all existing cases of a disease in a population measured at a given point whereas **incidence** is the number of new cases of a disease in a population over a given period of time.

Periodontal Diseases

Periodontal diseases can be defined as inflammatory diseases affecting the periodontium, which encompass the tissues that surround and support the teeth. Periodontal diseases involve progressive loss of the gingival tissues and alveolar bone around the teeth and, if left untreated, can lead to tooth mobility and subsequent loss of teeth. A convergence of bacteria and an overly aggressive immune response against these bacteria cause periodontal diseases. Although bacterial infections cause periodontal diseases, a variety of factors affects its severity.

Epidemiology

As most dental hygienists could anecdotally predict, many individuals experience gingivitis. (See Figure 17-1 ■.) The third National Health and Nutrition Examination Survey (NHANES III) found that 50 percent of adults have gingivitis on at least three or four teeth.[2] Refer to Table 17-1 ■ for additional information about the

---

BOX 17-1 Findings from the US Surgeon General's Report on Oral Diseases and Conditions

- Microbial infections, including those caused by bacteria, viruses, and fungi, are the primary cause of the most prevalent oral diseases. Examples include dental caries, periodontal diseases, herpes labialis, and candidiasis.
- The etiology and pathogenesis of diseases and disorders affecting the craniofacial structures are multifactorial and complex, involving interplay among genetic, environmental, and behavioral factors.
- Many inherited and congenital conditions affect the craniofacial complex, often resulting in disfigurement and impairments that may involve many body organs and systems and affect millions of children worldwide.
- Tobacco use, excessive alcohol use, and inappropriate dietary practices contribute to many diseases and disorders. In particular, tobacco use is a risk factor for oral cavity and pharyngeal cancers, periodontal diseases, candidiasis, and dental caries, among other diseases.
- Some chronic diseases, such as Sjögren's syndrome, present with primary oral symptoms.
- Oral-facial pain conditions are common and often have complex etiologies.

Source: US Department of Health and Human Services. *Oral health in America: A Report of the Surgeon General.* Rockville, MD: Department of Health and Human Services, National Institute of Dental and Craniofacial Research, National Institutes of Health; 2000.

Table 17-1   Prevalence of Periodontal Disease: Adults 20–64 Years of Age, 1999–2004

Characteristic	Periodontal Disease (percent)[a]	Moderate or Severe Periodontal Disease (percent)[b]
Age in Years		
20–34	3.84	NA
35–49	10.41	5.00
50–64	11.88	10.73
Gender		
Male	10.65	6.74
Female	6.40	3.46
Race and Ethnicity		
White, non-Hispanic	5.82	4.15
Black, non-Hispanic	16.81	8.30
Mexican American	13.76	6.43
Poverty Status (*income compared to federal poverty level*)		
Less than 100 percent	19.95	9.92
100 percent–199 percent	15.34	9.42
More than 200 percent	5.96	3.50
Education		
Less than high school	17.33	11.64
High school	9.34	5.65
More than high school	5.78	3.11
Smoking History		
Current smoker	14.74	11.14
Former smoker	7.61	4.62
Never smoked	5.94	2.34
Overall	8.52	5.08

[a]Periodontal disease is defined as having at least one periodontal site with 3 millimeters or more of attachment loss and 4 millimeters or more of pocket depth.

[b]According to CDC-American Academy of Periodontology definitions: Moderate periodontal disease is defined as having at least two teeth with interproximal attachment loss of 4 millimeters or more *or* at least two teeth with 5 millimeters or more of pocket depth at interproximal sites. Severe periodontal disease is defined as having at least two teeth with interproximal attachment loss of 6 millimeters or more *and* at least one tooth with 5 millimeters or more of pocket depth at interproximal sites.

Source: The National Health and Nutrition Examination Survey (NHANES). Tables 1–4. http://www.nider.nih.gov/DataStatistics/FindDataByTopic/GumDisease/PeriodontaldiseaseAdults20to64

FIGURE 17-1 Gingivitis

Source: Centers for Disease Control.

prevalence of periodontal diseases for adults. The facts have been well documented that only 5 to 15 percent of any population suffers from severe generalized periodontitis and that older adults, African-American and Hispanic adults, current smokers, and those with lower incomes and less education are more likely to have periodontal disease.[2,3,4]

Risk Factors

The host response is important in severe periodontal disease. Risk factors for periodontal diseases are numerous (see Box 17-2■). Although the majority of the population does not have severe periodontal disease, most have a mild to moderate form. Risk factors can be summarized including smoking, genetic predisposition, (probably) psychological stress, diabetes, and several uncommon systemic diseases.[5]

DENTAL HYGIENE SPOTLIGHT:
Lt. Comm. Angela Girgenti, RDH, BS

Lieutenant Commander Angela Girgenti of the US Public Health Service (USPHS) currently is a senior public health analyst with the Health Resources and Services Administration (HRSA), Office of Performance Review, Regional Division, Dallas, Texas. She is a graduate of the Texas Woman's University Dental Hygiene Program in Denton and is currently enrolled in the master's of public health program at the University of North Texas Health Science Center in Fort Worth. Lt. Comm. Girgenti, the recipient of two PHS commendation medals, has worked in a variety of public health settings and has spoken about and presented programs on numerous topics.

I asked for her comments on several professionally related topics.

Why did you decide to go into dental hygiene?

I started in dentistry as a volunteer for the Red Cross in Fort Ritchie, Maryland. I received free training as a dental assistant from the Red Cross and the Fort Ritchie Army dental clinic in exchange for 200 hours of volunteer work at the dental clinic. This was my first exposure to the field of dentistry, which heightened my interest in working in health care. After I completed the volunteer hours, I was hired as a dental assistant in a private practice where I continued to learn more about dentistry and dental hygiene. I loved working with patients and knew a career in dental hygiene would suit me well. After returning to Texas, I enrolled at Texas Woman's University and was accepted into the school of dental hygiene.

How did you get into dental public health? Did you need additional education?

The opportunity to work in a public health setting began with an internship with the USPHS I completed between my junior and senior years of hygiene school. The internship allowed me to work at a federal prison, providing care to federal inmates under the supervision of the chief dental officer. This introduced me to the possibility of a full-time career in the uniformed services and public health. I learned about the various ways dental hygienists could work with underserved populations in the Federal Bureau of Prisons and in other federal agencies, such as the Indian Health Service. After graduation, I was offered a full-time position at the federal prison and received my commission as an officer in the USPHS.

What are your current positions?

Currently, I am a public health analyst for Health Resources and Services Administration in Dallas. HRSA, part of the US Department of Health and Human Services, is the primary federal agency for improving access to health care services for people who are uninsured, isolated, or medically vulnerable. Information about HRSA and its programs can be found at www.hrsa.gov. I continue to serve HRSA as an officer in the USPHS. My role is to provide guidance to federal grantees and assist them in improving performance and increasing health care access to the underserved and uninsured. I also continue to provide dental hygiene services at the federal prison on a regular basis to stay clinically active and fulfill my desire to provide patient care.

Can you discuss any particularly interesting experiences you have had in your dental public health positions?

My career in the USPHS has been both extremely exciting and rewarding. I am grateful for the experience I gained as a new hygienist at the Bureau of Prisons. I learned to work with culturally diverse populations and underserved populations. Many of my patients never had the opportunity to have dental care; I was their first dental provider. This experience allowed me to grow as a clinician and health educator.

After Katrina, the USPHS deployed hundreds of officers to the Gulf Coast to assist in stabilizing the region. I was sent to Baton Rouge temporarily and served in an administrative role on the Emergency Response Team of the Secretary of Health and Human Services. This was my first deployment as a commissioned officer, and I learned a great deal about the operations of federal, state, and local governments in times of disaster. I felt fortunate to serve the Gulf Coast residents in this capacity and was impressed by the dedication of my fellow officers.

One of the most unique experiences of my career was in 2007 when I was deployed on the Navy hospital ship the *USNS Comfort*. Four teams of USPHS officers were invited to participate in the US Training and Humanitarian Assistance Mission to Latin and South America. I spent an entire month onboard the ship and provided direct care to residents of Nicaragua, El Salvador, and Peru. I was amazed by the overwhelming crowds that gathered to receive care. I was also touched by the kindness and hospitality we were shown in each country. Most of all, I was proud of those I served alongside on the *USNS Comfort* and how well they represented our country.

What type of advice would you give to a practicing hygienist who is thinking of doing something different?

Continuing my education has proven to be a success. Looking back, most of my opportunities came from internships, other school activities, and volunteering. I am currently finishing my master's degree in public health, which was essential in obtaining my current position at HRSA. Also, having a variety of mentors is extremely helpful. Along the way, I have had wonderful mentors who helped me succeed and encouraged me to continually grow. For those who are looking for a change, don't be afraid to embrace new opportunities and have confidence in your abilities. Hygienists are excellent teachers, problem solvers, and promoters of change. Our skills are not strictly clinical. Last, volunteering is an excellent way to network and meet other professionals. The need for dental care in this country is overwhelming, and volunteering in alternative settings can help increase access to care for those who need it most and positively impact your career.

Source: Christine Nathe writes the Public Health Column in RDH magazine published by Pennwell Publishing.
For more public health spotlights please see RDH magazine online at http://www.rdhmag.com/index.html.

BOX 17-2 Risk Factors for Periodontal Diseases

- **Age:** Risk increases with age.
- **Gender:** Diseases are more prevalent in males than females.
- **Socioeconomic Status:** Lower socioeconomic status increases risk.
- **Genetics:** Research continues.
- **Plaque:** Plaque and gingivitis increase risk.
- **Tobacco:** Smokers have an increased risk.
- **Systemic Conditions:** Diabetes and other systemic stressors increase risk.

Increase in probing depth over a period of years is the strongest predictor of future periodontal disease activity.

Did You Know?

Dental hygienists focus attention on periodontal diseases for good reason. Most individuals experience some stage of periodontal infection during their lifetime.

Tooth Loss

By maintaining a healthy dentition and receiving regular dental hygiene care, most people have the ability to keep their teeth throughout their lives. The prevalence of both partial and total tooth loss in adults has decreased from the early 1970s through the latest (1999–2004) National Health and Nutrition Examination Survey. In spite of this improvement, significant disparities remain in some population groups.[6]

Epidemiology
See Table 17-2 ■ for information about tooth loss for adults age 20 to 64 years and other selected population groups. Only 3.75 percent of adults in this age group have no remaining teeth although most adults have had tooth loss. The same populations that suffer from severe generalized periodontitis have fewer remaining teeth than other populations.

Risk Factors
Risk factors for tooth loss include dental caries. In addition, tooth loss can be caused by periodontal diseases associated with the risk indicators of age, male gender, smoking, lack of professional maintenance, inadequate oral hygiene, diabetes mellitus, hypertension, rheumatoid arthritis and anterior tooth type. Trauma can also lead to tooth loss. Maintaining a healthy dentition and wearing athletic mouthguards during sporting events are the best ways to avoid tooth loss.

Dental Caries

Dental caries, commonly referred to as *tooth decay,* is one of the most common of all diseases, second only to the common cold. It usually occurs in children and young adults, but any person can experience it. It is a common cause of tooth loss in young people. Bacterial plaque converts all foods, especially sugar and starches, into acids that subsequently dissolve the enamel surface of the tooth, called *demineralization.* If left untreated, demineralization progresses to form a "cavity."

Did You Know?

Many individuals believe that if one of their parents lost all of their teeth, they are destined for the same fate, but as noted, only a very small percentage of the US population experiences total tooth loss.

Epidemiology
Dental caries remains the most prevalent chronic disease in both children and adults even though it is largely preventable. Although caries has significantly decreased for most Americans over the past four decades, disparities remain among some population groups. In addition, this downward trend has recently reversed for young children, who can be afflicted with early childhood caries. All populations can suffer from occlusal and interproximal carious lesions. (See Table 17-3 ■ for untreated dental decay and urgent need for dental care in children and Figure 17-2 ■ for early childhood caries.)

Did You Know?

Early childhood caries, also known as *baby bottle caries* and *nursing bottle decay,* is a syndrome characterized by severe decay in the teeth of infants or young children. Frequent and prolonged drinking from a bottle (especially at bedtime) increases the risk of this disease, which first effects the maxillary primary anterior teeth.

Table 17-2   Percentage of Tooth Loss for Adults Aged 20-64 Years in U.S., by State

Characteristic	Mean Number of Permanent Teeth	Percentage with no Remaining Teeth
Age in Years		
20–34	26.90	NA
35–49	25.05	2.63
50–64	22.30	10.13
Gender		
Male	25.06	3.79
Female	24.90	3.72
Race and Ethnicity		
White, non-Hispanic	25.23	3.96
Black, non-Hispanic	23.68	4.14
Mexican American	25.32	1.51
Poverty Status (*income compared to federal poverty level*)		
Less than 100 percent	23.52	9.28
100 199 percent	23.64	6.48
More than 200 percent	25.48	2.35
Education		
Less than high school	23.10	8.07
High school	24.35	5.41
More than high school	25.76	1.66
Smoking History		
Current smoker	23.47	7.79
Former smoker	25.12	3.57
Never smoked	25.67	1.55
Overall	24.98	3.76

Source: The National Health and Nutrition Examination Survey (NHANES). Tables 1–4. Total Tooth Loss Among Persons Aged Greater Than or Equal to 65 Years—Selected States, 1995-1997.

Table 17-3   Percentage of Third Grade Students with Untreated Tooth Decay

| State | School Year | Percent with Untreated Tooth Decay | | Response Rate[1] (%) | Percent eligible for free and reduced-cost lunch program[2] | | |
| | | | | | Sample | | |
					Schools[3]	Students[4]	State
Alaska	2007–2008	%	**26.2**[5]	48	42	NR	46
		CI	(23.2–29.3)				
		N	826				
Arizona	1999–2002	%	**39.4**	NR	53	NR	52
		CI	(34.9–44.0)				
		N	3189				
Arkansas	2001–2002	%	**42.1**[5]	86	55	NR	45
		CI	(38.4–45.8)				
		N	815				
California	2004–2005	%	**28.7**	52	64	NR	57
		CI	(27.0–30.4)				
		N	10444				
Colorado	2006–2007	%	**24.5**	79	40	NR	41
		CI	(23.0–26.1)				
		N	3012				
Connecticut	2006–2007	%	**17.8**	81	37	NR	35
		CI	(14.8–20.8)				
		N	8755				
Delaware	2001–2002	%	**29.9**	43	37	41	40
		CI	(25.3–34.4)				
		N	1032				
Georgia	2004–2005	%	**27.1**	51	52	53	51
		CI	(26.0–28.3)				
		N	2861				
Idaho	2000–2001	%	**27.3**	71	50	NR	39
		CI	(24.4–30.2)				
		N	3126				
Illinois	2003–2004	%	**30.2**	66	54	NR	47
		CI	(27.9–32.6)				
		N	6630				
Iowa	2005–2006	%	**13.2**[5]	68	35	31	36
		CI	(11.2–15.2)				
		N	1126				
Kansas	2003–2004	%	**27.6**[5]	32	NR	NR	NR
		CI	(24.9–30.4)				
		N	3375				
Kentucky	2000–2001	%	**34.6**	64	52	NR	NR
		CI	(31.9–37.4)				
		N	3244				

(continued)

Table 17-3   Percentage of Third Grade Students with Untreated Tooth Decay (continued)

| State | School Year | | Percent with Untreated Tooth Decay | Response Rate[1] (%) | Percent eligible for free and reduced-cost lunch program[2] | | |
| | | | | | Sample | | State |
					Schools[3]	Students[4]	
Maine	1998–1999	%	20.4[5]	51	NR	31	32
		CI	(18.3–22.6)				
		N	1297				
Maryland	2000–2001	%	25.9	50	NR	28	36
		CI	(21.6–30.2)				
		N	2482				
Massachusetts	2006–2007	%	17.3[5]	46	NR	28	32
		CI	(14.0–20.7)				
		N	2211				
Michigan	2005–2006	%	25.0	68	37	40	38
		CI	(21.4–28.6)				
		N	1586				
Mississippi	2004–2005	%	39.1	62	70	NR	70
		CI	(37.7–40.5)				
		N	2824				
Missouri	2004–2005	%	27.0	49	45	NR	46
		CI	(26.0–28.0)				
		N	3535				
Montana	2005–2006	%	28.9[5]	90	41	NR	35
		CI	(26.1–31.9)				
		N	957				
Nebraska	2004–2005	%	17.0	92	34	NR	34
		CI	(13.6–20.4)				
		N	2057				
Nevada	2005–2006	%	44.0	22	44	NR	41
		CI	(37.6–50.3)				
		N	794				
New Hampshire	2000–2001	%	21.7[5]	78	NR	NR	NR
		CI	(14.3–29.1)				
		N	410				
New Mexico	1999–2000	%	37.0[5]	47	NR	NR	NR
		CI	(32.3–41.6)				
		N	2136				
New York	2001–2003	%	33.1	38	NR	48	51
		CI	(29.6–36.6)				
		N	10895				
North Dakota	2004–2005	%	16.9[5]	73	31	NR	29
		CI	(14.7–19.4)				
		N	1015			(continued)	

Table 17-3   Percentage of Third Grade Students with Untreated Tooth Decay (continued)

| State | School Year | Percent with Untreated Tooth Decay | | Response Rate[1] (%) | Percent eligible for free and reduced-cost lunch program[2] | | |
| | | | | | Sample | | State |
					Schools[3]	Students[4]	
Ohio	2004–2005	%	25.7	53	37	38	33
		CI	(23.9–27.5)				
		N	14029				
Oklahoma	2002–2003	%	40.2[5]	74	NR	NR	41
		CI	(35.8–44.7)				
		N	495				
Oregon	2006–2007	%	35.4	76	47	NR	47
		CI	(31.4–39.4)				
		N	1259				
Pennsylvania	1998–1999	%	27.3	NR	NR	NR	NR
		CI	(23.9–30.6)				
		N	1767				
Rhode Island	2007–2008	%	28.2[5]	66	46	NR	42
		CI	(22.5–33.9)				
		N	1303				
South Carolina	2007–2008	%	22.6[5]	38	56	56	51
		CI	(21.0–24.3)				
		N	2657				
South Dakota	2005–2006	%	32.9	66	NR	24	NR
		CI	(29.9–35.9)				
		N	643				
Utah	2000–2001	%	23.0[5]	51	NR	NR	NR
		CI	(21.0–25.0)				
		N	800				
Vermont	2002–2003	%	16.2	68	31	NR	31
		CI	(12.9–19.5)				
		N	409				
Washington	2004–2005	%	19.1	77	38	NR	40
		CI	(16.7–21.5)				
		N	3633				
Wisconsin	2007–2008	%	20.1	89	36	NR	37
		CI	(18.9–21.3)				
		N	4413				

% Percentage
CI 95% Confidence Interval
N Number of students in sample
NR Not Reported

[1]Survey response rates differ among states. Differential nonresponse can bias the estimates. Response rates, the percent of selected children who actually participated, are presented to help the reader judge the potential for bias.

[2]Untreated tooth decay may be associated with income. Eligibility for the free and reduced-cost lunch program is presented to help the reader assess whether the survey sample is representative of all 3rd graders in the state.

[3]The percent eligible for the free and reduced-cost lunch program among students attending schools that participated in the survey.

[4]The percent eligible for the free and reduced-cost lunch program among students who participated in the survey.

[5]The percent with untreated tooth decay reported by this state has not been adjusted for nonresponse.

Source: http://apps.nccd.gov/nohss/IndicatorV.asp?Indicator=3. Accessed June 25, 2009.

FIGURE 17-2   Early Childhood Caries

Source: Courtesy of Dr. Lezley McIleveen, Department of Dentistry, Children's National Medical Center, Washington, DC.

Adults experience dental decay, and because many of them have exposed root surface(s), they experience root caries. Approximately 85 percent of adults in the United States has at least one tooth with decay (untreated or treated.) (See Table 17-4 ■.) Root caries affects approximately 50 percent of adults seventy-five years and older.

Risk Factors

Risk factors for dental caries include susceptibility of teeth and age. The use of dental sealants and fluoride decreases the risk for dental caries. Specifically, dental sealants create a barrier to protect fissures and pits from demineralization. Fluoride protects teeth from demineralization and actually can aid in the remineralization of demineralized tooth surfaces. See specific risk factors in Box 17-3 ■.

Oral and Pharyngeal Cancer

Oral and pharyngeal cancers occur in the oral cavity, lips, and/or pharyngeal tissues. An individual can have oral cancer, but certain risk factors seem to increase the likelihood of developing it. As with any cancer, treatments for oral and pharyngeal cancers are most effective when the cancer is diagnosed at an early stage.

Epidemiology

More than 34,000 Americans will be diagnosed with oral or pharyngeal cancer this year,[7] and it will cause more than 8000 deaths, killing roughly one person per hour, twenty-four hours per day.[7] Of those 34,000 newly diagnosed individuals, only half will be alive in five years, a percentage that has not significantly improved in decades.[7] **Mortality,** defined as the ratio of the number of deaths from a given disease or health problem to the total number of cases reported, from oral cancer is nearly twice as high in some minorities (especially African-American

---

BOX 17-3 Risk Factors for Dental Caries

Teeth Most Susceptible
- Molars (high incidence)
- Mandibular molars (attacked first)
- Higher incidence in pits and fissures

Socioeconomic Status
- Most powerful determinant

Age—Early Childhood Caries
- Low socioeconomic status
- Diet

Gender
- Incidence of decayed, missing, filled teeth (DMF index) higher for females than for males

Race/Ethnicity
- Heritage (Mexican-Americans, Native Americans, immigrants to the United States)

Environment
- Low socioeconomic status
- Family lifestyles and behaviors

Genetics
- Intrafamilial transmission of *S. Mutans* (ie, mother's transmission of pathogen to baby)

Diet
- Frequency and total intake of sugar
- Type of sugar

Table 17-4 Proportion of Adults* with Untreated Dental Caries, by Selected Age Groups and Demographic Characteristics

	Age 35–44 Years		Age 65–74 Years	
	United States[a] *(%)*	*<STATE>*[f] *(%)*	*United States (%)*	*<STATE>*[f] *(%)*
Healthy People 2010 **Target**	15	15		
TOTAL	26		19	
Race or Ethnicity				
American Indian or Alaska Native	68[b]			
Asian or Pacific Islander	DSU			
Asian	DNC			
Native Hawaiian and other Pacific Islander	DNC			
Black or African American	46[d]			
White	24[d]			
Hispanic or Latino	DSU			
Mexican American	34[c]		34[c]	
Not Hispanic or Latino	DNA			
Black or African American	47[d]		27	
White	23[d]		18[e]	
Sex				
Female	25[d]		14[e]	
Male	29[d]		24	
Education Level				
Less than high school	51[d]			
High school graduate	34[d]			
At least some college	16[d]			
Disability Status				
Persons with disabilities	DNA			
Persons without disabilities	DNA			

DNA = Data not analyzed

DNC = Data not collected

DSU = Data are statistically unreliable or do not meet criteria for confidentiality

*Excludes edentulous adults (persons without natural teeth).

[a]National data are for 1999–2000 unless otherwise indicated.

[b]Data are for areas served by Indian Health Service, 1999.

[c]National data are for Mexican Americans.

[d]Data from NHANES III, 1988–1994.

[e]Data are statistically unreliable.

[f]<State Data Source(s)>

Sources: Aged 35–54 years: U.S. Department of Health and Human Services. *Healthy People 2010, Progress Review, 2000.* Available at www.cdc.gov/nchs/ppt/hpdata2010/focusareas/fa21.xls. Aged 65–74 years: *Health, United States, 2004.* Table 80, p. 267. Available at www.cdc.gov/nchs/data/hus/hus04.pdf.

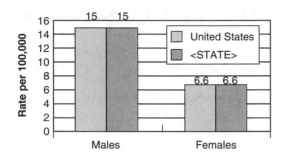

FIGURE 17-3   Oral and Pharyngeal Cancer Incidence Rate by Gender, United States, 2001

Source: http://www.cdc.gov/OralHealth/publications/library/burdenbook/pdfs/burden.pdf. Accessed June 22, 2009.

males) as it is in Caucasians. Methods used to treat oral cancers, such as surgery, radiation, and chemotherapy, cause **morbidity,** which is defined as the ratio of "sick" (affected) individuals to well individuals in a community, and are disfiguring and costly.[8] See Figures 17-3 ■ and 17-4 ■ for oral cancer information.

Most oral cancers start in squamous cells and form in any of three main areas: lips, oral cavity, and the oropharynx. (See Figure 17-5 ■.) Oral cancer is more common in men than in women, but the number of women in the United States diagnosed with tongue cancer has increased significantly over the past twenty years. In Western countries, including the United States, the most common areas for oral cancer are the tongue and the floor of the mouth. In parts of the world where chewing tobacco or betel nuts is common, oral cancer often forms in the retromolar area and buccal mucosa.[9] The human papillomavirus has also been linked to oral cancer.[10,11] Refer to Box 17-4 ■ for signs and symptoms of oral cancer.

Risk Factors

Approximately 75 percent of oral cavity and pharyngeal cancers are attributed to the use of smoked and smokeless tobacco. These cancers affect the mouth, tongue, lips, throat, parts for the nose, and larynx. Those who chew tobacco are at high risk for gum and cheek lesions that can lead to cancer. Alcohol consumption is another risk factor. Combinations of tobacco and alcohol are believed to be substantially higher risk factors than consumption of either substance alone. Other risk factors for these cancers are viral infections, immunodeficiencies, poor nutrition, exposure to ultraviolet light (a major cause of lip cancer), and certain occupational hazards, such as exposure to specific chemicals.[8]

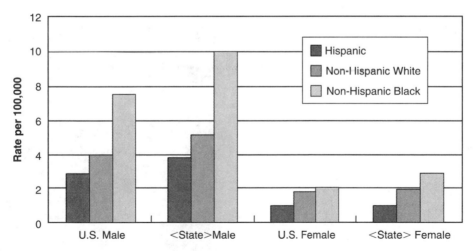

*Per 100,000, age-adjusted to 2000 U.S. population

FIGURE 17-4   Oral Cancer Death Rate* by Sex and Race/Hispanic Origin, and United States, 2001

Source: http://www.cdc.gov/OralHealth/publications/library/burdenbook/pdfs/burden.pdf. Accessed June 22, 2009.

FIGURE 17-5   Oral Cancer

Not engaging in the high-risk behaviors listed earlier is critical in preventing oral cancers. Early detection is key to increasing the survival rate for these cancers.

Mucosal Infections and Diseases

Large-scale population-based screening studies have identified the most common oral lesions as candidiasis, recurrent herpes labialis, recurrent aphthous stomatitis, mucocele, fibroma, mandibular and palatal tori, pyogenic granuloma, erythema migrans, hairy tongue, lichen planus, and leukoplakia.[12,13,14]

Epidemiology

Primary oral infection with the herpes simplex virus (HSV) typically occurs at a young age, is asymptomatic, and is not associated with significant morbidity.[12] After primary oral infection, HSV may persist in a latent state in the trigeminal ganglion and later reactivate as the more common herpes labialis, or cold sores.

Risk Factors

Common triggers for reactivation include ultraviolet light, trauma, fatigue, stress, and menstruation. These

---

BOX 17-4   Signs and Symptoms of Oral Cancer

- Mouth sore that fails to heal or that bleeds easily
- White or red patch in the mouth that will not go away
- Lump, thickening or soreness in the mouth, throat, or tongue
- Difficulty chewing or swallowing food.

---

lesions affect approximately 15 to 45 percent of the US population.[12,15] Infection with the oral herpes simplex virus has been related to socioeconomic factors; 75 to 90 percent of individuals from lower socioeconomic populations develop antibodies by the end of the first decade of life.[16] (See Figure 17-6 ■.)

Epidemiology

Recurrent aphthous stomatitis, or canker sores, is an oral ulcerative condition that is usually painful. Recurrent aphthous stomatitis has a prevalence ranging from 5 to 21 percent.[17] Recurrent aphthous stomatitis is characterized by recurring, painful, solitary, or multiple ulcers, typically covered by a white-to-yellow pseudomembrane and surrounded by an erythematous halo.[12]

Risk Factors

Although various host and environmental factors have been implicated, the precise pathogenesis remains

FIGURE 17-6   Herpetic Lesion

Source: University of New Mexico, Division of Dental Hygiene.

FIGURE 17-7 Oral Candidiasis

unknown. Smoking is associated with a lower prevalence, but other associations, such as nutritional deficiencies (eg, vitamin B_{12}, folate, iron), remain unclear.[17]

Epidemiology

Candidias, sometimes referred to as thrush, is a fungal infection of any of the *Candida* species, of which *Candida albicans* is the most common. As many as 60 percent of healthy adults carry *Candida* species as a component of their normal oral flora.[12] (See Figure 17-7 ■.)

Risk Factors

However, certain local and systemic factors may favor overgrowth: use of dentures or a steroid inhaler, xerostomia, endocrine disorders, human immunodeficiency virus (HIV) infection, leukemia, malnutrition, and reduced immunity based on age, radiation therapy, systemic chemotherapy, and use of broad-spectrum antibiotics or corticosteroids.[18–22]

Cleft Lip/Palate

Cleft lip and cleft palate are variations of a congenital deformity caused by abnormal facial development during gestation. Cleft lip is formed in the top of the lip as either a small gap or an indentation in the lip continuing into the nose. It can occur as unilateral or bilateral and is due to the failure of the maxillary and medial nasal processes to fuse. Cleft palate is a condition in which the two plates of the skull that form the hard palate are not completely joined. The soft palate in these cases also is cleft. In most cases, cleft lip is also present. Both deformities can be successfully treated with surgery soon after birth.

Epidemiology

Cleft lip and cleft palate are among the most common classes of congenital malformation. (See Figure 17-8 ■). In the United States, the prevalence for cleft lip with or without cleft palate is 2.3 to 11.7 per 10,000 births. Cleft palate alone results in a prevalence rate of 5.5 to 6.6 per 10,000 births.[23]

Risk Factors

Cleft lip and cleft palate are thought to be caused by a combination of genes and other factors. Smoking during

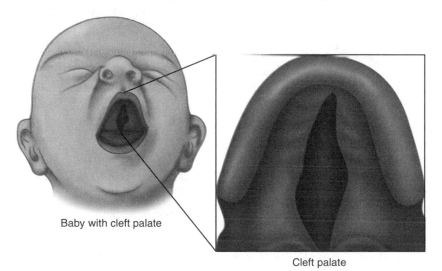

Baby with cleft palate

Cleft palate

FIGURE 17-8 Cleft Lip and Palate

pregnancy increases the chance of their occurrence, as can certain medications, changes in nutrition, and other factors.[24] Cleft lips/palates are more common in Native Americans than any other ethnic group.[25]

Injury

Many injuries to the dentition are complex and costly. Loosing incisor teeth or even fracturing teeth causes tremendous change to the dentition. Even more important is the fact that blows to the oral cavity can result in concussion due to the excessive physical force exerted during the arches occlusion.

Epidemiology

The leading causes of head and face injuries that result in emergency room visits are falls, assaults, sports injuries, and motor vehicle collisions.[1] The majority of dental trauma occurs to the anterior teeth.[26] Regardless of the patient's age, dental trauma can be emotional and painful. Cost of the repairs can also be a substantial economic burden. Individuals of all ages can be especially troubled psychologically because of unsightly fractures,[27,28] especially when the front teeth are adversely affected. Another burden is the amount of time involved in the healing process and in receiving treatment. Dental trauma's effects include tooth death, root resorption, tooth loss, and altered potential to develop permanent teeth.[29]

Risk Factors

Interestingly, 36 percent of all unintentional injuries to children and adults occurs during sports activities.[30] Prevention is a significant consideration because 20 million children age six to sixteen years are playing out-of-school sports, and 25 million youths are participating in competitive sports.[31] Although many orofacial injuries can be prevented during participation in athletic activities by using protective devices such as athletic mouth guards, many individuals do not use them. An athletic mouth guard, sometimes referred to as a mouth protector, is a removable oral appliance that protects the hard and soft tissues of the oral cavity and brain during contact sports. Mouth guards protect by absorbing energy during an impact, thus decreasing the likelihood of trauma.[32]

Toothaches

A toothache is a type of morbidity that causes pain. This pain can substantially impact the quality of life.

Epidemiology

Oral facial pain can greatly reduce quality of life.[1] Toothache pain can be caused by infection to the pulpal tissues or periodontium, dental caries infections, periodontal infections, trauma, mucosal sores, and temporomandibular joint (TMJ) disorder. In a six-month period, 22 percent of adults experience at least one type of oral facial pain.[33] Adults living in poverty are more likely to report toothaches than adults living above the poverty level.[34]

Risk Factors

Undoubtedly the major risk factor for toothache is untreated disease. Many times dental disease, whether it be carious lesions or periodontal infection, initially does not produce pain, so infection goes unnoticed. Many people may believe a stain on a tooth or bleeding gums are natural, the latter possibly caused by brushing too vigorously, rather than recognizing a problem. When pain does begin and is not treated, it can become severe.

Many individuals who have difficulty accessing dental care postpone seeking it until symptoms, such as severe toothache and facial abscess, become so debilitating that they seek care in hospital emergency and operating rooms. This is not cost effective and—most important—does not address dental disease management because few hospitals deliver comprehensive dental services.

Did You Know?

By preventing infection, dental hygiene is one solution to decreasing the painful toothaches many individuals experience.

PREVENTION BY USING DENTAL CARE

Dental Visits

Many individuals in the United States do not seek regular dental care. See Tables 17-5 ■ and 17-6 ■ for the percentages of adults over the age of eighteen who

Table 17-5 Adults aged 18+ who have had their teeth cleaned in the past year (among adults with natural teeth who have ever visited a dentist or dental clinic)

State	Yes (percent)	No (percent)	State	Yes (percent)	No (percent)
All States in United States	69.0	31.0	Montana	60.6	39.4
Alabama	69.3	30.7	Nebraska	75.0	25.0
Alaska	64.4	35.6	Nevada	63.2	36.8
American Samoa	—	—	New Hampshire	77.9	22.1
Arizona	65.9	34.1	New Jersey	74.8	25.2
Arkansas	57.7	42.3	New Mexico	66.3	33.7
California	67.9	32.1	New York	70.4	29.6
Colorado	69.6	30.4	North Carolina	69.5	30.5
Connecticut	79.1	20.9	North Dakota	67.6	32.4
Delaware	77.8	22.2	Ohio	71.1	28.9
DC	69.0	31.0	Oklahoma	59.4	40.6
Florida	67.2	32.8	Oregon	66.0	34.0
Georgia	66.6	33.4	Palau	—	—
Guam			Pennsylvania	69.6	30.4
Hawaii	—	—	Puerto Rico	70.6	29.4
Idaho	65.0	35.0	Rhode Island	78.8	21.2
Illinois	69.3	30.7	South Carolina	66.7	33.3
Indiana	67.1	32.9	South Dakota	70.2	29.8
Iowa	75.4	24.6	Tennessee	71.5	28.5
Kansas	75.0	25.0	Texas	58.7	41.3
Kentucky	73.3	26.7	Utah	69.3	30.7
Louisiana	66.6	33.4	Vermont	74.5	25.5
Maine	69.3	30.7	Virgin Islands	55.4	44.6
Maryland	73.6	26.4	Virginia	71.8	28.2
Massachusetts	79.0	21.0	Washington	69.3	30.7
Michigan	75.3	24.7	West Virginia	64.1	35.9
Minnesota	78.7	21.3	Wisconsin	75.7	24.3
Mississippi	56.6	43.4	Wyoming	64.7	35.3
Missouri	63.0	37.0			

Source: United States Department of Health and Human Services, Centers for Disease Control and Prevention, National Center for Chronic Disease Prevention and Health Promotion, Division of Oral Health. October 27, 2008. http://apps.nccd.cdc.gov/nohss/ListV.asp?qkey=6&DataSet=2 Accessed January 5, 2009.

Table 17-6   Adults 18+ Dental Visits (yes/no)

State	Yes (percent)	No (percent)	State	Yes (percent)	No (percent)
United States	69.0	31.0	Nebraska	74.3	25.7
Alabama	67.2	32.8	Nevada	62.0	38.0
Alaska	68.3	31.7	New Hampshire	76.2	23.8
American Samoa	—	—	New Jersey	74.4	25.6
Arizona	66.6	33.4	New Mexico	66.4	33.6
Arkansas	59.7	40.3	New York	70.0	30.0
California	68.7	31.3	North Carolina	67.7	32.3
Colorado	71.1	28.9	North Dakota	68.4	31.6
Connecticut	79.3	20.7	Ohio	71.3	28.7
Delaware	76.4	23.6	Oklahoma	60.5	39.5
DC	70.3	29.7	Oregon	67.1	32.9
Florida	66.4	33.6	Palau	—	—
Georgia	67.3	32.7	Pennsylvania	68.4	31.6
Guam	—	—	Puerto Rico	67.3	32.7
Hawaii	—	—	Rhode Island	77.3	22.7
Idaho	66.7	33.3	South Carolina	66.7	33.3
Illinois	71.4	28.6	South Dakota	71.3	28.7
Indiana	65.8	34.2	Tennessee	69.0	31.0
Iowa	74.1	25.9	Texas	59.2	40.8
Kansas	72.4	27.6	Utah	71.6	28.4
Kentucky	69.8	30.2	Vermont	73.2	26.8
Louisiana	66.3	33.7	Virgin Islands	59.0	41.0
Maine	68.7	31.3	Virginia	72.8	27.2
Maryland	74.8	25.2	Washington	70.0	30.0
Massachusetts	78.2	21.8	West Virginia	61.5	38.5
Michigan	75.9	24.1	Wisconsin	76.7	23.3
Minnesota	79.0	21.0	Wyoming	67.0	33.0
Mississippi	58.0	42.0			
Missouri	63.4	36.6			
Montana	64.7	35.3			

have had their teeth cleaned or visited a dental provider in a one-year period. Remember that these data do not necessarily reveal regular, consistent assessment and preventive care but identify dental care received only during the time period. Although most oral diseases are preventable, untreated dental disease remains prevalent throughout the United States. Disparities in oral health are most evident among populations with low income and educational levels, special needs, and those who live in communities without access to oral health services. Oral diseases have been associated with a number of systemic conditions and chronic diseases such as diabetes, cardiovascular disease, and preterm low birth-weight babies, underscoring the importance of oral health services for all individuals.[1]

Preventive Modalities

Dental sealants are highly effective in preventing dental caries that occur on the surfaces of teeth that have pits and fissures and increasingly have been used as a preventive modality. (See Figure 17-9 ■.) Fully retained sealants are 100 percent effective.[35,36] In examining the effectiveness of school-based or school-linked dental sealant programs, the *Guide to Community Preventive Services* documented a 60 percent decrease in tooth decay on the chewing surfaces of posterior teeth up to five years after sealant application.[37] School-based sealant programs also are cost efficient.[38] In 2002, the Task Force on Community Preventive Services strongly recommended school-based or school-linked sealant programs to prevent and control dental caries.[37]

Water fluoridation prevents tooth decay mainly through direct contact with teeth throughout life and when consumed by children during the tooth-forming years. The most inexpensive way to deliver the benefits of fluoride to all residents of a community is through water fluoridation. All water naturally contains some fluoride; when a community fluoridates its water, it adjusts the level in the water to an optimal level for preventing tooth decay.[39]

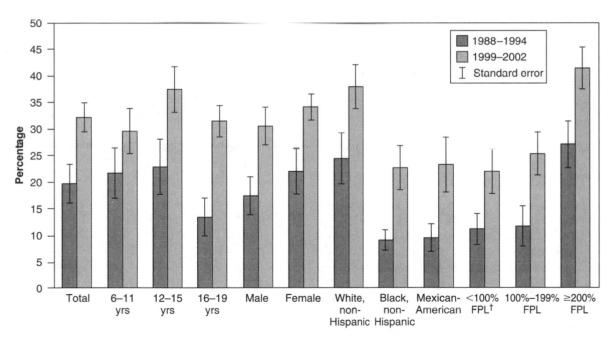

FIGURE 17-9 Prevalence of Dental Sealants in Children and Adolescents Age 6-19 Years

Source: http://www.cdc.gov/mmwr/preview/mmwrhtml/ss5403a1.htm.

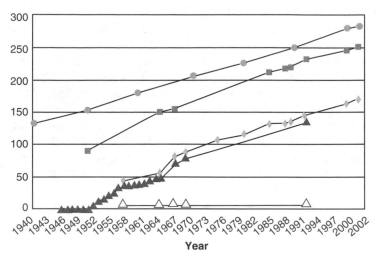

FIGURE 17-10 Fluoridation Growth, by Population, United States 1940–2002

Source: http://www.cdc.gov/nohss/images/fluoride_growth02.gif.

Nearly 70 percent of US residents whose water comes from public systems now have fluoridated water. The objectives of *Healthy People 2010,* which sets health goals for the nation for the year 2010, is 75 percent. Currently, more than 184 million people in the United States are served by public water supplies containing enough fluoride to protect teeth. (See Figure 17-10 ■.) Water fluoridation is a low-cost way to bring the benefits of fluoride to all residents of a community.[39]

SUMMARY

Although the fact that many oral health disparities are based on gender, race/ethnicity, age, and SES has been established, more information is needed in the field of oral epidemiology. Various oral diseases and conditions including periodontal diseases and dental caries are widespread in the United States and are major issues regarding the nation's health. These findings reflect the minor value that society in general places on oral health care. The dental hygienist must be aware of the epidemiology of all oral diseases, conditions, and manifestations and have a clear understanding of the need for and ways to provide dental care in the United States.

SELF-STUDY TEST ITEMS

1. Tobacco use, excessive alcohol use, and inappropriate dietary practices contribute to a number of diseases and disorders. In particular, tobacco use is a risk factor for oral cavity and pharyngeal cancers, periodontal diseases, candidiasis, and dental caries among other diseases.
   a. The first statement is true; the second statement is false.
   b. The first statement is false; the second statement is true.
   c. Both statements are true.
   d. Both statements are false.

2. Which gender do periodontal diseases affect the most?
   a. Males
   b. Females
   c. Neither
   d. Teen and elderly females

3. In which teeth are early childhood caries most evident?
   a. Permanent molars
   b. Permanent anteriors
   c. Primary anteriors
   d. Primary molars

4. Early detection frequently affects the outcome of
   a. Oral cancer treatment
   b. Cleft lip rates
   c. Cleft lip and palate rates
   d. None of the above

5. When toothaches are not prevented, which services might individuals seek?
   a. Medical
   b. Dental hygiene
   c. General dentistry
   d. Cosmetic dentistry

REFERENCES

1. US Department of Health and Human Services. *Oral Health in America: A Report of the Surgeon General.* Rockville, MD: US Department of Health and Human Services, National Institute of Dental and Craniofacial research, National Institutes of Health; 2000.

2. Oliver RC, Brown LJ, Loe H. Periodontal diseases in the United States population. *J Periodontol.* 1998;69:269–278.

3. US Public Health Service, National Institute of Dental Research. *Oral Health of United Sates Adults: National Findings.* Bethesda, MD: National Institute of Dental Research; 1987. NIH Publication No. 87-2868.

4. *Third National Health and Nutrition Examination Survey, 1988–1994.* Hyattsville, MD: Centers for Disease Control; 1997. Public Use Data File No. 7-0627.

5. Epidemiology of Periodontal Diseases: Position Paper. American Association of Periodontology Academy Report. *J Periodontol.* 2005;76:1406–1419.

6. *National Health and Nutrition Examination Survey, 1999–2004.* Hyattsville, MD: Centers for Disease Control, 2005.

7. Oral Cancer Facts. http://www.oralcancerfoundation.org/facts/. Accessed September 16, 2008.

8. Oral Cancer. http://www.cdc.gov/OralHealth/topics/cancer.htm. Accessed September 17, 2008.

9. What Is Oral Cancer? http://www.nidcr.nih.gov/OralHealth/Topics/OralCancer/. Accessed September 17, 2008.

10. Haddad RI. *Human Papilloma Virus Infection and Oropharyngeal Cancer.* Alexandria, VA: American Society of Clinical Oncology; 2007.

11. D'Souza G, Kreimer AR, Viscidi R, Pawlita M, Fakhry C, Koch WM, Westra WH, Gillison, ML. Case–Control Study of Human Papillomavirus and Oropharyngeal Cancer. *N Engl J Med.* 2007;356(19):1944–1956.

12. Gonsalves W, Chi AC, Neville BW. Common Oral Lesions: Part I. Superficial Mucosal Lesions. *Am Fam Physician.* 2007;75:501–507.

13. Shulman JD, Beach MM, Rivera-Hidalgo F. The prevalence of oral mucosal lesions in U.S. adults: Data from the Third National Health and Nutrition Examination Survey, 1988–1994. *J Am Dent Assoc.* 2004;135:1279–1286.

14. Bouquot JE. Common oral lesions found during a mass screening examination. *J Am Dent Assoc.* 1986;112:50–57.

15. Herpes simplex virus. In: Neville B, Damm DD, Allen CM, Bouquot J. *Oral and Maxillofacial Pathology.* Philadelphia, PA: Saunders; 2002:213–220.

16. Whitley, RJ. Prospects for vaccination against herpes simplex virus. *Pediatr Ann.* 1993a;22:726,729–732.

17. Rivera-Hidalgo F, Shulman JD, Beach MM. The association of tobacco and other factors with recurrent aphthous stomatitis in an U.S. adult population. *Oral Dis.* 2004; 10:335–345.

18. Fotos PG, Vincent SD, Hellstein JW. Oral candidosis. Clinical, historical, and therapeutic features of 100 cases. *Oral Surg Oral Med Oral Pathol.* 1992;74:41–49.

19. Candidiasis. In: Neville B, Damm DD, Allen CM, Bouquot J. *Oral and Maxillofacial Pathology.* Philadelphia, PA: Saunders; 2002:189–197.

20. Epstein JB, Gorsky M, Caldwell J. Fluconazole mouthrinses for oral candidiasis in postirradiation, transplant, and other patients. *Oral Surg Oral Med Oral Pathol Oral Radiol Endod.* 2002;93:671–675.

21. Ghannoum MA, Abu-Elteen KH. Pathogenicity determinants of Candida. *Mycoses.* 1990;33:265–282.

22. Abu-Elteen KH, Abu Elteen RM. The prevalence of *Candida albicans* populations in the mouths of complete denture wearers. *New Microbiol.* 1998;21:41–48.

23. Forrester MB, Merz RD. Descriptive epidemiology of oral clefts in a multiethic population, Hawaii, 1986–2000. *Cleft Palate-Craniofacial Journal.* 2004;41(6):622–628.

24. Cleft Lip and Palate Fact Sheet. http://www.cdc.gov/ncbddd/bd/cleft.htm. Accessed September 17, 2008.

25. Lowry RD, Thunem NY, Uh SH. Birth prevalence of cleft lip and palate in British Columbia between 1952 and 1986: Stability of rates. *Can Med Assoc J.* 1989;140(10):1167–1170.

26. Cuttrell G. Dental trauma. In Harris NO, Garcia-Godoy F, Nathe CN, eds. *Primary Preventive Dentistry.* 7th ed. Upper Saddle River, NJ: Pearson; 2008.

27. Slack GL, Jones JM. Psychological effect of fractured incisors. *Br Dent J.* 1955;99:386–388.

28. Cortes MI, Marcenes W, Shelham A. Impact of traumatic injuries to the permanent teeth on the oral health-related quality of life in 12- to 14-year old children. *Community Dent Oral Epidemiol.* 2002;30:193–198.

29. Douglass AB, Douglass JM. Common dental emergencies. *Am Fam Phys.* 2003;67(3):515.

30. Bijur PE, Trumbel A, Harel Y, Overpeck MD, Jones D, Scheidt PC. Sports and recreation injuries in US children and adolescents. *Arch Pediatr Adolesc Med.* 1995:149:1009–1016.

31. National Youth Sports Foundation. *Fact Sheet.* Needham, MA: National Youth Sports Foundation; 1994.

32. Nathe CN. Athletic Mouthguard. In Harris NO, Garcia-Godoy F, Nathe CN. *Primary Preventive Dentistry.* 7th ed. Upper Saddle River, NJ: Pearson; 2008.

33. Lipton JA, Ship JA, Larach-Robinson D. Estimated prevalence and distribution of reported orofacial pain in the United States. *J Am Dent Assoc.* 1993;4(10):113–121.

34. Vargas CM, Macek MD, Marcus SE. Sociodemographic correlates of tooth pain among adults: United States 1989. *Pain.* 2000;85(1–2):87–92.

35. National Institutes of Health. Consensus development conference statement on dental sealants in the prevention of tooth decay. *J Am Dent Assoc.* 1984;108:233–236.

36. Llodra JC, Bravo M, Delgado-Rodriguez M, Baca P, Galvez R. Factors influencing the effectiveness of sealants—A meta analysis. *Community Dent Oral Epidemiol.* 1993;21:261–268.

37. Task Force on Community Preventive Services. Recommendations on selected interventions to prevent dental caries, oral and pharyngeal cancers, and sport-related craniofacial injuries. *Am J Prev Med.* 2002;23(suppl 1):16–20.

38. Griffin SO, Griffin PM, Gooch BF, Barker LK. Comparing the costs of three sealant delivery strategies. *J Dent Res.* 2002;81:641–645.

39. Community Water Fluoridation Status Now Reaches Nearly 70 percent of US Population. http://www.cdc.gov/fluoridation/statistics/cwf_status.htm. Accessed September 17, 2008.

PEARSON

myhealthprofessionskit™

Multimedia Extension Activities

Use this address to access the interactive Companion Website created for this textbook. Simply select "Dental Hygiene" from the choice of disciplines. Find this book and log in using your username and password. To obtain a username and password, please register using the scratch-off access code on the inside front cover of this book.

Chapter 18

Biostatistics

Christine French Beatty, RDH, PhD

OBJECTIVES

After studying this chapter, the dental hygiene student should be able to:

- Define and describe data analysis and interpretation
- Identify data by their type and scale of measurement
- Define and describe descriptive, correlation, and inferential statistics
- Select and compute appropriate measures of central tendency and measures of dispersion for various types of data
- Describe and construct frequency distributions and graphs for various types of data
- Select appropriate inferential statistical tests for various types of data
- Interpret research results

KEY TERMS

Biostatistics
Causality
Correlation
Data analysis
Degrees of freedom
Descriptive statistics
Graphs
Inferential statistics
Interpretation
Measures of central tendency
Measures of dispersion

COMPETENCIES

After studying the chapter and participating in accompanying course activities, the dental hygiene student should be competent to do the following:

- Use evidence-based decision making to evaluate and incorporate emerging treatment modalities
- Assume responsibility for dental hygiene actions and care based on accepted scientific theories and research as well as the accepted standard of care

Normal distribution
Null hypothesis
p value
Parametric statistics/Nonparametric statistics
Reliability
Research (alternate) hypothesis

Scales of measurement
Skewed distribution
Statistical decision
Type I and Type II errors
Validity

The subject of **biostatistics,** the use of data analysis and interpretation in health care research, is a course unto itself, and fortunately for the dental hygienist in the twenty-first century, computer programs are available to do the computations.[1] Nevertheless, the dental hygienist must have a working knowledge of statistics to use these computer programs and interpret research results.

Upon completion of a research project or program evaluation, data must be analyzed in preparation for interpreting the results. **Data analysis** involves the application of statistical tests to the data in order to organize, describe, summarize, and analyze it to answer a research question or test a hypothesis.[2] When the data have been analyzed, the researcher must interpret these results. **Interpretation,** which is the explanation of results, requires that critical thinking be used to explain the meaning and application of the findings, identify possible factors that could have influenced the results, and draw inferences to the population.[2,3] Biostatistics is used to demonstrate response to dental hygiene therapy, to test products and treatment regimes used in dental hygiene therapy, to determine the needs of target populations, to evaluate oral health treatment, prevention, and educational programs, and to complete a variety of other purposes in relation to oral health care.[4] Although not every dental hygienist will conduct research studies or evaluate community programs, each and every dental hygienist must understand the research process, including data analysis and interpretation, to be able to critically analyze the results of published studies and understand the epidemiology of disease. This is essential for the dental hygienist to be able to practice therapies and implement programs that are based on scientific evidence.[5]

Students of research often reflect a bias that statistics are undependable because they can be used to "say whatever you want them to say."[4] However, the appropriate application of the sound principles of biostatistics will produce valid results and interpretations. For the researcher who is not familiar with statistical analysis, consultation with a statistician experienced in this field is highly recommended when planning a research project to avoid errors in research design and misinterpretation of results. If the number of subjects is insufficient, the study is not long enough in duration, incorrect measurement instruments or procedures are used, or the wrong statistical tests are used to analyze the data, the resulting conclusions will be invalid. Repeating the research study due to statistical errors is frustrating for the principal investigator and highly aggravating to the financial sponsors. A statistician also can be very helpful in interpreting the results and making inferences to the population.

> ### Did You Know?
>
> A foundation in biostatistics helps the dental hygienist understand literature and research reports.

DATA CATERGORIZATION

Data are the information that a researcher collects.[6] The word *data* actually is the plural term; the singular term is *datum.* Each piece of information is called an *item of data,* and a group of all data items collected is called a *data set.* Data can be quantitative or nonquantitative, sometimes referred to as *qualitative. Quantitative data* are numerical representations. For example, pocket depths, number of sealed teeth, and number of communities with water fluoridation can be expressed as counts, percentages, and means. Information that reflects the quality or nature of variables that cannot be measured numerically is referred to as *qualitative data.* The values of qualitative data are expressed as outcomes or states and can be counted for reporting. These variables can often be rank ordered as well.[7] An example is a list of clients' responses to what they liked most and least about their treatment visits to a dental clinic.

Variables are classified as continuous or discrete. A *continuous variable* is made up of distinct and separate units or categories and can be expressed by a large or infinite number of measures along a continuum.[7] These variables can be expressed in fractions and are considered quantitative. For example, height, weight, and time are continuous because they fall on a continuum and have value when expressed as fractions.

A *discrete variable* is also made up of distinct and separate units or categories, but it is counted only in whole numbers[7] and is quantitative because these data are represented numerically. An example of a discrete variable is the number of children. Logically, we cannot have fractions of children, although we might refer to having a mean of 2.3 children per family. The dental index, decayed, missing and filled teeth (DMFT) is also a discrete variable because it is not possible to have a fraction of a tooth. However, sometimes the distinction between discrete and continuous variables is unimportant in application because many discrete variables, especially those that have a high number of possible scores, can be treated meaningfully as continuous for statistical analysis.[8] For example, it is meaningful to express a mean of 2.5 on a DMF index, plaque index, gingival index, number of sealants, most other dental indices, and many rating scales.

A variable that has no numeric representation is a *categorical variable*.[7] Gender (male/female), color (red/blue/yellow), or rating (excellent/fair/poor) are examples of this type of variable. Religious preference and socioeconomic status (SES) are also categorical variables. Although categorical variables can be arranged logically and numbered accordingly, there is no meaning to the numeric representation. For example, an average religious preference or SES of 1.8 makes no sense. A *dichotomous variable* is a categorical variable that places data into only two groups, such as male/female, pass/fail, yes/no, or true/false.[6] Categorical and dichotomous variables are qualitative in nature.[6]

Data are also classified by the use of **scales of measurement.**[6] Four scales of measurement exist: nominal, ordinal, interval, and ratio. The higher the level of data, the more information it conveys about the differences among values. The scale of measurement is important because it determines which statistics and graphs can be used to represent and analyze the data.

The *nominal* scale of measurement organizes data into mutually exclusive categories, but the categories have no rank order or value, and there is no numeric relationship between the different classifications.[7] Ethnic group membership is an example. African American may be placed in category A, American Indian and Alaska native in category B, Asian in category C, native Hawaiian and other Pacific Islanders in category D, and White in category E.

The *ordinal* scale of measurement organizes data into mutually exclusive categories that are rank ordered based on some criterion, but the difference between ranks is not necessarily equal in value.[6] An example is the classification of level of difficulty of patients' needs in a dental hygiene clinic: Class 0, 1, 2, 3, and 4. The higher class reflects more difficulty, but the difference between class 1 and class 2 is not numerically equivalent to the difference between class 2 and class 3. Also, a class 4 is not necessarily twice as difficult as a class 2. Another common example is a five-point scale of ordered responses that range from strongly agree to strongly disagree to statements that evaluate the value of a program.

The *interval* scale of measurement has the characteristics of the ordinal scale but the distance between any two adjacent units of measurement is equal. However, there is no meaningful zero point.[6] In other words, the zero point is arbitrary, not determined by nature. An example is the Fahrenheit measurement scale. Scores on an interval scale can be added and subtracted meaningfully but not multiplied and divided. A one-degree difference is numerically equal all along the scale. However, because of the arbitrary zero point, we cannot say that 90°F is twice as hot as 45°F, although we can say that 90°F is warmer than 45°F.

The *ratio* scale of measurement contains all characteristics of the preceding scales and has an absolute zero point determined by nature.[6] Therefore, all arithmetic procedures can be applied. Blood pressure, height, weight, number of teeth, and number of sealants are examples of ratio variables. We can say that a person who weighs 150 pounds is twice as heavy as a person who weighs 75 pounds.

In general, categorical and dichotomous variables use the nominal and ordinal scales of measurement, and discrete and continuous data use the interval or ratio scales of measurement. However, several important points are necessary to understand that sometimes the rules for treating the various scales of data statistically vary. One point is that discrete and continuous data can be converted to nominal or ordinal data.[8] For example, subjects can be placed in nominal categories of "controlled BP" or "unncontrolled BP" according to their blood pressure, which is a continuous variable.

Another example is to categorize subjects' gingivitis as mild, moderate, or severe (ordinal scale) according to the number of bleeding points (discrete variable). Another point discussed previously is that when ordinal data consist of many ranks or categories, the data are customarily treated as continuous rather than discrete.[6,8] For example, ordinal attitude scales (eg, very satisfied, satisfied, neither satisfied nor dissatisfied, dissatisfied, very dissatisfied) are commonly treated as interval data.[6] A third point is that the distinction between interval and ratio data is insignificant for our purposes. Both types of variables are handled the same way when analyzing data.[9]

DESCRIPTIVE STATISTICS

Statistics are divided into two major categories: descriptive and inferential. **Descriptive statistics** consist of the procedures that are used to summarize, organize, and describe quantitative data.[7] Data are generally presented by describing and summarizing them with the use of descriptive statistics and tables and graphs rather than presenting all of the raw data. **Inferential statistics,** on the other hand, are used to make inferences or generalizations about a population based on data taken from a sample of that population.[6] This process is also called *making statistical decisions.* The application of descriptive statistics to a data set always precedes the use of inferential statistics. A data set can be summarized numerically with a measure of central tendency, a measure of dispersion, and a sample size. Use of tables and graphs displays the data to further enhance the understanding of the nature of the variable. Descriptive statistics include measures of central tendency, measures of dispersion, frequency distribution tables, and graphing techniques.

Measures of Central Tendency

The term **measures of central tendency** refers to measures of the central tendency of data within a research study. When describing statistics, the term *average* is rarely used. Instead, one of the three measures of central tendency (*mean, median,* or *mode*) is used, depending on the type of data the researcher is describing.[10] A summary of the measures of central tendency is presented in Table 18-1 ■.

The *mean* is what is commonly called the *average.* It is the arithmetic average of the data set. The symbol used to denote the mean is *x;* the symbol *M* is also commonly used in journal articles.[8] To arrive at the mean, one would add all scores and divide by the total number. The formula for the mean is $\Sigma x/n$. The uppercase Greek letter sigma (Σ) means "the sum of." If the letter *x* represents a single value in the distribution, then Σx means "the sum of all the values." The letter *n* represents the sample size or number of observations. For example, to compute the mean of the numbers 2, 3, 3, and 4, $\Sigma x/n = 12/4 = 3$. The mean is appropriate to use with interval and ratio data. It is also commonly used with ordinal data when they are treated as continuous data as previously described.

Did You Know?

The mean cannot be used to describe nominal data.

The *median* is the mid-point of the data, in other words, the point at which exactly half of the values are above and half are below.[10] The median of the scores 2, 2, 3, 4, and 5 is 3. If we have only the scores 2, 2, 3, and 4, the median is the average of the middle two scores, which in this case is 2.5. Note that the scores must be

Table 18-1 Measures of Central Tendency

Measure	Description	Appropriate Use
Mean	Arithmetic average	Ratio and interval data
		Ordinal data that are treated as continuous
Median	Middle score	Ordinal data
Mode	Most frequently occurring score	Nominal data

placed in ascending or descending order (called an *array*) to be able to determine the median manually. The median can be used to describe ratio, interval, or ordinal data, but not nominal data because they cannot be rank ordered.

The *mode* is the value that occurs most often in the distribution.[10] The mode of the scores 2, 3, 3, and 4 is 3. Some distributions may have more than one mode, which would be referred to as *bimodal* (two modes) or *multimodal* (more than two modes). The mode can be used to describe all types of data. When analyzing nominal data, such as gender and SES, the mode is the only measure of central tendency that can be used.[7]

Measures of Dispersion

A **measure of dispersion,** also called a *measure of variability,* communicates how much variation is present in a group of data.[11] It describes the distribution of data within a research study. Two distributions of data can have the same measure of central tendency and vastly different measures of dispersion. For example, a distribution could have a mean of 90 with a low score of 80 and a high score of 97, while another distribution could have a mean of 90 with a low score of 88 and a high score of 94. The distribution with the wider spread of scores has a higher measure of dispersion. Because of this, to report a measure of central tendency without a measure of dispersion can misrepresent the data.

The measures of dispersion are the range, variance, and standard deviation. The *range* is determined by subtracting the lowest score from the highest score. It is the simplest and least useful measure of dispersion because it is based only on the lowest and highest

scores.[11] Sometimes the range is reported as the distance between the lowest and highest scores, for example a range of 80 to 97 for a set of test scores. The range is usually reported with the median.[4]

> ### ─ Did You Know? ─
>
> At all times, it is important to look not only at the average or mean but also at the dispersion of the data.

The *variance* represents the average distance of each score from the mean, and the *standard deviation* (SD) is the square root of the variance. Because they are based on the average squared distances of values around the mean, these are the most common and useful measures of dispersion.[12] The variance or SD is usually reported with the mean. When analyzing normally distributed data, standard deviation can be used in conjunction with the mean in order to calculate data intervals.

The steps for computing a variance and SD are presented in Box 18-1 ■.[2] Although it is no longer necessary to compute these values manually, understanding the computation helps to understand the significance of the values.[12] Notice that each score in a distribution is used to compute the variance and SD. This makes them more accurate and useful measures of dispersion than the range. In the previous example of two distributions with a mean of 90, the distribution with a high score of 97 and a low score of 80 would have a wider variance and SD than the distribution with a high score of 94 and a low score of 88. In this way, the value of the variance or the SD in relation to the mean depicts the distribution of scores.

BOX 18-1 Steps in Computing the Variance and Standard Deviation (SD)

1. Calculate the mean for the distribution of scores.
2. Subtract the mean from each score (individual score – mean). This is called the *deviation.* When the mean is larger than the score, the result is a negative value.
3. The sum of the deviations always equals zero. Add the deviations to check this.
4. Square each deviation (individual score – mean)^2.
5. Add the squared deviations to determine the sum of squares (Σ[individual score – mean]^2).
6. Divide the sum of square by N – 1 (number of scores – 1). This resulting value is called the *variance.*
7. Take the square root of the variance. This resulting value is the *standard deviation.*

The Normal Distribution

Most occurrences in this world theoretically fall into a bell-shaped curve, called the **normal distribution** or *Gaussian distribution.*[7] Generally, the majority of subjects fall under the large part of the middle of the curve with a few low and high outliers. Grades are a good example of this tendency. If one looked at a group of people from the general population of college students who took a class in principles of chemistry, most of them would receive a grade of C with a few getting Bs and Ds and an even fewer receiving As and Fs. When researchers want to know whether an intervention has made a difference, they cannot just look at pure numbers. It is not enough that a group's mean score improved; the improvement also must be *statistically significant.* The normal distribution forms the theoretical foundation for these comparisons and in making statistical decisions.

This theoretical normal distribution yields a symmetrical, unimodal, bell-shaped curve.[6] This shape explains why random variables tend to be normally distributed.[11] The mean, median, and mode of the normal distribution are of equal value. The curve's extreme ends

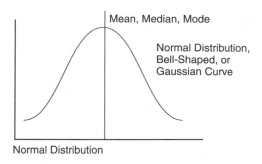

FIGURE 18-1 Standard Normal Distribution

(called *tails*) do not touch the abscissa (x-axis). See Figure 18-1 ■ for an example of standard normal distribution.

Use of the *empirical rule* estimates the spread of the data given the mean and the standard deviation of a data set that follows the standard normal distribution.[13] According to this empirical rule, for a normal distribution, approximately 68 percent of the data fall within 1 SD of the mean, 95 percent within 2 SD, and 99.7 percent within 3 SD.[11] See Figure 18-2■ for a graphic presentation of the empirical rule.

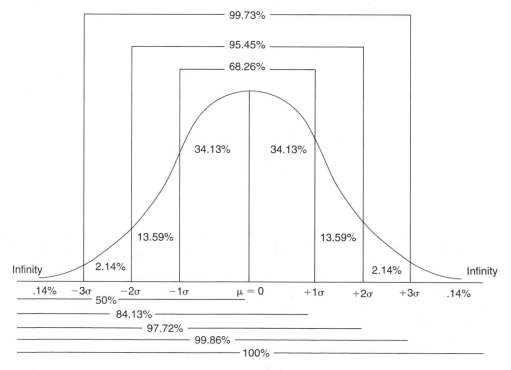

FIGURE 18-2 Empirical Rule of the Normal Distribution

Source: Darby ML, Bowen DM. *Research Methods for Oral Health Professionals: An Introduction.* St. Louis, MO: C. V. Mosby, 1980. Reprint. Pocatello, ID: McCann; 1993.

The normal distribution is also the foundation of the *central limit theorem*. Based on this statistical proposition, less sampling error will occur with a larger sample, and a sample size of thirty or more will estimate the population mean with reasonable accuracy.[10] The normal distribution can be used to study a wide variety of statistical problems.[10] According to the central limit theorem, if an infinite number of randomly selected samples are drawn from a population, the means of the samples tend to be normally distributed, and the average of the sample means is very close to the actual population mean. The SD of these sample means is called the *standard error of the mean*.[10] To calculate it, divide the SD by the square root of the sample size; hence, a larger sample size significantly reduces the standard error. The term *error* here does not signify an error made but indicates the fact that each sample mean is likely to vary somewhat from the population mean.[6]

Did You Know?

In dental studies it is important to have at least thirty subjects in a clinic trial study.

In contrast to a normal distribution, when a distribution of scores is asymmetrical, the curve is said to be distorted, or skewed, and the study is said to have a **skewed distribution.**[11] (See Figure 18-3 ■.) The skew is caused by a few extreme scores in the distribution. A skewed curve can be identified by the curve's appearance resulting from plotting the data. A skewed distribution also can be identified by comparing the mean and median of the distribution.[13] In a positively skewed (or upward or right-skewed) distribution, the infrequent or

extreme scores are on the right side of the *x* axis, the mean is larger than (to the right of) the median, and the tail is in a positive direction. In a negatively skewed (or downward or left-skewed) distribution, the infrequent or extreme scores are on the left side, the mean is smaller than (to the left of) the median, and the tail is in a negative direction. Vogt suggests a method to remember which skew is which.[6] Remember that a skewer is pointed. When the point is on the right, it is right skewed; when the pointed end is on the left, it is left skewed.[6] Because of the relative position of the mean and median, the skew of a curve can also be determined by examining the values of the mean and median of the distribution in relation to each other without seeing a curve that represents the plot of the data.

The mean is highly affected by extreme scores and is pulled in their direction; therefore, the median and mode more accurately represent central tendency in a skewed distribution.[11] For this reason, it is wise to examine all three values to determine the type of distribution represented by the data. The significance of recognizing a skewed sample distribution is that it may result from using small or homogenous samples or from failing to use random sampling or random assignment techniques.[2,5] In addition, for many of the statistical tests that are used to test a hypothesis to be reliable, the population must approximately follow a normal distribution.[10]

GRAPHING DATA

Data can be presented pictorially in graphs. The advantages of using graphs and tables include effective and economic communication of data, easier and quicker understanding and interpreting of data, and the ability to compare multiple distributions visually.[2]

Negatively skewed distribution

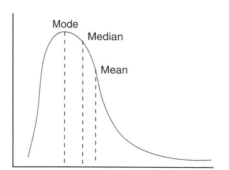

Positively skewed distribution

FIGURE 18-3   Skewed Distributions

Frequency Distribution Tables

A *frequency distribution table* presents data in a way that shows the number of times each score occurs in the group of scores.[7] For nominal and ordinal variables, the categories are listed in a natural order and then the frequency for each category is tabulated. Table 18-2 ■ illustrates a frequency distribution table for ordinal data, that is, age category of patients treated in a dental hygiene clinic.

For interval and ratio data, the values are first arranged in an array, which is an ordered display of a set of observations.[6] For these types of data, the frequency can be expressed in four ways:

1. The actual frequency or count for the category
2. The relative frequency or percent calculated by dividing the frequency by the total number in the data set
3. The cumulative frequency, which is the total up to and including that value
4. The cumulative relative frequency or cumulative percent, which is also known as the percentile rank

Frequency distribution tables can be ungrouped or grouped.[7] An *ungrouped frequency* distribution includes all the scores in the distribution. It is recommended for small samples with less than 30 observations. With a large data set (more than 30 observations), a grouped frequency distribution can be constructed by grouping the data into class intervals. Also, if the difference between the maximum and minimum values is more than 15, a grouped frequency distribution is recommended.[6] However, it is important to note that when the scores are widely dispersed, grouping the data can cause loss of detail in the scores reported.

To construct a *grouped frequency distribution,* group a set number of scores into mutually exclusive intervals called *class intervals* also known as *collapsing the data.*[6] Try to choose an interval and a starting point that are divisible by 5. To determine the number of intervals, consider the total number of measurements. It is equally inappropriate to have just one or two measurements in several intervals and to have a large number of measurements in only a few intervals. About 5–10 intervals are appropriate for most distributions.[14] See Table 18-3 ■ for an ungrouped frequency distribution for ratio data and Table 18-4 ■ for a grouped frequency distribution for the same data. Note how much easier it

Table 18-2 Frequency Distribution Table of Nominal Data

Number of Patients Treated in Dental Hygiene Clinic in Fall 2006 by Age Category

Patient Type	Number	Percent
Child	55	11%
Adolescent	62	12
Adult	173	34
Geriatric	216	43
Total	506	100%

Table 18-3 Ungrouped Frequency Distribution for Ratio Data

X	f	X	f	X	f	X	f
100	0	90	0	80	0	70	0
99	2	89	4	79	1	69	1
98	1	88	2	78	3	68	0
97	1	87	2	77	1	67	0
96	0	86	0	76	4	66	0
95	1	85	0	75	1	65	0
94	3	84	3	74	2	64	1
93	1	83	4	73	0	63	0
92	1	82	2	72	0	62	0
91	1	81	1	71	0	61	0

Table 18-4 Grouped Frequency Distribution

Class Interval	f	Cumulative f
95–99	5	45
90–94	6	40
85–89	8	34
80–84	12	26
75–79	10	14
70–74	2	4
65–69	1	2
60–64	1	1

is to understand the data in the grouped frequency distribution table.

Types of Graphs

A frequency distribution can also be displayed in a **graph,** which is a diagram showing the variation of a variable in comparison with one or more other variables; it is also called a *chart*. A graph showing frequency distribution is usually constructed by representing the variable on the horizontal (*x*) axis and the frequency on the vertical (*y*) axis, although the axes can be reversed. The vertical axis should have a height of one-half to three-fourths the width of the graph.[8] This prevents expanding or collapsing the *x* and *y* scales and minimizes misrepresentation and misinterpretation of the data.[2] Computers

have facilitated the construction of graphs. Some computer programs, for example, Excel, label graphs as charts. Some of the most commonly used graphs are the bar graph, histogram, polygon, frequency polygon, scattergram, and pie chart.

A *bar graph* (or bar chart) is used to present categorical data.[6] A space separates the bars to emphasize the discrete nature of the data. The length of each bar corresponds to the frequency of the value it represents. See Figure 18-4 ■ for an example of a bar graph. Each bar represents a reason for a missed appointment. Two or more distributions can be compared by using a cluster bar graph (Figure 18-5 ■).

A *histogram* is similar to a bar graph, but the bars appear side by side, that is, touching. It is appropriate for showing interval or ratio variables and sometimes ordinal variables that are treated as continuous data.[7] Both ungrouped and grouped frequencies can be represented in a histogram. Computer programs are handy for experimenting with the number and height of bars and the width of the intervals so that you can meet the goal of constructing a graph with a smooth appearance that accurately represents the data. See Figure 18-6 ■ for an example of a histogram.

A *frequency polygon* is a line graph that represents frequency data that are continuous in nature and drawn by connecting the midpoints of the bars of a histogram and then extending the line at both ends to imaginary midpoints at the right and left of the histogram. This extension of the line ensures that the total areas of both graphs are equivalent.[8] As with histograms, frequency polygons can be used to represent ungrouped or grouped frequency distributions and can present frequency, percent, cumulative frequency,

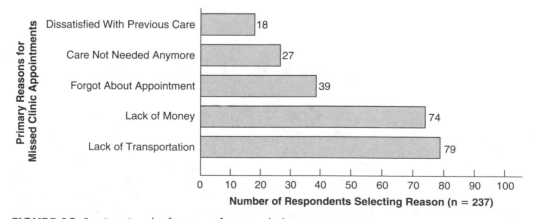

FIGURE 18-4 Bar Graph of Reasons for Missed Clinic Appointments

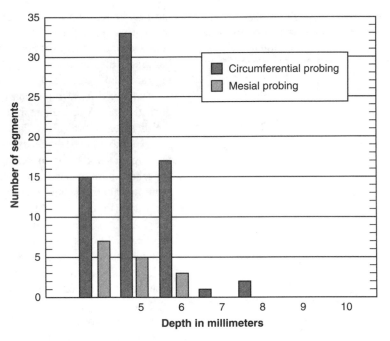

FIGURE 18-5 Cluster Bar Graph

FIGURE 18-6 Histogram

FIGURE 18-7 Frequency Polygon Comparing Two Distributions

or cumulative percent. They are especially useful for comparing two or more distributions visually by superimposing them in one graph as in Figure 18-7 ■.

A *polygon* (line graph) can also be used to plot a variable over time.[2] Refer to Figure 18-8 ■ for an illustration of such a polygon that depicts the change in mean plaque scores over a series of periodontal therapy appointments.

A *scattergram* shows the relationship between two variables. For each subject, the level of one variable is plotted on the *x* axis against the level of the other variable on the *y* axis.[11] The resulting scattergram shows how the level of one variable varies as the level of the other variable changes. See Figure 18-9 ■ for scattergrams that depict different relationships between variables.

Mean Plaque Index Scores of Perio Patients over Four Weeks, Spring 2004 (*n* = 26)

FIGURE 18-8   Polygon

A *pie chart* represents parts of a whole. Its use is more acceptable with lay audiences than in scientific or technical publications and presentations. When used, the percentage represented by each part of the pie should be labeled for clarity.[15] See Figure 18-10 ■.

Did You Know?

Pie charts are helpful to use when describing the demographics of study participants.

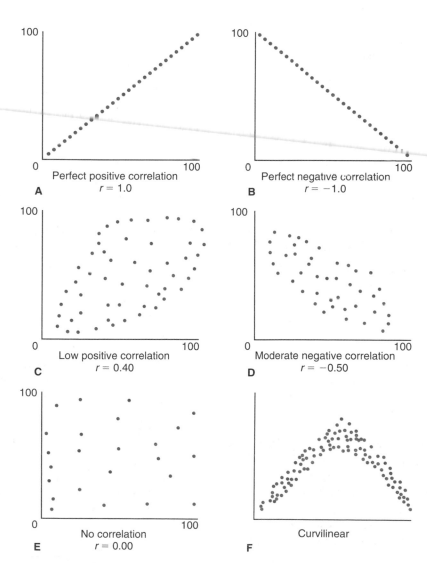

A Perfect positive correlation *r* = 1.0

B Perfect negative correlation *r* = −1.0

C Low positive correlation *r* = 0.40

D Moderate negative correlation *r* = −0.50

E No correlation *r* = 0.00

F Curvilinear

FIGURE 18-9   Scattergrams Demonstrating Relationships of Data

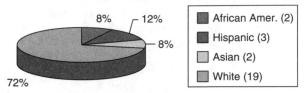

Ethnic Groups Represented in Dental Hygiene Class of 2004

| African Amer. (2) |
| Hispanic (3) |
| Asian (2) |
| White (19) |

8% 12%
8%
72%

FIGURE 18-10 Pie Chart

Tables and graphs facilitate our understanding and interpretation of the data. They help us quickly spot the shape of the distribution, where the data cluster, and how the data scatter around the clustering points, outliers, and gaps in the data.[8] Data presented in tables and graphs should be understandable even without the written discussion of the data. See Box 18-2 ■ for characteristics of effective tables and graphs and appropriate ways to achieve them.[2,6,8,15]

CORRELATION

Correlational techniques are used to study relationships among variables. The term correlation is used in everyday language to mean relationship. In statistics, **correlation** refers to a relationship or association between variables that can be measured mathematically.[11] The null hypothesis in a correlation analysis is one of no association between the variables.

The statistic used to measure correlation is the *correlation coefficient,* signified by *r,* which is expressed as a number between −1 and +1. The value of *r* communicates both the direction and strength of the association.[11] The sign (+ or −) determines the direction of the relationship. In a positive relationship, both variables vary in the same direction. In other words, as one increases in value, the other also increases in value. In the same way, as one decreases in value, the second also decreases in value. An example is the relationship between periodontal disease and heart disease. Heart disease and periodontal disease increase and decrease together in the population. In a negative relationship, the variables vary in opposite directions, so as one variable increases in value, the other decreases, and vice versa. This is also described as an *inverse relationship.*

Did You Know?

Another example of inverse relationship would be that as the consumption of fluoridated water increases, the caries rate decreases, and as the consumption of fluoridated water decreases, the caries rate increases.

BOX 18-2 Characteristics of Effective Tables and Graphs and Ways to Achieve Them

1. **Accuracy.** Enter data carefully. Follow basic principles for construction of tables and graphs. Select the type of table or graph considering the type of data being presented. Construct graphs that will not be misleading or open to misinterpretation. Begin the vertical axis at zero with a break drawn in, if necessitated by a high frequency of scores. Make the height of the vertical axis one-half to three-fourths of the horizontal width of the graph.

2. **Simplicity.** Present data in a straightforward manner. Highlight only the major points of information. Minimize the use of grid lines, tics, unusual fonts, and showy patterns.

3. **Clarity.** Make data easy to understand and self-explanatory. Use brief but clear titles and headings, and label all axes and variables including type of frequency (count, percent, cumulative).

   Carefully choose intervals. Include information on when and where data were collected, if appropriate, and the size of the groups. Communicate exclusions of observations from the data set including the reasons and criteria for their exclusion. Include the basis for the measurement of rates. Use textbooks on statistics and graphing, scientific writing style manuals, and samples of tables and graphs in journal articles to guide your construction.

4. **Appearance.** Pay attention to the construction so that the final result is neat and appealing.

5. **Well-Designed Structure.** Emphasize the important points visually. Use dark bars and light grid lines and horizontal lettering when possible.

Table 18-5   Guide to Interpretation of *r*

Value of **r**	Strength of Association
0.00–0.25	Little if any
0.26–0.49	Weak
0.50–0.69	Moderate
0.70–0.89	High
0.90–1.00	Very high

Source: Munro BH, *Statistical Methods for Health Care Research.* 5th ed. Philadelphia, PA: Lippincott; 2007.

The value of *r* indicates the strength of the relationship. As the value moves closer to +1.0 or −1.0, it indicates a stronger relationship; as it moves closer to 0, it indicates a weaker relationship. This means that a value of +0.90 is just as strong as a value of −0.90. A value of +1.0 or −1.0 indicates a perfect relationship, and a value of zero indicates no relationship. Refer to Table 18-5 ■ for a general interpretation of *r*. In oral health when two variables are associated, the relationship generally is not perfect because other variables are also associated with the variables being correlated. For example, the association between fluoride and dental caries is not perfect because of the role of diet and plaque bacteria in the development of caries.

Several correlation techniques are available. The selection is based on the number of variables to be correlated, the nature of the variable (discrete or continuous), the measurement scale, and the linearity of the relationship between the variables,[16] which is depicted by the scattergram. (See Figure 18-9.)

The most common correlation coefficient is the *Pearson product moment correlation coefficient.* Pearson *r* is used when both variables are continuous, are at least interval scaled, and have a linear relationship.[11] The linearity of the relationship is determined by plotting the scores on a scattergram. In Figure 18-9, scattergrams A, B, C, and D demonstrate linear relationships, E demonstrates no relationship, and F demonstrates a curvilinear relationship.

The *Spearman rank-order correlation coefficient* (also called *Spearman rho*) is a variation of *r* used to correlate two ordinal variables.[11] Other correlation techniques

are available for data that are nominally scaled, for data with curvilinear relationships, for relating more than two variables, and for other purposes.[8] Correlation techniques are also used to determine reliability of data collection instruments, intrarater reliability, and interrater reliability.[11] Statistical significance of correlation can also be determined to rule out the possibility that the correlation we observe is due to chance alone.

Regression analysis, like correlation, can be used to quantify the relationship of two variables. However, unlike correlation, it expresses the functional relationship between the variables.[13] It is used to predict the score of one variable (dependent variable referred to as *y*) based on the score of another (independent variable referred to as *x*).[11] For example, regression can be used to predict an individual's score on the National Board based on GPA in the program. Multiple regression analysis goes a step further to provide a mathematical model that gives the strength of the ability of two or more variables (independent variables) to predict another variable (dependent variable). For example, the strength of the ability of GPA, Scholastic Aptitude Test scores, and other factors to predict success on the National Board could be tested with multiple regression analysis.

Correlation does not necessarily equal causality, otherwise known as a *cause-and-effect relationship.*[11,17] Simply, **causality** means that a certain exposure will result in a particular outcome. Causality in epidemiology depends on the strength of the association of the variables, the consistency of their association in repeated observations, the specificity of the relationship (not dependent on other factors), the occurrence of the causal factor at a point in time prior to the outcome, evidence of a dose-response curve in the relationship, plausibility of causality, agreement with current knowledge of the disease or condition, and analogy to causal relationships previously established.[18]

Correlation provides much of the evidence in oral epidemiology because it establishes risk, which is the probability that a specified event will occur but not necessarily through a causal chain.[17] In other words, a strong significant correlation between two variables does not mean that one necessarily has caused the other. For example, caries and fluorosis are highly correlated, but fluorosis is not the cause of caries and caries does not cause fluorosis. Fluoride is the causal factor for both fluorosis and low caries rates. It is also a mistake to think that two correlated variables cannot be causally related or that correlation provides no evidence whatsoever for cause.[6]

Remember that the first evidence of a cause-and-effect relationship between caries and fluoride was correlation. Additional research demonstrated that there was indeed causation. When correlation techniques indicate that two variables are associated, further longitudinal observational research and/or experimental research are indicated to provide more evidence of causality.[5,17]

STATISTICAL DECISION MAKING

The **null hypothesis** is an initial negative statement of belief about the value of a population parameter, for example, that two groups do not differ as to a variable.[11] Basically, a null hypothesis is accepted unless the statistical test indicates it should be rejected. The **research (alternative) hypothesis,** also called the *positive hypothesis,* is the logical opposite of the null hypothesis and can indicate a direction of difference. (See Chapter 14.) For example, the null hypothesis is that the retention rate of one brand of sealants does not differ from the retention rate of a second brand. The accompanying research hypothesis can be that the retention rates differ (no direction of difference specified) or that the first brand has a higher retention rate than the second (directional hypothesis). The object of hypothesis testing is to decide whether it is reasonable to continue believing that the null hypothesis is true or to reject this belief in favor of the research hypothesis.

A **statistical decision** is made about the null hypothesis based on the results of inferential statistics.[10] Remember that inferential statistics (more later) is the category of statistics used to make inferences or generalizations about a population based on data taken from the sample. These statistics are used to test a hypothesis or to estimate a population parameter based on the sample data, for example, to estimate the mean satisfaction score of dental hygienists in the United States based on the mean satisfaction score of a representative sample surveyed.

The statistical decision to reject or accept the null hypothesis is based on probability at a set significance level, also known as the *alpha α level.* It is expressed as a probability value or *p* **value,** or the probability that the findings from a study are due to chance. The *p* value commonly accepted as statistically significant in oral health research is equal to or smaller than 0.05 ($p \leq .05$).[11] We see *p* values of .05, .01, and .001 in research reports. A low *p* value signifies greater statistical significance of the result. When the *p* value is larger than .05, the results are said to be not statistically significant, or NS. Simply stated, a result of hypothesis testing reported as $p = .05$ means that the probability of this result occurring by chance alone equals 5 percent. The *p* value is the final arithmetic solution obtained by using the calculated test statistic, the sampling distribution of the test statistic, and the size of the sample. Regardless of the inferential statistic used, the statistical decision is made this same way by using the *p* value to determine statistical significance.

A caution regarding the interpretation of a *p* value is appropriate at this point. A *p* value is not simply the probability that the null hypothesis is true. Rather, the *p* value is the probability that the data have a sampling error and the null hypothesis is true. When reacting with disbelief about the null hypothesis because the *p* value is small, it does not necessarily mean that a false null hypothesis has been detected. There is a possibility of error when either rejecting or accepting a null hypothesis because the statistical decision is based on probability.[10]

A **Type I error** (also called *alpha α error*) occurs when the null hypothesis is rejected but it is actually true and should have been accepted.[10] (See Table 18-6 ■.) The probability of a Type I error is the same as the alpha α level. For example, in a study comparing the retention rates of two sealants, a Type I error would be made if the statistical decision indicated that one sealant had a better retention rate than the other when in actuality their retention rates were equivalent. Setting an alpha level at .05 denotes a willingness to take a 5 percent chance of making an alpha error. A large sample size can lead to a Type I error,[6] but a randomly selected representative sample and a good study design help to avoid making it.[14] The researcher can also control a Type I error by setting the alpha level low.

A **Type II error** (also called *beta β error*) occurs when the null hypothesis is accepted, but it is actually

Table 18-6 Type I and Type II Errors Made When Rejecting and Accepting the Null Hypothesis

	Decision About the Null Hypothesis	
	Accepted	*Not Accepted*
True	No error made	Type I error (α)
Not true	Type II error (β)	No error made

false and should have been rejected.[10] (See Table 18-6.) Using the same example of a study to test the retention of sealants, a Type II error would be made if the statistical decision was that the retention rates of the two sealants did not differ when in fact one had better retention than the other. Unlike the probability of a Type I error, the exact probability of computing a Type II error is generally unknown. Using too small a sample, unreliable measuring devices, or imprecise research methods increases the probability of making a Type II error.[9]

The *power* of a test is its ability to reject a false null hypothesis or to detect relationships among variables. By increasing power, we decrease the Type II error rate. A power of .80 is considered reasonable.[6] Power can be improved by increasing the sample size, improving the measuring device, increasing the α level, or choosing a different study design.[9,10] Power is critically important in clinical trials using a positive control because the differences in the groups are likely to be slight.[5] For example, if a test fluoride dentifrice is compared with a positive control of a standard fluoride dentifrice, differences in caries rates between the two groups will likely be small. In this case, group sizes have to be extremely large. A power analysis is a technique used to determine the appropriate sample size considering the statistic being used, the α level, and characteristics of the data.[8]

The probability of Type I and Type II errors is inversely related; that is, the smaller the risk of one, the greater the risk of the other. However, if the sample size is large enough, the researcher has the ability to decrease the risk of making a Type II error at the same time the risk of a Type I error is small.

Committing a Type I error can be more costly than a Type II error.[5] Type I errors lead to unwarranted change while Type II errors maintain status quo. For example, with a Type I error, a patient could receive incorrect treatment but with a Type II error, a patient could not receive treatment that could have been helpful, even life saving. The degree of risk of a Type I or Type II error relates directly to the level of significance. When planning a research project, the Type I and Type II error rates should be considered regarding the particular research problem and which error type is more serious for the situation.[5] Because it is not possible to know whether a Type I or Type II error has occurred, it is important to conduct replication studies to increase the confidence that results are valid.[5] Guidelines for the conduct of oral research should be followed to avoid both Type I and Type II errors.[19,20]

Degrees of freedom (*df*) refers to the number of values or observations that are free to vary when computing a statistic, that is, the number of measurements taken minus 1 for each population parameter estimated.[17] The number is necessary to interpret inferential statistical tests. Degrees of freedom is based on the sample size so the larger the *df*, the easier it is to obtain a statistically significant result.

> ## Did You Know?
>
> Statistics textbooks contain clear rules for calculating and using *df* to interpret a statistic.

INFERENTIAL STATISTICS

The purpose of inferential statistics is to generalize between the sample being studied and the population that it represents.[7] Computing inferential statistics and analyzing the results require a more sophisticated understanding of statistics. Some of these are fairly easy to compute using a computer program. Others are more complex, and the use of computers and consultation with a statistician are advised when these statistics are used.

Confidence Interval

A *confidence interval* is a statistical technique used to infer the true value of an unknown population parameter, for example, the mean from the sample statistic.[7] Typically, 95 percent and 99 percent confidence intervals are used, and the standard error of the mean is used to calculate the intervals. The use of a 95 percent confidence interval is acceptable in oral health research. For example, if the 95 percent confidence interval for the mean Plaque index of 1.16 in a representative sample of school children is 1.08 to 1.24, we can be 95 percent certain that the mean Plaque index of the population is between 1.08 and 1.24.

Parametric Statistics

Inferential statistics used to test a hypothesis are classified as either parametric or nonparametric. **Parametric statistics** are used for hypothesis testing when the data meet certain assumptions.[7] (See Box 18-3 ■.) One of these assumptions is that the data are classified as continuous. This includes ratio and interval data as well as ordinal data that approximate the continuous nature.

BOX 18-3 Assumptions Required for Use of Parametric Statistics

- Data are continuous.
- Adequate sample size is used.
- Population distribution is normal.
- Group variances are equal.

Recall our previous discussion about continuous and discrete data. Discrete variables that have a large number of possible scores can be treated as continuous data, for example, DMF, Plaque index, Gingival index, most other dental indices, and many rating scales. The *t*-test and ANOVA will be discussed here.

Student *t*-test

The *t*-test is used to compare two mean scores to determine whether a statistically significant difference exists.[10] Formally known as the *Student* t-*test,* it is named after its inventor who published under the pseudonym Student. It is used to test a null hypothesis of differences, for example, "the mean sealant retention rates for the two groups do not differ." There are two versions of the *t*-test. First, let's consider the t-*test for independent samples,* also called the *nonpaired* t-*test.* It is selected when the mean scores are from two groups drawn independently from a population, that is, two different and unrelated groups of subjects.[10] For example, a dental hygienist might want to test the effectiveness of a new model of electric toothbrush compared with the existing older model of the same toothbrush. In this case, the dental hygienist would have one group of patients use the new model and the second group use the older model. At the end of the study, the mean improvement of the two groups could be compared using the *t*-test for independent samples. The statistical decision to reject or accept the null hypothesis is based on the resulting *p* value. Today, computers make the task easier for the statistical computation, comparison to the *t* distribution, and determination of the *p* value.

In this same study of a new electric toothbrush model, assume that the dental hygienist wanted to compare the pretest and posttest plaque scores for only the group that used the new model. In this case, the groups of data (pretest and posttest) are not mutually exclusive or independent, thereby violating one of the assumptions described earlier. To accommodate, the dental hygienist would use the t-*test for correlated samples,* also known as the t-*test for paired samples.* This *t*-test is used when the two mean scores are derived from the same group of subjects as described or when the experimental and control groups are matched on the basis of a variable known to be correlated with the independent variable.[10] For example, in fluoride dentifrice studies, the experimental and control groups are frequently matched for baseline DMF, age, and gender because these variables correlate with dental caries. The *t*-test for correlated samples would be used to compare the difference in caries improvement of the two groups. The results of the *t*-test for correlated samples would be interpreted the same way as the *t*-test for independent samples.

Analysis of Variance (ANOVA)

In this same example of the study testing the new model of electric toothbrush, suppose that a third group of patients is using a manual toothbrush for comparison purposes. In this case, three mean improvement scores would be compared. ANOVA is the parametric statistic used to determine whether statistically significant differences occur when comparing more than two mean scores.[10] Sometimes similar studies are reported in journals in which the data are analyzed using the *t*-test to perform multiple comparisons with different combinations of mean scores, two at a time. This is an incorrect application of the *t*-test because the Type I error rate will increase exponentially by the number of combinations of the *t*-test conducted.[4,8] When more than two mean scores are being analyzed, the ANOVA should be used.

Various forms of the ANOVA statistic are used according to the number of independent variables: one-way ANOVA for one independent variable and two-way ANOVA for two independent variables.[8] It can also be used as multivariate analysis of variance (MANOVA) to analyze the effects of the independent variable(s) on two or more dependent variables within the same test to increase power, limit Type I errors, and control for a relationship among the dependent variables. Analysis of covariance (ANCOVA) is another variation that controls for the effect of an extraneous variable that equally affects all groups, called a *covariate.*

ANOVA is used to analyze the differences within each group, the differences between or among groups, and the interactions. The data are presented in a complex table that describes these various comparisons. The result of the ANOVA test is an *F* ratio, which tells us whether a difference exists among the groups. However, it does not tell us which group mean significantly differs from the others.

For example, when comparing the means of three groups, all three means could differ from each other significantly, or two means could be similar while the third mean differs significantly.[13] To determine which mean is significantly different, a post hoc analysis follows the ANOVA analysis by using one of a variety of available tests, including Tukey, Scheffe, Duncan, and Newman-Keuls.[6]

Using the previous example of the study testing the effectiveness of a new electric toothbrush model, the use of the ANOVA allows comparison of the mean improvement of plaque scores from the three groups: new model electric brush, older model electric brush, and manual brush. The F and corresponding p values suggest that the improvement of one group is statistically different from the others, and the post hoc analysis tells us which group has the statistically different improvement. Now assume that some of the patients are regular flossers while others are not, and we want to make sure that this extraneous variable does not affect our results. In this case, we would use ANCOVA. Finally, to measure the effect of the different brushes on plaque and gingivitis (two dependent variables that are correlated), the MANOVA is the test of choice.[10]

Nonparametric Statistics

When variables are discrete, sample size is small, population distributions are not normal, or group variances are not equal, **nonparametric statistics** should be used for hypothesis testing.[10] There is a variety of nonparametric statistics to test a range of null hypotheses from a question about relationships among variables to a question about group differences in outcome measures.

Chi-Square Test

The chi-square test (χ^2), the most commonly used nonparametric statistic,[8] is utilized to determine whether a significant difference exists between frequency counts of nominal (categorical or dichotomous) data by comparing the observed frequencies to expected frequencies.[11] It can be used to compare two or more data sets from different sample groups (χ^2 test of the independence of categorical variables) or to compare the observed frequencies in one group to the expected frequencies (goodness of fit). Use of the chi-square test requires that a group be composed of at least five.

This example illustrates two uses of chi-square for the same study of the new model electric toothbrush. The

researcher crossed over the groups so that by the end of the study, all patients had used each of the toothbrushes. Then each subject was asked which was the preferred brush to use. Thus, the three groups formed one group of 90 who scored their toothbrush preference. According to probability theory, the normal (or expected) preference frequencies would be equal for each toothbrush. With 90 subjects in the study, 30 would be expected to prefer the new electric model, 30 to prefer the old electric model, and 30 to prefer the manual brush. The observed frequencies, which are the patients' reported preferences, are 40 for the new electric model, 30 for the old electric model, and 20 for the manual. The goodness of fit χ^2 test would reveal whether the observed preference for the new model is statistically significant compared with the expected preferences. Another example is to conduct the same study in two offices, one a family practice and the other a periodontal practice. The observed frequencies for the family practice patients are 40, 30, and 20 as in the previous example. The observed frequencies for the periodontal practice patients are 47 for the new electric mode, 38 for the old electric model, and 5 for the manual brush. The χ^2 test of independence reveals whether the different preferences of the patients in the two offices are statistically significant.

Other Nonparametric Tests

Various other tests provide nonparametric equivalents to parametric statistics. The *Fisher test* is used for nominal data in place of the chi-square when group sizes are less than five.[10] The *sign test for paired comparisons* and the *Wilcoxon matched pairs signed-rank test* are used to compare ordinal or higher data from two paired measures and are considered to be nonparametric equivalents of the paired t-test.[7,10,14] The Wilcoxon matched pairs signed-rank test is more powerful than the sign test because it considers the magnitude of the differences between observations as well as the direction of the difference.[14] *McNemars's test* is used for the same purpose for nominal data, that is, to compare distributions of two paired data sets such as from the same sample.[10,14] The *Mann-Whitney rank-sum test* is used to test whether two independent groups have been drawn from the same population and is an alternative to the t-test for independent samples with ordinal variables. The *Kruskal-Wallis* and the *Friedman matched-pairs tests* are nonparametric equivalents of two forms of ANOVA.[8] See Table 18-7 ■ for a summary of nonparametric equivalents to parametric tests.

Table 18-7 Nonparametric Equivalents of Parametric Tests

Nonparametric Test	Type of Data	Application	Equivalent Parametric Statistic
Chi-square	Nominal	Compare observed to expected frequencies of two or more groups of 5 or more	t-test for independent samples
Fisher	Nominal	Compare observed to expected frequencies of two or more groups of less than 5	t-test for independent samples
McNemar	Nominal	Compare frequencies of two or more measures from same group	Paired t-test
Sign	Ordinal	Compare two measures in same group	Paired t-test
Wilcoxon signed-rank	Ordinal	Compare two measures in same group	Paired t-test
Mann-Whitney rank-sum	Ordinal	Compare two measures from different groups	t-test for independent samples
Kruskal-Wallis	Ordinal	Compare three or more measures from different groups	ANOVA
Friedman	Ordinal	Compare three or more measures in same group	ANOVA

INTERPRETATION OF DATA AND RESEARCH RESULTS

When the research project has been concluded, the subjects dismissed, and the statistical analysis completed, the researcher must interpret the results and draw conclusions from the study. This requires the researcher to critically think and rethink about the meaning of the results in an unbiased manner. Interpretation should answer the questions presented in Box 18-4 ■.[2]

Interpretation requires taking a close look at the course and events of the research project that could have impacted the results. Important factors to examine include subjects who dropped out and other unforeseen occurrences such as subject death, subject noncompliance, contaminated samples, and uncontrolled variables. These and other elements of the study must be scrutinized in regard to how they might have affected the study's internal and external **validity**. *External validity* means that the results of the study can be inferred to the

---

BOX 18-4 Questions That Should Be Answered by Interpretation of Data

1. What could these results mean?
2. What factors might be contributing to these results?
3. Were these results expected based on the theoretical framework of the study and what is known in the field?
4. Do these results agree or disagree with other researchers' findings related to the same subject area?
5. Are there any known limitations or threats to internal and external validity that could have contributed to the results?
6. To what conclusions do these results lead?
7. How do the findings relate to, contribute to, advance, or have implications for the current knowledge or practice in the field?
8. In what populations, conditions, or settings would these same results hold true?
9. What additional research questions did these research results identify?
10. What additional research is needed to further answer this research question?

Source: Darby ML, Bowen DM. *Research Methods for Oral Health Professionals: An Introduction.* St. Louis, MO: C. V. Mosby, 1980. Reprint. Pocatello, ID: McCann; 1993.

general population and depends on how well the sample represents the population.[18] On the other hand, *internal validity* means that the study measured what it was supposed to measure. (See Chapter 15.) Use of valid and reliable instruments, control of intra- and interrater reliability, standardization of procedures among groups, use of a control group, and randomization are examples of procedures that affect the study's internal validity.[5] A research study should be reliable and valid. **Reliability** refers to the degree to which the study would yield the same results within the same population every time the study is repeated. Reliability focuses on the consistency of the study.

The researcher should avoid the temptation to make speculative deductions and conclude more than the numerical data indicate. Also, replications and effect size computations are more important than results from a single study that conclude only with a *p* value and a statistical decision about its statistical significance. A single research project rarely answers a question definitively but requires many types of studies with different sample populations over time to do so. These replication studies are necessary to provide results that can be used to make evidence-based practice decisions.[5] Results based on one sample do not provide enough evidence to warrant changes in practice.

Most often research projects reflect the need for continued research and give rise to new questions.[10] Each carefully planned and executed research study is valuable because the additional scientific evidence can provide new insight into the results of previous studies and increase the overall understanding of this study's topic. Results of a study should be discussed in relation to those of previous studies conducted on the same or related topics.[5] In this way, much like a jigsaw puzzle, each bit of research provides a small clue to solving the big picture.

It is possible that results of a study can have statistical significance but not have *clinical* or practical *significance*.[4,5] In other words, research that may or may not be inherent in the statistical results can have practical implications. When study groups are large, even trivial differences in disease increments can be statistically significant,[3] which can be misleading when they have no clinical importance. Also, the actual reductions in disease or health-related conditions should be scrutinized. One example of statistical versus clinical significance is a study comparing the time that it takes two tooth-bleaching products to whiten teeth. The statistical decision may reveal that one product whitens teeth in less time than the other product. However, the actual difference in time could be clinically meaningless or negligible. In this case, although the statistical significance is real, it is not useful in clinical application. Another example is the evaluation of an oral hygiene regime with a group of residents in a state mental health residential facility. If their baseline plaque score was 90 percent and was reduced throughout the program by one-fourth, at the end of the program the residents would still have 67.5 percent plaque. Even if these results were statistically significant, the remaining plaque status would still reflect compromised oral hygiene, which will likely lead to continuing oral disease. Although it may be worthwhile to continue the oral hygiene regimen tested, it would be wise also to seek other measures to further reduce the group's plaque status. Critically interpreting research results before applying them to dental hygiene practice is important for professionals.

One of the responsibilities of the ethical researcher is to disseminate research results to the profession and the appropriate public.[21] Without the distribution of research results, practicing dental hygiene professionals will not be able to fulfill their professional responsibility for continued competence and lifelong learning.[22,23] Incorporating new knowledge and techniques into daily practice can benefit both the public's oral health and dental hygienists' occupational health. Reported research should include not only a description of the project and the results but also a candid discussion of the interpretation of the results including the study's limitations.[5,11,24] This allows the consumer of research to apply the results intelligently to professional practice.

Quality research is disseminated through peer-reviewed formats intended to provide reliable sources of quality research results.[25] The peer review process is designed to protect the consumer of research by controlling the quality of published research results. By depending on peer-reviewed publications and presentations to gain new knowledge, the practitioner can be more confident of the information's validity. Nevertheless, it is important for dental hygienists to be able to recognize, interpret, and apply good quality research to their evidence-based practice.[26] Through this mechanism, laboratory science and epidemiology become the art of oral care.

DENTAL HYGIENIST SPOTLIGHT:
Elmer Gonzalez, RDH

Immediately after graduating as a dental hygienist, Elmer Gonzalez began his dental public health career in a clinic that serves patients with developmental disabilities. He had worked as an aide to individuals with developmental disabilities before becoming a dental hygienist. Now, Mr. Gonzalez is also pursuing his graduate degree in dental hygiene and was recently selected to attend a premier workshop for health providers treating patients with developmental disabilities.

Why did you decide to go into dental hygiene?

I became very interested in dental hygiene when I was working at the group home of a local agency in Albuquerque. I saw many oral health problems in people with disabilities, such as poor oral hygiene, bad breath, and dry mouth. The oral conditions of the people I was working with opened my eyes to a new world. I felt the need to help them; unfortunately, there was not much I could do nothing more than trying to brush their teeth the best I could. I was then an undergraduate at the University of New Mexico pursuing a degree in Spanish and psychology. My cousin was an undergraduate at the same time. She said she was pursuing a degree in dental hygiene. It sounded interesting, and I began to take prerequisites for that program. Dental hygiene is the tool I was looking for to better serve the needs of people with disabilities.

How did you get into dental public health? Did you need additional education?

Following my admission to the University of New Mexico dental hygiene program, I became interested in working as a public health hygienist, particularly somewhere to serve people with developmental disabilities or any other underserved groups. My interests were clearly prominent throughout my dental hygiene training. While in school, I was able to be an intern at Carrie Tingley Hospital Dental Clinic (CTHDC), serving children and adults with disabilities or "special needs." The internship was a wonderful experience, and my desires to work serving a special population increased. After graduation from the dental hygiene program at the University of New Mexico, I was offered the available dental hygiene position at CTHDC.

As a public health hygienist, I felt the need to pursue higher education in order to be able perhaps to make a greater impact and to advocate for people with disabilities or any other underserved population. I was admitted to the master's program in dental hygiene at the University of New Mexico. The program has allowed me to experience new horizons and to expand the body of knowledge I acquired in the undergraduate program. In the master's program, I was able to serve an interdisciplinary training at the New Mexico Leadership Education in Neurodevelopmental Disabilities (LEND) program, which is part of the Center for Development and Disability (CDD) at the UNM School of Medicine, Department of Pediatrics. As part of the requirements of the master's program as well as a personal goal, I received a certificate in developmental disabilities.

What is your current position?

I am the dental hygienist at Carrie Tingley Hospital Dental Clinic, which serves individuals who have developmental disabilities. I teach in the junior clinic and also teach students who rotate through the clinic.

Can you discuss any particularly interesting experiences you have had in your dental public health career?

Working as a public health hygienist at CTHDC is challenging both physically and mentally; however, the rewards I receive after each and every patient goes home in a better oral health condition than when he or she came really makes a difference and gives me strength to keep going.

The best reward and experience I've had at CTHDC has come from those patients who are very challenging to provide care for and struggle in every step of the treatment process: Those who scream obscenities when asked to open their mouth, constantly move their head from side to side so that the instrument doesn't go in their mouth, but yet give me a hug, apologize, and thank me after finishing the treatment.

What type of advice would you give to a practicing hygienist who is thinking of doing something different?

I personally believe that some hygienists are interested only in working in the usual private practice environment; however, I would like to encourage a hygienist who wants to experience something new to face the challenges as they come and to never ever give up their dream to be the hygienist they've always wanted to be.

There is no doubt that knowledge is a powerful tool that helps accomplish a goal. Goals are sometimes remote thoughts, but they're there, and transforming them into reality requires perseverance, dedication, education, and lots of passion and hard work.

Source: Christine Nathe writes the Public Health Column in RDH magazine published by Pennwell Publishing. For more public health spotlights please see RDH magazine online at http://www.rdhmag.com/index.html.

SUMMARY

Volumes have been written on research, biostatistics, and even various types of statistics and specific statistical tests. The information presented in this chapter is intended to serve as a guide for conducting research, assessing communities, evaluating community programs, and understanding the oral health literature. However, planning and interpreting complex research projects requires more information and consultation with a statistician. In this way, solid research results will be disseminated to the professional and the appropriate public for the benefit of both.

SELF-STUDY TEST ITEMS

1. Which variable is made up of distinct and separate units or categories but is counted only in whole numbers?
   a. Quantitative
   b. Qualitative
   c. Continuous
   d. Discrete

2. Which scale of measurement contains all of the characteristics of all scales and has an absolute zero point determined by nature?
   a. Interval
   b. Ordinal
   c. Ratio
   d. Numerical

3. Which type of correlational relationship would the following statement indicate? As the consumption of fluoridated water increases, the caries rate decreases.
   a. Positive
   b. Inverse
   c. Strong
   d. Weak

4. The research hypothesis, also called the *alternative* or *positive hypothesis,* is the logical opposite of the null hypothesis. The research hypothesis can indicate a direction of difference.
   a. The first statement is true; the second statement is false.
   b. The first statement is false; the second statement is true.
   c. Both statements are true.
   d. Both statements are false.

5. The chi-square test (χ^2) is the most commonly used nonparametric statistic. It is used to determine whether a significant difference exists between frequency counts of nominal (categorical or dichotomous) data by comparing the observed frequencies to expected frequencies.
   a. The first statement is true; the second statement is false.
   b. The first statement is false, the second statement is true.
   c. Both statements are true.
   d. Both statements are false.

REFERENCES

1. Darby ML, Walsh MM. *Dental Hygiene Theory and Practice.* 2nd ed. Philadelphia, PA: W. B. Saunders; 2003.
2. Darby ML, Bowen DM. *Research Methods for Oral Health Professionals: An Introduction.* St. Louis, MO: Mosby, 1980. Reprint. Pocatello, ID: McCann; 1993.
3. Wassertheil-Smoller S. *Biostatistics and Epidemiology, A Primer for Health and Biomedical Professionals.* 3rd ed. Bronx, NY: Springer; 2004.
4. Rose L. Overview of biostatistics. In: Gluck GM, Morganstein WM. *Jong's Community Dental Health.* 5th ed. St. Louis, MO: Mosby; 2003.
5. Burt BA, Eklund SA. *Dentistry, Dental Practice, and the Community,* 6th ed. St. Louis, MO: Elsevier Saunders; 2005.
6. Vogt WP. *Dictionary of Statistics & Methodology: A Nontechnical Guide for the Social Sciences.* 3rd ed. Thousand Oaks, CA: Sage Publications; 2005.
7. van Belle G, Fisher LD, Heagerty PJ, Lumley T. *Biostatistics, A Methodology for the Health Sciences.* 2nd ed. Hoboken, NJ: John Wiley; 2004.
8. Munro BH. *Statistical Methods for Health Care Research.* 5th ed. Philadelphia, PA: Lippincott; 2007.
9. Wright DB. *Understanding Statistics: An Introduction for the Social Sciences.* London, UK: Sage Publications; 1996.
10. Glantz SA. *Primer of Biostatistics.* 6th ed. New York, NY: McGraw Hill; 2005.
11. Hebel JR, McCarter RJ. *A Study Guide to Epidemiology and Biostatistics.* 6th ed. Boston, MA: Jones and Bartlett; 2006.
12. Gerstman BB. *Basic Biostatistics: Statistics for Public Health Practice.* Sudbury, MA: Jones & Bartlett; 2008.
13. Plonsky M. *Psychological statistics.* 2006. http://www.uwsp.edu/psych/stat/. Accessed June 26, 2007.
14. Weintraub JA, Douglass CW, Gillings DB. *Biostats: Data Analysis for Dental Health Care Professionals.* Chapel Hill, NC: CAVCO; 1985.
15. Good PI, Hardin JW. *Common Errors in Statistics (And How to Avoid Them).* 2nd ed. Hoboken, NJ: Wiley/Jossey Bass; 2006.
16. Darby ML. Community oral health planning and practice. In: Darby ML. *Mosby's Comprehensive Review of Dental Hygiene.* St. Louis, MO: Mosby; 2006.
17. Jewell NP. *Statistics for Epidemiology.* Boca Raton, FL: Chapman and Hall/CRC; 2004.
18. Friis RH, Sellers TA. *Epidemiology for Public Health Practice.* 3rd ed. Boston, MA: Jones and Bartlett; 2004.
19. Fédération Dentaire Internationale, Commission on Classification and Statistics for Oral Conditions. Principal requirements for controlled clinical trials in periodontal diseases. *Int Dent J.* 1977;27:62–76.
20. Fédération Dentaire Internationale, Commission on Oral Health, Research and Epidemiology. Principal requirements for controlled clinical trials of caries preventive agents and procedures. *Int Dent J.* 1982;32:292–310.
21. Brunson D. Social responsibility. In: Geurink KV. *Community Oral Health Practice for the Dental Hygienist.* 2nd ed. St. Louis, MO: Elsevier Saunders; 2005.
22. Daniel SJ, Harfst SA, Wilder RS. *Mosby Dental Hygiene Concepts, Cases, and Competencies.* 2nd ed. St. Louis, MO: Mosby Elsevier; 2008.
23. Wilkins EM. *Clinical Practice of the Dental Hygienist.* 10th ed. Philadelphia, PA: Lippincott Williams & Wilkins; 2009.
24. Weil SA. Research. In: Geurink KV. *Community Oral Health Practice for the Dental Hygienist.* 2nd ed. St. Louis, MO: Elsevier Saunders; 2005.
25. Wilder R. The importance of peer review. *J Dent Hyg.* 2006;80(3):1–2.
26. Forrest JL, Miller S. A practical guide for incorporating evidence into dental hygiene practice. *Access,* 2007; 21(10):12–18.

Chapter **19**

Evaluation of Scientific Literature and Dental Products

OBJECTIVES

After studying this chapter, the dental hygiene student should be able to:

- Describe how to evaluate dental care products
- Defend the dental hygienists' value in advocating the use of effective dental care products and treatment modalities
- Educate the public in evaluating dental care products
- Effectively critique dental research reported in dental and lay publications

KEY TERMS

Abstract
Peer reviewed
PubMed
Refereed
Regulation
Sample size
Statistical significance

COMPETENCIES

After studying the chapter and participating in accompanying course activities, the dental hygiene student should be competent to do the following:

- Use evidence-based decision making to evaluate and incorporate emerging treatment modalities
- Assume responsibility for dental hygiene actions and care based on accepted scientific theories and research as well as the accepted standard of care

Dental hygienists are recognized as advocates in health care today because of the valuable information they provide patients concerning dental hygiene treatment philosophies, oral health behavioral education, and dental care products.[1] The recent branding campaign conducted for the American Dental Health Association (ADA) indicated that most patients seek advice first and foremost from their dental hygienist regarding dental care products.[2] Dental hygienists working in any aspect of health care are required to understand and effectively critique published research reports.

A few decades ago, supermarkets and drug stores had only a small portion of shelves available for dental care products; now they generally dedicate an entire aisle to oral health. This increased availability underscores the need for professionals who are able to provide consumers with valuable information about these products. For these reasons, the dental hygienist must have a background in research to be able to recognize effective and ineffective dental care products, product ingredients, and treatment modalities.

REGULATION OF DENTAL CARE PRODUCTS

Currently dental products are under the **regulation,** that is, the rule or order, of the Food and Drug Administration (FDA) in the Department of Health and Human Services.[3] See Figure 19-1 ■ for information concerning the regulation of dental care products. The FDA's responsibility is to ensure that food, cosmetics, and radiation-emitting products are safe and that medicines and medical devices are safe and effective. It has the authority to encourage a company that violates its enforceable laws to voluntarily correct the problem or to recall a faulty product from the market. If a company cannot or will not correct a public health problem, the FDA can bring legal sanctions to bear and impose criminal penalties, including imprisonment, if warranted.

Did You Know?

Regulation of dental care products governs the control and guidelines of the products for safety and efficacy.

Periodically, the FDA provides dental professionals information concerning various oral health products through the *FDA Medical Bulletin.* It also publishes

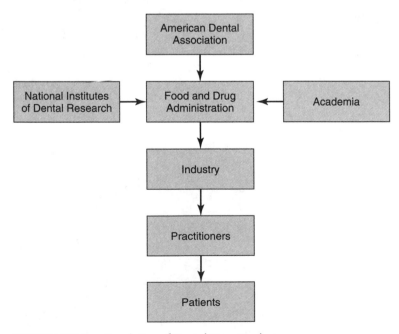

FIGURE 19-1 Regulation of Dental Care Products

monographs concerning therapeutic products. FDA approval of drug products is mandated by law; without FDA approval, a manufacturer may not legally market a product.[4,5]

The ADA offers guidelines for testing and advertising products through its ADA Seal of Acceptance Program.[6] Although the program is strictly voluntary, not government regulated, many companies participate in it. The ADA's Council on Scientific Affairs and staff scientists review oral care products and declare them safe, effective, and worthy of the ADA seal, which is generally awarded for a three-year period. A manufacturer that applies for the seal must meet specific guidelines and, upon its expiration, reapply to continue using it. In some instances, the ADA may conduct or request additional product testing.[6]

The ADA reviews all advertising claims for a product bearing the seal. A product with the ADA Seal featured in an advertisement often promotes dentists as the experts rather than dental hygienists. This omission may be due to the ADA recommendations for the advertisement and promotion of dentists, not dental hygienists, as experts in dental hygiene recommendations.

As a health care professional, the dental hygienist should recommend a product or treatment modality based on documented evidence rather than a product seal, which is not always a reliable gauge of safety or effectiveness. For example, toothbrush manufacturers sued the ADA for failing to adequately warn people about the possible dangers of brushing. Specifically, the lawsuit sought damages on behalf of anyone who suffers from toothbrush abrasion.[7] The ADA is not a government entity but represents the interests of the dental profession. The dental professional consequently must base recommendations on scientific literature and reported product findings. This is a good rule to follow regardless of the organization involved.

Dental hygienists must be able to understand advertisement mechanisms and effectively critique published research so that the public receives accurate information.

— Did You Know? —

The ADA Seal is not mandatory for any dental care product and does not imply the superiority of that product to other products on the market.

RESEARCH SOURCES FOR DENTAL CARE PRODUCTS

Sales representatives are definitely knowledgeable about the products they carry and frequently about competitors' products, but it is important to remember the bias that sales representative may have towards their products. However, this contact can be especially helpful in gathering clinical reports and published articles that are **peer reviewed,** that is, have been reviewed for content and accuracy by other dental health researchers. Companies generally make articles pertinent to their products easily accessible. (See Box 19-1 ■.)

Dental hygienist and dental schools can be great sources of information. Faculty members could be researching certain products or techniques and may have access to scientific information not available to clinical providers. Many faculty members have contacts around the world and can be a great resource.

Another way to gather information is by attending courses or seminars for continuing education, which most states require. Although some courses may not provide the desired information, collegial contacts and distributed resources often be helpful in obtaining it.

The Internet provides a great deal of information regarding dental health care. Most Internet sites are not peer reviewed, however, so information gleaned from them should be used with caution. One reliable source is **PubMed,** http://www.ncbi.nlm.nih.gov/pubmed/, a Web site from the US National Library of Medicine (NLM) that includes more than 17

BOX 19-1 Sources of Information on Dental Care Products

- Colleagues
- Continuing education courses/professional meetings
- Dental hygiene and dental schools
- Lay magazines
- Library
- Internet
- Patients
- Professional magazines, journals, and newsletters
- Sales representatives
- Television

BOX 19-2 Questions to Ask When Assessing Scientific Information Found on the Internet

- Who is(are) the author(s) of the material? What are the author's(s') affiliations, qualifications, and biases?
- Is the source peer reviewed or edited?
- Is the site authored by an organization? What are its affiliations, qualifications, and biases?
- What is the domain name? (ie, .gov, .edu, .org, .net, .com, .mil)
- Does the author list sources or citations?
- Can the information be verified elsewhere?
- Does the site reflect a particular bias or viewpoint?
- Are obvious errors in spelling or grammar present?

- Why and for whom was this Web site created?
- Is there advertising on this Web site?
- When was the site first presented and last updated? Has it been revised?
- When was this Web site reviewed by a professional organization?
- Are the links current, good, and helpful? Are any links dead?
- Is the Web site comprehensive?
- Is the site easy to read?
- Is the color easy on the eyes?
- Are the site and the material well organized?

Source: Beatty CF. Presentation at: 6th Annual Dental Public Health Educator's Workshop. University of New Mexico, Division of Dental Hygiene; October 4, 2007; Albuquerque, NM.

---

million citations from MEDLINE (the National Library's medical literature analysis and retrieval system online) and life science journals for biomedical articles back to the 1950s.[8] Furthermore, PubMed brings together authoritative information from NLM, the National Institutes of Health (NIH), and other government agencies and health-related organizations.

Internet sites are usually reliable if they originate from well-established, reputable professional organizations, government agencies, accredited universities, and community foundations and agencies. Often the information found on sites hosted by companies selling their products is unreliable. A dental hygienist should research Web sites to determine the accuracy of their information. Some simple questions, such as those in Box 19-2 ■, can be asked to help make decisions on information quality.

Did You Know?

It is always important to thoroughly research products. Reading information from the top Googled companies is not enough.

Patients often alert the dental hygienist to products and therapies available, but their information may have been obtained at the local supermarket or from a magazine advertisement. Therefore, it is important for the dental hygienist to keep up-to-date on advertisers' claims and advise patients as to their accuracy.

EVALUATION OF ADVERTISEMENTS

The dental hygienist should be able to effectively critique both published studies and lay magazine advertisements and infomercials in order to be a good consumer advocate. This role is becoming increasingly important with the proliferation of advertising in print, electronic, and nontraditional formats, such as brand placement in movies. The dental hygienist needs to be aware of what advertisements may be implying or promoting to people.

One example of an influential advertisement claim is that a mouthwash is the number one choice of hospitals. This advertisement has been notably effective, yet it says nothing about the product's effectiveness or method of efficacy. What does that claim mean to dental hygienists? They generally recommend a product that meets the needs of individual patients or groups. A patient who has questions about mouthwash selection is not likely to contact a local hospital but would more likely ask the dental hygienist and/or dentist during a dental visit.

In addition, it is important to realize the influence advertisements have on patients. For instance, many patients now think they should buy toothpastes with tartar control. Does an advertised tartar control remove plaque more effectively or prevent the accumulation of

Table 19-1 Toothpaste Constituents

Ingredient	Percentage
Abrasives	20–40%
Water	20–40
Humectants	20–40
Foaming agent (soap or detergent)	1–2
Binding agent	Up to 2
Flavoring agent	Up to 2
Sweetening agent	Up to 2
Therapeutic agent	Up to 5
Coloring or preservative	<1

Source: Zayan M. Dentifrices, Mouthrinses, and Chewing Gums. In: Nathe C, ed. *Primary Preventive Dentistry.* 7th ed. Upper Saddle River, NJ: Prentice Hall; 2008.

calculus? Certainly not, but advertising causes many patients to believe this and other myths.

Making information about dental products available to patients is another way to help them assess the validity of manufacturers' claims. The dental hygienist should be familiar with common ingredients used in dental care products, such as those in Tables 19-1 ■ and 19-2 ■.

EVALUATION OF SCIENTIFIC LITERATURE

Dental hygienists rely on scientific literature such as published research reports, literature reviews, and commentaries to gather information about products and treatment modalities, but for the information to be useful, the hygienists must be able to assess the credibility of such data. In the past decade, many periodicals that include literature reviews have been started; their articles examine pertinent studies conducted on a particular topic and provide current theories and paradigms for dental hygiene practice. The literature review should contain an introduction stating the

Table 19-2 Some Agents Added to Chewing Gums

Agent	Purpose/Claim	US Example(s)
Aspirin	Relieve pain	Aspergum
Caffeine	Increase alertness	Stay Alert
Calcium carbonate	Neutralize stomach acid	Chooz
Casein phosphopeptide–amorphous calcium phosphate	Remineralize and strengthen teeth	Trident Advantage
Chlorhexidine	Prevents plaque, gingivitis	None
Dimenhydrinate	Prevents motion sickness	None
Fluoride	Prevents caries	None
Sodium bicarbonate	Freshens breath	Dental Care
	Whitens teeth	Trident Advantage
	Reduces plaque	
Xylitol	Prevents caries	Trident
		BreathRx
		Theragum

Source: Zayan M. Dentifrices, Mouthrinses, and Chewing Gums. In: Nathe C, ed. *Primary Preventive Dentistry.* 7th ed. Upper Saddle River, NJ: Prentice Hall; 2008.

significance of the topic, a main body describing advantages and disadvantages of the study results, and a summary. These reviews can be valuable in helping the dental hygienist stay current with ever-changing technological advances but normally are merely summaries of the current literature available on a particular topic, are not the report of actual research.[9]

The need for hygienists to be savvy, consumer-oriented professionals has never been greater and underscores the need to critically review scientific literature to be able to assess evidence found in it when making decisions. Evidence-based practice requires being able to critique information appropriately. Specifically, it entails the use of multiple resources. Basing practice on available evidence includes using information derived from a body of knowledge as opposed to a single study. A study's effectiveness also depends on its characteristics, basically a hierarchy of evidence (see Table 19-3 ■) and methods based on causation and control of evidence.

Knowing the components of a well-written study is the first step in assessing a study's quality. See Box 19-3 ■ for the current *Journal of Dental Hygiene* guidelines for reporting original research.

Table 19-3 Levels of Evidence

Level	Evidence
1	Systemic reviews, meta-analysis, and randomized controlled trials
2	Case–control studies
3	Case series
4	Traditional narrative reviews (no critical appraisal)
5	Studies that do not involve human subjects

Source: Beatty CF. Presentation at: 6th Annual Dental Public Health Educator's Workshop. University of New Mexico, Division of Dental Hygiene; October 4, 2007; Albuquerque, NM.

Did You Know?

When "abstracting" the key concepts from a published study, it is necessary to identify its purpose; the problem investigated; the methodology, materials, and equipment used; the results obtained; and the conclusions drawn.

BOX 19-3 *Journal of Dental Hygiene* Guidelines for Original Research Reports

Reports of basic, clinical, and applied studies that provide new information, applications, or theoretical developments typically include an abstract, introduction, review of the literature, methods and materials, results, discussion, and summary or conclusion.

- **Abstract:** Approximately 250 words in length. Use the headings "Purpose" (purpose), "Methods" (design, subjects, procedures, measurements), "Results" (summary of findings), and "Conclusion."
- **Introduction:** Briefly orient the reader to the given subject with an overview of the research problem studied with enough detail to ensure clarity.
- **Review of the Literature:** Cite a variety of relevant, current studies. Compare findings, clearly indicating all sources of concepts and data. When a source is quoted, use quotation marks. Note the current status of the topic, and if further study is needed, provide a sound case for it. Define the variables, the hypotheses or research objectives, and how this study relates to previous research.

- **Methods and Materials:** Describe the research instruments, equipment, procedures, and method of data analysis. Specify the measurements and statistical tests used as well as their significance. Furthermore, assure the reader that all pertinent federal and state regulations concerning the protection of the rights and welfare of all human and animal subjects have been adhered to.
- **Results:** Summarize all relevant data including statistics and data characteristics.
- **Discussion:** Evaluate and interpret the findings. Compare them with those of other related studies. Discuss study limitations and the study's implications to dental hygiene practice, education, and research, and recommendations/plans for further study.
- **Conclusion:** State the conclusions, theories, or implications that may be drawn from the study. Discuss how they relate to the dental hygiene practice, profession, education, and research. Include overall health promotion and disease prevention, clinical and primary care for individuals and groups, and basic and applied science.

BOX 19-4 Questions to Ask When Judging a Research Report

- When was the work published?
- Where was it published?
- Are the authors' qualifications appropriate?
- Is the purpose clearly stated?
- Is the experimental design clearly described?
- Have the possible influences on the findings been identified and controls instituted?
- Has the sample been appropriately selected?
- Has the reliability of the scoring been assessed?

- Is the experimental therapy compared appropriately to the control therapy?
- Is the investigation of sufficient duration?
- Is the statistical analysis appropriate to answer the research questions or hypotheses?
- Have the research questions or hypotheses been answered?
- Do the interpretations and conclusion logically follow the experimental findings?

Source: McCann A, Schneiderman E. Interpreting and evaluating a research report. *Dent Hyg News.* 1997;5:5–10.

Knowing how to assess each part of a study equips the dental hygienist with the tools to evaluate a study's quality. See Box 19-4 ■ for details of specific areas of research reports that the dental hygienist should consider. Some of these aspects are discussed in the following sections.

Abstract

The abstract is a study section that basically outlines its content by concisely stating its purpose, intent (why the study is so significant), previous findings, methodology, results, and suggestions for future studies in no more than 250 words. The abstract gives an overview of the entire project so that readers can decide whether the article is of interest to them.

Introduction

The introduction should provide a clear, concise statement of purpose for the research study. Its importance cannot be stressed enough. To illustrate how it can affect study results and uses, consider the following scenario. Suppose a company is promoting information that its plaque-removing, brushing prerinse product removes excess plaque when compared with brushing without the rinse. The study on which the promotion is based may have clearly delineated that rinsing and brushing together does in fact remove more plaque than just brushing without rinsing. Common sense would lead us to believe in the validity of this statement. To dental hygienists, however, it is evident that this study was designed to promote the product, not necessarily to support its claims with a scientific base.

Literature Review

The literature review should include a brief, detailed outline of previous research, clinical care standards, landmark studies, and commentaries, which address specific issues and controversies that impact the current study. It is important to have current information, although the use of landmark studies or historical benchmarks sometimes is appropriate to help explain phenomena and provide a historical context for current studies results regarding diseases or treatments. The research also should be from a reputable journal; although information in lay or dental hygiene magazines may be appropriate for identifying practice trends or controversies, it generally should not be included in a literature review.

Methodology

This research report section describes the methods and materials used for the study. Many of these are discussed in detail in Chapters 14 and 15 of this text. Important considerations when evaluating the quality of a study's methodology follow:

Sample Selection. Randomization ensures that subjects in the study are selected by chance.

Sample Size. The sample needs to be large enough to be representative of the population.

Ethical Considerations. The study must be free of plagiarism, copyright, or patent infringement; falsifying or fabricating data; misrepresenting data; and conflict of interest. Participation must be voluntary.

Research Design. A double-blind study requires neither the researcher nor the subjects participating in it to know who receives placebos, but this is not always possible.

Product Usage. Uses of the researched product need to be defined, including patient education

DENTAL HYGIENIST SPOTLIGHT:
Michele Hair

A dental hygienist who has a diverse background in public health, Michele Hair was the Golden Scaler award recipient in the Wayne County Community College Dental Hygiene Program in 1988 and went on to receive her bachelor's degree in dental hygiene from the University of Detroit. She is currently working with Head Start and Early Head Start as an oral health coordinator. She finds her career in dental public health to be fulfilling.

Why did you decide to go into dental hygiene?

I always enjoyed going to the dentist as a child; however, I had never "been" to a dental hygienist because my dentist did not have a dental hygienist working at his office. I wanted to become a hygienist because one had come to my elementary school. I loved getting fluoride treatments (which I guess was odd), and I think I knew then that this is what I wanted to do. I did well in science classes in high school, so I wanted to have a career that focused on science.

How did you get into dental public health? Did you need additional education?

I worked in public health during a student rotation at the Detroit Institute for Children, which treated special needs children. In 1993, I applied for a summer job working for the Colorado migrant health program as a dental hygienist providing fluoride treatments, sealants, and education to children attending the migrant school. This was when I realized that I was passionate about this type of dental hygiene.

I went on to work as the supervisor/coordinator of the migrant health program in Denver the following year. In this position, I supervised dental professionals located throughout Colorado. Then I created a full-time dental hygiene position in Colorado Springs at the Community Health Center (now Peak Vista).

What are your current positions?

Currently, I am the oral health program coordinator for Head Start and Early Head Start children enrolled through Community Partnership for Child Development (CPCD) in Colorado Springs. Head Start and Early Head Start are programs of the US Department of Health and Human Services that provide comprehensive education, health, nutrition, and parent involvement services to low-income children aged zero to five and their families. Head Start was created in 1965 and is the longest-running program to address systemic poverty in the United States.

I am responsible for developing and implementing the oral health program serving approximately 1,135 Head Start and Early Head Start children. I provide clinical assessment and preventive therapies to children and give presentations on the oral health issues concerning pregnant women, infants, and young children to the dental and medical community. I also coordinate dental volunteers who provide dental education to parents during parent center meetings.

Can you discuss any particularly interesting experiences you have had in your dental public health positions?

There are so many rewards to working for CPCD. Head Start has clear goals that are set by the federal government but with the opportunity for each program to be creative in meeting those goals. The comprehensive program that CPCD offers to children and families provides a well-rounded approach to success. I also appreciate the fact that CPCD works with the community as a whole, not only the children and families that it serves through its programs.

What advice would you give someone in choosing a career in public health?

If you are interested in public health, my advice would be to pursue opportunities that allow you to work in it. Contacting your local and state health departments may lead you to areas that have public health opportunities. Everyone has gifts and talents, so if you enjoy clinical hygiene work, then work in that area where you make a difference. If you enjoy public health, you might have to do something other than dental public health initially, but it could lead later to a dental public health opportunity. Don't give up! Again, I feel that public health is not more or less valuable than clinical hygiene. What is important is what excites you.

Source: Christine Nathe writes the Public Health Column in RDH magazine published by Pennwell Publishing. For more public health spotlights please see RDH magazine online at http://www.rdhmag.com/index.html.

protocols and the number and specific times the product was used. The study duration should be at least six months. The longer the study period, the more valid are its results.

Quality of Examiners. The examiners should be calibrated and the same one used throughout the study.

Statistical Significance. The result is unlikely to have occurred by chance. In the scientific community, a $p \leq .05$ is considered the cutoff point for **statistical significance,** meaning that an obtained result could happen by chance only five times or less in 100 instances.

Results and Discussion

The results and discussion section discusses the study itself and its findings. In this section, the researcher compares the findings with those of related studies; discusses study limitations, implications for dental hygiene practice, education, and research; and suggests needs for further study.

Results may be published in peer-reviewed **(refereed)** publications. To be accepted for publication, several other researchers review the report and agree with its content. See Box 19-5 ■ for a list of peer-reviewed publications germane to the dental hygiene science. Reviewers at one time were generally not told who conducted the study, so peer review was sometimes referred to as *blind review;* however, this practice is not as common today. Studies that contain valid research results are occasionally published in nonpeer-reviewed publications.

BOX 19-5   Peer-Reviewed Dental Hygiene Periodicals

- *Journal of Dental Hygiene*
- *International Journal of Dental Hygiene*
- *Contemporary Oral Hygiene*
- *Journal of Practical Hygiene*
- *Dimensions in Dental Hygiene*
- *Dental Health*
- *Probe*
- *Compendium of Continuing Education in Dental Hygiene*
- *Dental Hygienist News*

Conclusion and Recommendation

This section states the study's conclusion and addresses its implications. The conclusion discusses theories that relate to dental hygiene practice, the profession, education, and research and suggests recommendations for further studies.

SUMMARY

Dental hygienists should be able to understand and evaluate published research reports and educate consumers regarding dental care products. Clearly understanding the principles of research methods will enhance dental hygienists' decision-making skills when treating patients and recommending dental care products. Practicing professionals must always be consumer advocates and stay current with contemporary products and modalities.

SELF-STUDY TEST ITEMS

1. The ADA Seal of Approval program is regulated by the FDA. It is mandatory for all over-the-counter dental care products.
   a. The first statement is true; the second statement is false.
   b. The first statement is false; the second statement is true.
   c. Both the statements are true.
   d. Both the statements are false.

2. PubMed is a service of the US National Library of Medicine (NLM). It includes more than 17 million citations from MEDLINE and other life science journals for biomedical articles back to the 1950s.
   a. The first statement is true; the second statement is false.
   b. The first statement is false; the second statement is true.
   c. Both the statements are true.
   d. Both the statements are false.

3. Which of the following is/are part of a research report's methods and materials section?
   a. Research design
   b. Ethical considerations
   c. Sample size
   d. All of the above

4. Which of the following terms defines the review of manuscripts by experts for content and accuracy before they can be included in refereed journals?
   a. Critique
   b. Double Blind
   c. Primary evaluation
   d. Peer reviewed

5. *Statistical significance* means that the result was not caused by
   a. Control
   b. Chance
   d. Placebo effect
   a. Sugar pill

REFERENCES

1. *Roles of the Dental Hygienist. Bylaws American Dental Hygienists' Association.* Chicago: American Dental Hygienists' Association; 2007.
2. ADHA Branding Campaign [video]. Presented at: New Mexico Dental Hygienists' Scientific Session; October 15, 2007; Albuquerque, NM.
3. US Department of Health and Human Services: What We Do. http://www.hhs.gov/about/whatwedo.html/. Accessed September 15, 2008.
4. How a drug is approved. US Food and Drug Administration. http://www.fda.gov/cder/info/consumer_approved.htm. Accessed September 15, 2008.
5. Rippere J. FDA regulation of OTC oral health care drug products. *Journal of Public Health Dentistry.* 1992;52: 329–332.
6. Whall C. The how and why of the ADA's evaluation program for dental therapeutic products. *Journal of Public Health Dentistry.* 1992;52:338–342.
7. Toothbrush abrasion spurs suit. *Albuquerque Journal,* 1998.
8. About Medline Plus. http://www.nlm.nih.gov/medlineplus/aboutmedlineplus.html. Accessed September 15, 2008.
9. McCann A, Schneiderman E. Interpreting and evaluating a research report. *Dent Hyg News.* 1997;5–10.

PEARSON
myhealthprofessionskit™

Multimedia Extension Activities

Use this address to access the interactive Companion Website created for this textbook. Simply select "Dental Hygiene" from the choice of disciplines. Find this book and log in using your username and password. To obtain a username and password, please register using the scratch-off access code on the inside front cover of this book.

Unit **IV**

Practical Strategies for Dental Public Health

The dental hygiene profession is responsible for expanding the public's opportunities to receive quality dental hygiene care. This final unit discusses the current careers available in dental public health and explains how a practitioner can work in a governmental position. This unit also presents information on how a dental hygienist could effectively create a dental hygiene position in an organizational setting or a private dental hygiene practice. This entrepreneurial endeavor will undoubtedly increase the underserved populations' access to dental hygiene care.

The final chapter serves as a review of dental public health principles germane to dental hygiene. Test-taking strategies and an overview of the topics and sample test items on National Dental Hygiene Examination Boards are presented to assist students preparing for examinations.

Chapter **20**

Careers in Dental Public Health

OBJECTIVES

After studying this chapter, the dental hygiene student should be able to:

- Describe dental public health careers
- Identify various governmental careers in dental public health
- Define dental hygiene positions in a variety of settings

KEY WORDS

Civil service employment
COSTEP program
Independent contractor
National Health Service Corps
United States Public Health Service
  Commissioned Corps
US Public Health Service (PHS)

COMPETENCY

After studying this chapter and participating in accompanying course activities, the dental hygiene student should be competent to do the following:

- Provide community services in a variety of settings

FEDERAL GOVERNMENT DENTAL PUBLIC HEALTH CAREER OPPORTUNITIES

Dental hygienists are eligible to practice in dental public health with an entry-level associate's degree or certificate, a bachelor's degree, a master's degree, or a doctoral degree. A plethora of positions exists in dental public health from clinical dental hygiene to administrative posts in governmental agencies. Examples of employment for dental hygienists by the federal government follow:

- Contract with Navy to provide clinical and educational services to military personnel in a military dental clinic
- Work with the National Institutes of Dental and Craniofacial Research as a lead researcher in a study on the relationship of periodontal diseases to systemic conditions/diseases
- Hold an administrative position with the Centers for Disease Control and Prevention, overseeing the agency's agenda on water fluoridation.
- Initiate dental hygiene services as an entrepreneur

US Public Health Service

The **US Public Health Service (PHS)** is a part of the US Department of Health and Human Services with eight agencies dedicated to improving and advancing the health of this country's people. It offers career opportunities in dental public health among other areas. As a major division of the Department of Health and Human Services, the PHS encompasses all federal civil service employees including the personnel of the PHS Commissioned Corps. See Box 20-1 ■ for the goals of the PHS.[1] As one of the seven uniformed services in the United States, the **United States Public Health Service Commissioned Corps** provides highly trained and mobile health professionals who conduct programs to promote the health of the nation, understand and prevent disease and injury, ensure safe and effective drugs and medical devices, deliver health services to federal beneficiaries, and provide health expertise in time of war or other national or international emergency. As one of the seven uniformed services of the United States, the PHS Commissioned Corps is a specialized career system designed to attract, develop, and retain health professionals who may be assigned to federal, state, or local agencies or international organizations to accomplish its mission.

The PHS Commissioned Corps with approximately 6000 officers is led by the Surgeon General. See Figure 20-1 ■ for a PHS officer in uniform.

> **Did You Know?**
>
> The first Surgeon General was appointed in 1871 to head the Marine Hospital Service, itself established in 1798 to minister to sick and injured merchant seamen. It was reorganized as the US Public Health Service in 1912.

BOX 20-1   Goals of US Public Health Service Agencies/Programs

To accomplish the mission of the PHS, its agencies/programs are designed to:

- Help provide health care and related services to medically underserved populations: Americans, American Indians, Alaska Natives, and other population groups with special needs
- Prevent and control disease, identify health hazards in the environment and help correct them, and promote healthy lifestyles for the nation's citizens
- Improve the mental health of all populations in the United States
- Ensure that drugs and medical devices are safe and effective, food is safe and wholesome, cosmetics are harmless, and electronic products do not expose users to dangerous amounts of radiation

- Conduct and support biomedical, behavioral, and health services research and communicate research results to health professionals and the public
- Work with other nations and international agencies on global health problems and their solutions

US Public Health Service Health Services Category Coin

Source: www.usphs.gov. Accessed August 18, 2009.

FIGURE 20-1   US PHS Officers in Uniform

Dental hygienists serve as health services officers (HSOs), a category that represents approximately 10 percent of all PHS commissioned officers. The majority of HSOs are assigned to the agencies listed in Box 20-2 ■. Eligiblity requirements for obtaining a commissioned officer position with the PHS include the following:

- Be a US citizen
- Be under forty-four years of age (but may be offset by prior active duty uniformed service time and/or civil service experience in a PHS agency at a PHS site at a level commensurate with the duties of a commissioned officer)
- Have served less than eight years of active duty if a current or previous member of another uniformed service
- Meet medical requirements
- Pass an initial suitability test

In addition, the candidate must have earned a qualifying bachelor's degree from a program accredited at the

---

BOX 20-2   Government Agencies Employing Dental Health Professionals

Department of Health and Human Services
- Indian Health Service
- Centers for Disease Control and Prevention
- Food and Drug Administration
- Health Resources and Services Administration
- National Institutes of Health

Department of Justice
- Bureau of Prisons

Department of Defense
- Military Bases

---

time the degree was conferred by the acceptable accrediting body. A current, unrestricted, and valid dental hygiene license in any of the fifty states, the District of Columbia, the Commonwealth of Puerto Rico, the US Virgin Islands, or Guam may be required. Compensation varies, depending on factors such as grade/rank, years of training and experience (T&E) in the candidate's profession, base pay entry data, specialty pay, geographic location of the duty station, and dependency status. T&E credit is determined by undergraduate education, graduate training, and experience considered to be professionally qualifying for appointment to the particular category. This credit is earned for time spent after receipt of the qualifying degree in degree-related activities. This could be

- Employment in dental hygiene (paid or volunteer)
- Research
- Further training in the field (clinical practice, etc.)
- Teaching at the postsecondary level
- Allied and relevant graduate studies and/or research

Did You Know?

US PHS dental hygienists have career ladder opportunities that often are not available in the private sector.

Civil Service Positions

The US Civil Service includes all appointed positions in the executive, judicial, and legislative branches of the federal government other than military positions. It offers a number of opportunities to dental hygienists in many government agencies and institutions, including federal prisons, Veteran's Affairs (VA) hospitals, and military bases.[2,4] A candidate must apply to a specific vacancy announcement, which may be used to fill a single vacancy or multiple vacancies over a period of time. Vacancies can change every two weeks or so, the candidate should visit the USAJOBS Web site frequently. Vacancy announcements on the Web site provide information on specific duties, qualification requirements, ranking factors, and application forms and procedures. Required application materials and instructions regarding submission of the application vary from announcement to announcement. Dental hygiene positions require copies of transcripts, licenses, and/or certifications. In addition, almost all civil service positions in the US Department of State require at least a secret security clearance. Evaluation procedures vary and are specified in each announcement. In all cases, the evaluation is based on the application material submitted.

National Health Service Corps

The **National Health Service Corps** (NHSC) is a part of the Health Resources and Services Administration (HRSA), a PHS agency. According to its mission statement, the NHSC "is committed to improving the health of the nation's underserved by uniting communities in need with caring health professionals and supporting communities' efforts to build better systems of care"[3] and works closely with state programs for underserved areas. (See Box 20-3 ■.) Working with other HRSAQ bureaus and programs, the NHSC recruits primary care clinicians to provide comprehensive team-based health care that bridges geographic, financial, cultural, and language barriers.

Dental hygienists may work as clinicians with the NHSC, and those with qualifying educational loans may be eligible to compete for repayment of those loans if they choose to serve in a community of greatest need. In addition to loan repayment, these clinicians receive a competitive salary, some tax relief benefits, and a chance to have a significant impact on a community.

Veteran's Administration

The Department of Veteran's Affairs (VA) was created to treat veterans' ongoing disabilities incurred during military service.[4] Comprehensive care is delivered primarily at 172 medical centers and 55 outpatient clinics located nationwide. They offer a full range of primary, acute, chronic, and inpatient and outpatient health care services.

VA dental services are an integral part of this health care system. Dental services are offered in each medical center and in most of the major outpatient clinics. The VA employs dentists, dental hygienists, and dental assistants and other support personnel. Dental hygienists are employed as civil service employees.

Service on Military Bases

Dental hygienists can practice in any military branch dental clinic as a civil service employee, independent contractor, professional dental management company employee, or active duty military personnel. In this setting, the dental hygienist usually works with a variety of

---

BOX 20-3 National Health Service Corps (NHSC) Strategies for Meeting the Mission

- Form partnerships with communities, states, educational institutions, and professional organizations
- Recruit caring, culturally competent clinicians for communities in need
- Provide opportunities and professional experiences to students through Scholarship and Loan Repayment Programs and the SEARCH (Student/Resident Experiences and Rotations in Community Health) program

- Establish systems of care that remain long after an NHSC clinician departs
- Shape the way clinicians practice by building a community of dedicated health professionals who continue to work with the underserved even after their NHSC commitment has been fulfilled

dentists and specialists and frequently works with other health care providers.[5] These opportunities vary from base to base.

Did You Know?

Dental hygienists who work for the federal government often have the opportunity to expand their scope of practice based on the most permissive state's practice act. For example, if a dental hygienist is licensed in a state that does not permit the provision of local anesthesia, that dental hygienist could, after taking a course on local anesthesia, provide local anesthesia in a federal employment setting because other states permit that practice.

Federal Prisons

It is the mission of the US Bureau of Prisons to protect society by confining offenders in the controlled environments of prisons and community-based facilities that are safe, humane, cost efficient, appropriately secure, and to provide work and other self-improvement opportunities to assist offenders in becoming law-abiding citizens.[6] The Health Services Division coordinates the Bureau of Prisons' medical, dental, and mental health services to federal inmates. Dental hygienists provide routine and advanced prophylactic and therapeutic dental care to the inmate population and plan and direct the preventive dental health program. Qualified applicants must be currently licensed to practice as dental hygienists in a state or territory of the United States or the District of Columbia and must possess specialized experience performing oral prophylactic care and provide oral health education services to patients. They must also have experience performing advanced oral prophylactic, therapeutic, and preventive procedures in cases of periodontal diseases or inflammation or on patients with other medical or dental problems; placing temporary fillings; and finishing amalgam restorations. Dental hygienists can be hired as civil service employees, independent contractors, US PHS officers, or employees of a professional dental management firm.

INDEPENDENT CONTRACTORS

Dental hygienists who are **independent contractors,** also known as consultants, freelancers, self-employed, entrepreneurs, and business owners, work for themselves.

They earn their livelihoods from their own independent businesses instead of working for employers. Dental hygienists may provide clinical, consultative, and educational services. Independent contracting dental hygienists usually earn more than those who work for employers but receive no benefits.

There is no single, clear-cut test for classifying workers as employees or independent contractors. Various government agencies use different legal tests for granting independent contractor positions including these:

- Internal Revenue Service
- US Labor Department
- National Labor Relations Board
- State unemployment compensation insurance agencies
- State workers' compensation insurance agencies
- State tax departments

Each of these agencies is involved with worker classification for different reasons, and each has different policies and practices. Each agency normally makes classification decisions independently, which means that one agency might classify a person as an independent contractor but another would not. If opportunities exist, dental hygienists can work as independent contractors for the Bureau of Prisons, the military, and various community dental clinics.

DENTAL STAFFING AGENCY EMPLOYEE

A number of professional management firms act as agencies to find health care personnel for federal dental and medical facilities throughout the United States.[7] These companies hire a dental hygienist as an employee and then place the person in a government dental clinic. Although the dental hygienist works in a government dental clinic, the person is still an employee of the professional management firm. The government agency pays the company a set fee for supplying a dental hygiene employee, and the firm the pays the dental hygienist. These professional firms usually provide a variety of benefits for their dental hygiene employees.

DPS, Inc., is a professional management firm that has administered more than ninety-four health care service contracts with the Air Force, Army, Coast Guard, Navy, and Bureau of Prisons. The firm finds employment for dentists, dental hygienists, dental assistants, and dental lab technicians at federal facilities. DPS recruits

DENTAL HYGIENIST SPOTLIGHT:
Diann Bomkamp, RDH, BSDH

Diann Bomkamp, RDH, BSDH, is president the American Dental Hygienists' Association. She is a wonderful inspiration for dental hygienists working in private practice who really treasure their practices and patients but are interested in promoting oral health in the public health arena. She has been a leader of her local and state associations and has served in multiple roles for the ADHA—the list is truly astounding.

Ms. Bomkamp is a member of Sigma Phi Alpha, the national dental hygiene honor society, and has received numerous awards from her state association and prestigious ADHA awards including the Warner-Lambert Excellence in Dental Hygiene Award, the Alfred C. Fones Award, and the Distinguished Alumni Award. She has a community dental health certificate, which she received from Wisconsin Northeast Technical College.

She answered some questions about her interesting career in dental hygiene.

Why did you decide to go into dental hygiene?

My uncle Jack, a general dentist, asked me to work for him as a dental assistant when I was sixteen years old. I had thought about becoming a nurse, but I loved dentistry right from the beginning. My uncle was a wonderful mentor to me. He would perform procedures and continually explain what he was doing and why. His enthusiasm was contagious. Back then, he also employed one of the few dental hygienists in St. Louis, who also influenced me to go into dental hygiene. When I first graduated with a diploma in dental hygiene from Marquette University, I worked for my uncle and then continued my education by earning a bachelor of science degree in dental hygiene. Even after having practiced as a clinical dental hygienist for thirty-nine years, I still have a passion for dental hygiene.

How did you get into dental public health? Did you need additional education?

I became interested in dental public health through my many activities with ADHA and the Missouri Dental Hygienists' Association. The access to care agenda has been on the radar screen for many years, and I wanted to play a more active role in helping consumers who did not have easy access to oral health care. So, I enhanced some of my public health skills by obtaining a community dental health certificate. Because the Missouri Department of Health and Senior Services (DHSS) Oral Health Program was restructuring to utilize dental hygienists as oral health consultants, I applied for one of the positions and was hired on a part-time basis. Although additional education was not required for my current position, I think it was extremely helpful for me. There is a different mindset in looking at the community as the patient rather than the individual in private practice. I would recommend more public health education for anyone working in a public health venue. I cannot pretend to be an expert in all aspects of public health; this would likely require a Master's in Public Health degree or more. But I can say that I have enjoyed working where dental hygiene began—in the community.

What are your current positions?

I also work as a clinical dental hygienist in a private periodontal office. I had to take a leave of absence from my clinical job and resigned my public health position due to my position as current ADHA president. However, let me explain my public health position. Our Missouri DHSS oral health team consists of five dental hygienists, including a dentist, Dr. Bonnie Branson, who is our oral health project manager. In addition, it has an MPH dentist consultant from University of Missouri–Kansas City

School of Dentistry, wonderful staff support, the Chief of the Office of Primary Care and Rural Health, and a dental advisory board.

As one of five oral health consultants, I mostly work with our DHSS Oral Health Preventive Services Program (PSP). This program is in place to improve the oral health status of Missouri's children. It is our belief that oral health will improve best when the community takes an active role in improving it, so we try to recruit lots of community help. PSP has four parts: surveillance by a licensed dentist or dental hygienist to determine the current oral health status, oral health education, prevention and intervention utilizing two fluoride varnish applications per year for any child in Missouri, and referral to a dentist. Go to www.mohealthysmiles.com and see our Web site. The consultants have also worked hard to develop a K–12 oral health educational curriculum. You can see it at http://www.dhss.mo.gov/oralhealth/OralHealthEducation.html.

Can you discuss any particularly interesting experiences you have had in your dental public health positions?

I have enjoyed working with the school nurses tremendously. They are the ones who see the effects of poor oral health every day. I love helping them see that we can turn some of this dental disease around with better prevention and routine care. I try to refer them to cost-effective sources of care, and when we find it, I believe that I have made a difference, even if it is in a small way. I feel good by educating them about oral health and enhancing their roles in improving total health. I think they are learning more about dental hygienists and the contributions we make.

Another highlight involved working at a recent workshop with Dr. Francisco Ramos-Gomez, who presented information on infant oral health to dental professionals and Head Start staff. We were able to visit a Head Start center and apply what he taught us by assessing caries risks and setting practical goals for parents at the center. Stressing the value of early oral health prevention with the community was invaluable.

What type of advice would you give to a practicing hygienist who is thinking of doing something different?

See what is available in the public health arena in your state or community. Call your state or local dental health program and find whether there are opportunities in public health. In addition, check out the public health section of the ADHA's Web site (http://www.adha.org/publichealth/index.html) to learn about continuing education options and its CareerCenter (http://careers.adha.org) to see whether it lists any public health positions.

Source: Christine Nathe writes the Public Health Column in RDH magazine published by Pennwell Publishing. For more public health spotlights please see RDH magazine online at http://www.rdhmag.com/index.html.

highly competent, qualified individuals who will be assets to a professional health care team. Its minimally requires employees to

- Hold an unrestricted license to practice in any one of the fifty states, the District of Columbia, the Commonwealth of Puerto Rico, Guam or the Virgin Islands
- Have experience in their field in a clinical setting for at least twelve months within the preceding twenty-four months or be a recent graduate of an accredited program within the past twelve months
- Have a current CPR certification

STUDENT DENTAL PUBLIC HEALTH OPPORTUNITIES

In 1948, the PHS established a summer employment program for medical students and in 1955 added other health disciplines to the program.[1] Finally, in 1956 the Commissioned Officer Student Training and Extern Program (COSTEP) was formally established. **COSTEP** enables students to enhance their educational background and provides hands-on experience to those with a commitment to future employment. It also introduces them to health disciplines for potential PHS careers. Students assigned to the Federal Bureau of Prisons receive hands-on training in correctional medicine, policies, and procedures.

The Senior COSTEP program was established to attract qualified students in accredited health care programs into the Commissioned Corps and service in the PHS. Effective the first day of formal studies for the last academic year, selected students are called to "active duty for training." They will be paid the salary of an ensign for that year.

To be eligible for appointment to the Senior COSTEP program, an interested student must

- Be a citizen of the United States under age 44
- Meet the medical fitness standards prescribed for appointment and active duty as a career officer
- Be enrolled in good standing in an accredited school of medicine, osteopathy, nursing, physician assistant training, medical records administration, pharmacy, sanitary science, computer science, dietetics, occupational therapy, physical therapy, dentistry, dental hygiene, or engineering
- Be eligible to enroll in the senior or final year of that school and begin formal studies required as part of the curriculum for the senior or final year on the date of entry on active duty
- Agree in writing to serve on active duty as a commissioned officer with PHS for twice the period of training sponsored by PHS as stated in Section F of the Commissioned Corps Personnel Manual
- Be free of any obligation or commitment that would conflict with extended active duty as a commissioned officer in PHS (eg, not be a member of a reserve or active duty component of any other uniformed service)
- Agree to waive any entitlement they may have to financial assistance (stipend or scholarship) in their final year of study other than assistance from the Senior COSTEP

The Senior COSTEP participant incurs a two-for-one commitment. For every month that the selecting agency funds the student during the final year of study, that person commits to a two-month obligation for service in that agency.

Did You Know?

The Junior COSTEP provides students an opportunity to become acquainted with the organization and mission of the PHS and with health-related career opportunities in various participating agencies, the Senior COSTEP then prepares the students to become US PHS Commissioned Officers.

Junior COSTEP participants are commissioned as ensigns in the PHS Commissioned Corps. Assignments may range from 31 to 120 days throughout the year and are scheduled to be convenient with college enrollment. To be eligible for appointment to the Junior COSTEP program, an interested student must

- Have completed at least one year of study in medical, dental, or veterinary school or at least two years of study in a professionally accredited baccalaureate program in dietetics, engineering, medical record administration, physician assistant training, nursing, pharmacy, sanitary science, computer science, occupational therapy, or physical therapy or be enrolled in a master's or doctoral program in a health-related field
- Expect to return to college or to a postgraduate program in a commissionable profession immediately following participation in COSTEP
- Be in a program of study accredited by an appropriate body
- Be free of any obligation or responsibility that would conflict with extended active duty as a commissioned officer in the PHS (eg, not be a member of a reserve or active duty component of any other uniformed service)
- Qualify for appointment in the PHS (be a US citizen, under 44 years of age, and able to meet the Corps' physical standards)

Participants in the Junior COSTEP program incur no obligation for future service with the PHS or the selecting agency.

STATE OPPORTUNITIES

Many state health departments employ dental hygienists to work as clinicians, educators, administrators, or researchers. Additionally, some states contract with private companies and/or independent dental hygiene contractors to provide clinical care and consulting. In many states, a dental hygienist with additional education and experience can be employed as the state dental director.

INTERNATIONAL OPPORTUNITIES

Dental hygienists have the opportunity to work in many different countries. In fact, only twenty-five countries educate dental hygienists, so opportunities for dental hygienists to initiate dental public health programs and dental hygiene educational programs in most of the world are available. The companion Web site for this book lists many opportunities for the dental hygienist overseas, including opportunities with the US Peace Corps.

SUMMARY

Dental hygienists have opportunities to work in various government positions in the United States. Various employment situations are available in these positions as a member of the US Public Health Service Commissioned Officer Corps, a civil servant, an independent contractor, and an employee of a professional dental management firm. Opportunities for student employment in the dental hygiene field exist with the US Public Health Service. For more information on these areas, please see the Website.

SELF-STUDY TEST ITEMS

1. Dental hygienists initially are eligible to be a US PHS Commissioned Office with which of the following credentials?
   a. Certificate in dental hygiene
   b. Associate's degree in dental hygiene
   c. Bachelor's degree in dental hygiene
   d. Master's degree in dental hygiene

2. Civil service agencies fall under the State Department. Many times hygienists are employed at VA hospitals as a civil service employee.
   a. The first statement is true; the second statement is false.
   b. The first statement is false; the second statement is true.
   c. Both statements are true.
   d. Both statements are false.

3. Students are eligible for the COSTEP program during their dental hygiene education. The COSTEP program is part of the US Department of Defense health care system.
   a. The first statement is true; the second statement is false.
   b. The first statement is false; the second statement is true.
   c. Both statements are true.
   d. Both statements are false.

4. Dental hygienists can work on military bases in the United States as
   a. Military officers
   b. PHS Officers
   c. Contract employees
   d. None of the above

5. Which of the following is a goal of the US Public Health Services?
   a. Prevent and control disease
   b. Identify health hazards in the environment
   c. Help provide health care to Native Americans
   d. All of the above

REFERENCES

1. www.usphs.gov
2. www.state.gov
3. http://nhsc.bhpr.hrsa.gov
4. www.va.gov
5. www.defenselink.gov
6. www.bop.gov
7. www.dpsjobs.com

PEARSON
myhealthprofessionskit™

Multimedia Extension Activities

Use this address to access the interactive Companion Website created for this textbook. Simply select "Dental Hygiene" from the choice of disciplines. Find this book and log in using your username and password. To obtain a username and password, please register using the scratch-off access code on the inside front cover of this book.

Chapter 21

Strategies for Creating Dental Hygiene Positions in Dental Public Health Settings

OBJECTIVES

After studying this chapter, the dental hygiene student should be able to:

- List the populations most in need of dental hygiene care.
- Describe the paradigm for creating a dental hygiene position.
- Develop protocol for a newly developed dental hygiene position.

KEY TERMS

Blueprint
Legislative initiatives
Marketing
Practice management
Proposal
Public relations

COMPETENCIES

After studying the chapter and participating in accompanying course activities, the dental hygiene student will be competent to do the following:

- Promote the values of oral and general health and wellness to the public and organizations within and outside the profession
- Assess the oral health needs of the community and the quality and availability of resources and services
- Provide screening, referral, and education to bring consumers into the health care delivery system
- Provide community oral health services in a variety of settings
- Facilitate client access to oral health services by influencing individuals and/or organizations regarding the provision of oral health care
- Evaluate reimbursement mechanisms and their impact on a patient's access to oral health care
- Evaluate the outcomes of community-based programs and plan for future activities

Although dental hygiene initially began as a profession focused on public health initiatives, the professional has long been positioned primarily in the private dental office. In this setting, dental hygienists frequently have little control over the delivery of dental hygiene care, but this is changing because society is demanding a more appropriate delivery system for dental hygiene services.[1]

Not all individuals in our society are able to visit a dentist's office for a variety of reasons such as a disability, chronic illness, lack of funds, or rural location. Refer to Box 21-1 ■ for a list of populations who frequently need dental hygiene services. For these populations, access to dental hygiene services has been virtually unattainable. This situation is especially significant because those who have the least access to dental hygiene services are the ones who would likely benefit most from care that emphasizes prevention.[2]

Members of the public, government agencies, and other health care professionals as well as the dental hygiene profession itself have shown significant interest in establishing dental hygiene programs in settings other than private dental offices. In some of these offices, the dental hygienist may be required to establish a distinct dental hygiene business.

Although most states have a difficult time containing health care costs while delivering quality care to all members of the population, access to preventive health care should undoubtedly improve overall costs while increasing autonomy for the dental hygiene practitioner. Moreover, having educated dental hygiene professionals should improve the quality and accountability of care. Few would argue that the practitioner specifically educated in dental hygiene sciences best provides the optimum level of dental hygiene care.[3] This chapter focuses on the strategies for implementing dental hygiene positions within the health care delivery systems.

LEGISLATIVE PERSPECTIVE

Some states do not allow the public the opportunity to subscribe to dental hygiene services in any way other than from a private dental practice. In fact, a few states require that dental hygienists work only in a private dental setting and be directly supervised by a dentist. Proposals to change or enact laws called **legislative initiatives** may be necessary to increase the accessibility of dental hygienists to the entire population.

Did You Know?

Legislative initiatives are what led to so many states permitting dental hygienists to practice outside of a private dental practice.

Forty-five states allow the dental hygienist to work in a variety of settings without a dentist present. By providing dental hygiene care in alternative settings, dental hygienists are able to interact with those population segments currently underserved.

PROPOSED PLAN FOR ACTION

The process for establishing a dental hygiene position should follow the dental public health program planning paradigm discussed in Chapter 12. It is important to identify the various aspects that an alternative delivery of dental hygiene care would entail and to establish the parameters for setting up a dental hygiene position.

Assessment

During the assessment phase, the dental hygienist proposing the new position should conduct a needs assessment of the population at hand, facilities, and funding. Information to be obtained may include the number, ages, and medical needs of individuals within the population; specific dental needs of the population; administrative support and values of dental hygiene care; and facility space, staff support, and reimbursement mechanisms. Involving entities within the organization can help identify current unmet dental needs and demands.

BOX 21-1 Populations Needing Dental Hygiene Care

- People who are homebound
- People who live in institutions
- Populations with disabilities
- Residents of rural areas
- Population with dental phobia
- Populations who have language or cultural barriers
- Prison inmates
- Patients without financing

The assessment should identify whether dental hygienists in the specific state can be reimbursed directly by Medicaid, CHIPS, and/or dental insurance companies. If not, ask the following questions to determine how this avenue of reimbursement can be achieved: Does it require legislation or a rule change? Is the organization amenable to hiring a dental hygienist as an employee and completing all collection services?

As a dental hygienist, never underestimate the importance of understanding which organizations will value dental hygiene services. Many individuals still do not know what a dental hygienist is, and many do not value preventive dental care. For these reasons, the dental hygienist must be clear in defining what services will be "sold."

Dental Hygiene Diagnosis

At this stage, the dental hygienist should develop a comprehensive dental hygiene diagnosis for the target population. For example, consider a dental hygiene diagnosis directed at a population employed by a major company (4000 employees). The company survey revealed that only 25 percent of the employees were currently seeking dental treatment (dental demand), either preventive or restorative, and that more than 500 days were lost to sick days due to toothaches (dental need). In addition, the company's on-site registered nurse calculated that 25 percent of visits made to her were for dental problems (dental need). A diagnosis of the population would therefore state that the population has tremendous dental needs (toothaches) but has a low dental demand because 75 percent were not seeking dental care.

Planning

The planning stage requires the prioritization of goals and objectives and the development of strategies and a program blueprint. This stage would address issues such as support of staff, space availability, reimbursement mechanisms, patient management systems, and dental health promotional activities. During the planning stage, **public relations,** the practice of managing the dispersion of information between an organization and its public, should also be made. Evaluation mechanisms such as the use of dental indexes, dental records, surveys, and interviews, should be developed. Meeting with administrators and/or other interested parties contributes to effective and efficient planning. See Table 21-1 ■ for a detailed business plan of action for dental hygienists starting their own business.

Did You Know?

Public relations is the process of strengthening ties with the population by promoting the value of a program through education.

Table 21-1 American Dental Hygienists' Association's Business Plan

Business Plan	What It Really Means
Service development	Continually refining what you are providing/selling to meet the changing needs of your potential clients
Marketing	Continually taking action to become more aware of your clients' needs and informing your potential clients why to use your service
Sales	Talking face-to-face with your potential clients and getting them to retain your services
Operations	Doing the work of the business, everything from answering the telephone to working directly with patients
Personnel	Managing the people who work with you
Finance	Measuring the financial results of your business, comparing them with your desired results, and using this comparison to identify critical business issues
Management	Making sure the preceding six areas are working in concert to meet your goals for the business

Source: http://members.adha.org/script/content/fetch.cfm?file=ADHA_marketing_workbook.pdf. Accessed July 2, 2009.

Table 21-2   The Four Ps of Marketing Adapted to a Dental Hygiene Practice

Product/Service	*Price*
• Quality dental hygiene services • Decrease in patients' plaque, acute pain, and dental diseases • Increase the value of dental health • Obtain positive feedback from patients and institution	• Assist in reimbursement mechanisms • Compete with local private dental practices • Have policies and procedures describing all types of reimbursement mechanisms
Distribution Plan	*Promotion*
• Specify practice location and hours • Schedule appointments • Identify labor force • Establish flexible conditions within an institution	• Describe quality image of program • Use creative and legal advertising techniques • Engage in publicity • Promote dental health education and strategies

Source: Kotler P. *Marketing for Nonprofit Organizations.* Upper Saddle River, NJ: Prentice Hall; 1982.

Practice promotion occurs when the practice effectively markets its service. **Marketing** is an organized approach to selecting and servicing markets and informing the public of a service as distinct from an impromptu approach to selling a service. The purpose of marketing a dental hygiene practice is to have patients select it for their care and then to service them. The four Ps of marketing include products/service, price, plan for distribution, and promotion. See Table 21-2 ■ for more information on marketing strategies for a dental hygiene practice.[4]

Implementation

Implementation refers to carrying out a plan. It involves the actual program operation and generally includes constant revisions. During implementation, the dental hygienist should manage the program, which can entail collaborating and sometimes supervising people. See Box 21-2 ■ for specific management skills needed. Evaluation during this process helps focus on the plan.

Evaluation

During evaluation, which should be continuous, the program's intended outcomes are measured and possibly revised. Measurement is performed by using dental indexes, records, and surveys. Moreover, other entities within the organization can be helpful at providing information concerning continuing unmet needs.

Providing administrators with documented written and oral reports concerning the measurement of the program's outcomes and revisions is vital. These reports emphasize the importance of the dental hygiene program and maintain its visibility and testify to its value. Ongoing communication and reporting to patients and

---

BOX 21-2 Skills Involved in Managing Programs

- Leadership
  - Coordinating effective change
  - Motivating personnel
  - Making logical, effective decisions
- Management
  - Coordinating all operations
  - Providing comprehensive resource management
  - Implementing personnel evaluation and supervision
  - Using effective problem solving
  - Using effective conflict resolution
- Planning
  - Performing long-term strategic planning
  - Performing short-term strategic planning
  - Formulating policies and procedures
  - Determining evaluation measurements
  - Planning for effective and logical decision-making practices by all

DENTAL HYGIENIST SPOTLIGHT:
C. Austin Risbeck, RDH

C. Austin Risbeck, RDH, is experiencing a fulfilling career that combines private practice and public health opportunities. Although he works in a progressive private practice, he has formed his own company to promote public health and has won several awards related to it. He has spoken throughout the country and published numerous articles in various dental hygiene periodicals. Mr. Risbeck has decided to respond to a number of challenges in dental hygiene, and the public is certainly benefiting.

Why did you decide to go into dental hygiene?

At the age of nineteen, I joined the Army to become a dental assistant. After a few years as a dental assistant, my next step up the military career ladder was dental hygiene school. At the time, I thought it was a way to get promoted. I had no idea what my future as a dental hygienist would entail.

How did you get into dental public health? Did you need additional education?

During National Dental Hygiene Month in 2000, the ADHA theme was "Want Some Life-Saving Advice? Ask Your Dental Hygienist," stressing the importance of oral health to total health. I was not prepared to educate my patients about the oral–systemic connection, so I ordered a copy of *Oral Health in America: A Report of the Surgeon General.* This publication opened my eyes to the ongoing research regarding the connection between chronic oral infections and other health problems including heart disease, diabetes, and adverse pregnancy outcomes. One major theme in this publication is "Lifestyle behaviors that affect general health such as tobacco use, excessive alcohol use, and poor dietary choices affect oral and craniofacial health as well." As a health care provider, I assumed the responsibility of promoting healthy lifestyles by incorporating tobacco cessation and nutritional counseling into my clinical practice. I want my patients to benefit from the research regarding the connection between periodontal disease and systemic conditions. I emphasize the importance of maintaining periodontal health.

We don't need additional education to improve and promote oral health. We need to work together with other health care providers to broaden the public's understanding of the importance of oral health and its relevance to systemic health. However, I am planning to pursue a master's degree in public health soon.

What are your current positions?

I serve as a member of the ADHA Council on Public Health, ADHA Tobacco Cessation Task Force, and California Dental Hygienists' Association (CDHA) Public Health Council, as a California Tobacco Cessation liaison, and I am a consultant to the Smoking Cessation Leadership Center and a continuing education provider. I am owner of a consulting firm that provides tobacco cessation, nutrition resources, and other educational information to local, state, and national organizations. I currently work at The Center for Aesthetic Dentistry in San Francisco as a clinical dental hygienist three days a week and as a consultant from home the rest of the week. This includes weekend work sometimes, but it's worth it! My firm provided the resources and helped with the design of the ADHA's "Ask. Advise. Refer." Web site. In 2004 and 2005, I designed several Web pages as part of CDHA's public health Web site to provide dental hygienists the resources to help their patients quit using tobacco, eat better, and manage their diabetes and to help hygienists include oral cancer, diet, and blood pressure screening as part of their dental hygiene appointments.

Can you discuss any particularly interesting experiences you've had in your dental public health positions?

In April 2004, I attended and provided a poster for the second national Steps to a HealthierUS Prevention Summit in Baltimore, Maryland. This national summit created by former Secretary of the Department of Health and Human Services Tommy Thompson focused on chronic disease prevention and health promotion. It featured presentations on obesity, diabetes, heart disease, stroke, and cancer as well as lifestyle choices including tobacco use, nutrition, and physical activity. The Steps to a HealthierUS program aims to help Americans live longer and healthier lives by reducing the burdens of diabetes, overweight, and obesity and through tobacco cessation, healthy eating, and physical activity.

As the only dental hygienist at this national summit with more than 1,400 participants, I was asked by two participants, "What is a dental hygienist doing at a prevention summit?" and "Why does a dental hygienist need to know about nutrition?" I loved these questions. I answered that dental hygienists are now involved in treating tobacco use and dependence and have long been involved in nutritional counseling and blood pressure screening. By providing these services and obtaining a comprehensive health history, dental hygienists can establish the presence or risk of chronic disease and refer those who are at risk to an appropriate medical provider.

I gathered my information from many sources that suggest:

- "Dental hygienists have more interaction time with their patients than other health-care providers, and their patients visit them two to four times per year as they perceive themselves as healthy."
- "Dental hygienists can expand their role to help other health professionals with the responsibility of achieving and maintaining the total health of the public."
- "Dental hygienists can expand health promotion and chronic disease prevention efforts by incorporating tobacco cessation, nutritional counseling, and blood pressure screening into their practices."
- "Many diabetics, or those at risk for diabetes, do not regularly visit a primary care provider but may seek the services of a dental hygienist."

- "Dental hygienists are well positioned to deliver prevention messages, communicate the need for metabolic control, and facilitate multidisciplinary diabetes care."
- "By all of us working together and sharing our expertise and experiences, we can all improve quality of life and reduce the burden of chronic diseases in America."

These two participants replied that they had no idea.

At the Steps to a HealthierUS Summit, Secretary Thompson released Prevention: A Blueprint for Action. This US Department of Health and Human Services' Steps to a HealthierUS Initiative outlines simple steps that people can take to promote healthy lifestyles. I brought this blueprint to the CDHA leadership, who implemented an effective weight-reducing initiative and continued to promote a smoking cessation initiative called The New California Gold Rush. CDHA is committed to informing and educating individuals about the importance of healthy eating, regular physical activity, disease screening, and avoiding risky behaviors such as tobacco use to promote health and prevent chronic disease.

What advice would you give a practicing hygienist who is thinking of doing something different?

Dental hygienists are teachers and educators. An exciting way to teach colleagues and the public is by publishing articles in scientific and peer-reviewed journals and taking continuing education courses.

Source: Christine Nathe writes the Public Health Column in RDH magazine published by Pennwell Publishing. For more public health spotlights please see RDH magazine online at http://www.rdhmag.com/index.html.

---

other health care providers is equally necessary so that needed revisions can be made.

PRACTICE MANAGEMENT

During the planning stage, issues involving the effective ongoing operation of a dental hygiene practice—known as **practice management,** which is the process of planning, organizing, and managing resources to bring about the successful completion of specific project goals and objectives—should be defined and then further refined during the implementation and evaluation stages. These issues can include tracking patients, scheduling appointments, promoting practice, and collecting fees. Written patient records are

extremely important in dental hygiene treatment. Information in these records should be comprehensive and include patient contact information (address, phone numbers, and other pertinent information); health history; dental hygiene assessments, diagnoses, planning, implementation, and evaluative documentation; and financial records. Maintaining accurate records enhances the operation.

Did You Know?

Practice management deals with issues involving a program's effective ongoing operation.

Effective appointment scheduling improves practice operations by decreasing patients' wait time and increasing productivity. Appointment scheduling could become more complicated in health care settings if patients have made arrangements for health care treatment a number of times during the day. Therefore, it could be beneficial to integrate appointment scheduling procedures within the institution.

PROPOSAL DEVELOPMENT AND PRESENTATION

Refer to Box 21-3 ■ for an example of a **proposal**—a written description of a planned program or project—for example, a dental hygiene position in a nursing facility—intended to motivate an entity such as the administrators or other decision makers to adopt a program or project,

---

BOX 21-3   Proposal to Fones Nursing Facility for the Establishment of a Dental Hygiene Program

Introduction

This proposal addresses the recognition of the oral health care needs of elderly people, the institution of a preventive dental program, and the addition of a contract dental hygienist. Dental hygienists have the scientific background and clinical skills to initiate dental programs in long-term care facilities; therefore, it is the intention of this proposal to clarify the procedures necessary to establish a dental hygiene position.

Significance

Certain physiological changes occur in the oral cavities of elderly people, including loss of teeth, recession of gums, and teeth that are becoming brittle and more prone to chipping and cracking. Due to the loss of muscle tone about the face and mouth, other conditions such as cheilosis (cracking in the corners of the mouth), flacid tongue, and epulis fissuratum (growths due to ill-fitting dentures) occur. As a result of aging or certain medication, xerostomia, or drying of the oral tissues, also can exist, causing discomfort, difficulty in speaking, loss of taste sensations, high incidence of gum-line cavities, and discomfort in denture wearers, to mention only a few problems.

In addition, dentures may cause serious conditions if they do not fit properly and can be a factor in oral cancer, which comes from the continual irritation of the soft tissue. The importance of examining the soft tissues of the face, neck, lips, and the structures inside the mouth cannot be adequately stressed. The incidence of oral cancer among elderly people is alarming. Early detection and prompt treatment make a significant difference in the prognosis of this disease.

Dental Hygiene Program

As a member of the health team and in collaboration with the dentist, the dental hygienist performs necessary procedures for total patient care. These services include counseling and instructing patients, conducting regularly scheduled in-service programs for the nursing staff, and providing preventive clinical services such as intra- and extraoral examinations, scaling (teeth cleaning), nonsurgical periodontal therapy, radiographs, fluoride treatments to desensitize exposed roots, denture care, denture labeling, and referral either to the patients' private dentist or to the facility's dental consultant. Moreover, the dental hygienist formulates a recall system by which annual and admission exams are regularly performed to meet federal and state health requirements.

A dental hygienist registered in New Mexico may be licensed to work in collaboration with a dentist. Therefore, employing a dental hygienist in a nursing home is legally permissible in New Mexico and ethical. Many dental hygienists are employed in nursing homes in different states. A contract dental hygienist may be reimbursed through Medicaid or fees charged directly to the patient for services provided, thus decreasing cost to the nursing home.

Conclusion

The quality of care provided to the residents of an institution is a priority of both the administration and staff. However, dental care often is not a priority and sometimes neglected. The dental hygienist contracted to work would improve and expand the quality of care, which would be beneficial to the staff, administration, and, most importantly, the residents of a nursing facility. This contract position, which provides necessary preventive dental care, can become an integral part of existing interdisciplinary comprehensive services.

such as to open a dental hygiene position. The proposal should always include an introduction stating the dental hygiene program's purpose and a statement of the significance of the suggested dental hygiene position.

A program's **blueprint**—a skeletal framework developed before implementing a program—should include a detailed budget and financing section. Specific teaching strategies will help the dental hygienist effectively present the proposal. The reader should be able to read a paragraph or two and understand the program's basic premise. The conclusion should summarize the important points and "sell" the reader on the need for this specific program.

Generally, ten to fifteen minutes are allowed for this presentation. Using a proposal handout and slides or transparencies can greatly enhance the attractiveness of the position. To sell the service, dental hygienists must be prepared and organized in addition to using effective and appropriate media. See Chapter 7 for more tips on effective presentation strategies.

DENTAL HYGIENE CONSULTATION AND POLICIES

See Box 21-4 ■ for a sample agreement or contract between a dental hygienist and nursing facility for the dental hygienist's services at a fixed price. This example should be helpful when developing a contract. Box 21-5 ■ is a sample policy statement for providing dental hygiene

---

BOX 21-4   Employment Agreement—Dental Hygienist

This agreement entered into on this _____ day of _____, _____, between _____, registered under the dental laws of this state, hereinafter referred to as the Registered Dental Hygienist (RDH), and the Fones Long-Term Care Facility, hereinafter referred to as Facility.

Whereas Facility desires to employ the services of RDH and whereas RDH is desirous of offering certain services, it is therefore mutually agreed that Facility does employ and RDH agrees to offer services on the following mutual terms and conditions:

A. Facility assumes the professional responsibility and administrative responsibility for services rendered.

B. RDH will perform services within the realm of the dental hygiene profession for Facility.

C. Insurance (individual terms to be determined).

D. As compensation, therefore, Facility agrees to pay RDH a salary of _____.

E. Irene Newman, RDH, is the licensed dental hygienist for Fones Long-Term Care Facility.

F. The RDH in conjunction and cooperation with the dental consultant is responsible for:

1. Formulating, establishing, and continually revising the policies for dental services in her role as a member of the Dental Advisory Board.

2. Coordinating and implementing in-service programs designed for the staff, which will include daily oral hygiene care for the residents, discussion of nutritional requirements related to dental health, and identification of pathology relevant to geriatric patients.

3. Recording and/or updating residents' dental history, maintaining one copy in the dental facility and placing one copy in the resident's medical file.

4. Evaluating the residents' oral health status by completing intra- and extraoral examinations.

5. Providing written quarterly reports and recommendations and plans for the implementation of those recommendations to the administration.

6. Assisting the nursing staff in carrying out the dental consultants' and RDH's recommendations.

7. Retaining on a continuing basis proper membership credentials in the American Dental Hygienists' Association and other affiliated associations. She is required to maintain the highest level of affiliation for the profession, including periodic participation in special workshops and continuing education, particularly those related to the dental care of geriatric patients.

G. Nursing personnel are responsible for notifying dentist/dental hygienist of any resident with a dental problem. A request for their services is left in the Nursing Office.

H. In cooperation with the Facility, the RDH, when necessary, will arrange for residents to be brought to the dental facility.

Source: Modified from Employment Agreement, Suzann C. Chenery, RDH, BS, Ashlar of Newtown, CT; 1990.

BOX 21-5 Policy for Dental Hygiene Services

Fones Long-Term Care Facility has arrangements to assist residents in obtaining emergency and routine dental care.

The dental hygienist will hold office hours on a designated day each week or more often if necessary.

Services provided by the dental hygienist are:

A. Obtain medical clearance from resident's physician prior to treatment.
B. Relieve pain in emergencies and/or to: examine the resident clinically and/or radiographically in the absence of the dental consultant, and refer the resident for immediate treatment to private dentist, dental consultant, or physician.
C. Perform periodic oral cancer screenings on all residents.
D. Compile dental indexes for all residents and submit results to the administration in report form with the quarterly report.

E. Document all examinations and treatment rendered.
F. Maintain communications between the nursing staff (especially the nurse's assistants), the dental consultant, and herself.
G. Initiate and reevaluate the dental recall system.
H. Render appropriate preventive clinical services, i.e.:

1. Obtain medical clearance and review medical history.
2. Record dental history.
3. Perform intra- and extraoral exam.
4. Design a treatment plan.
5. Take radiographs if necessary.
6. Perform oral prophylaxis: removal of calculus (tartar), dental plaque, and stains from natural teeth and/or artificial teeth by scaling and polishing.

Source: Modified from Dental Hygiene Services, Suzann C. Chenery, RDH, BS, Ashlar of Newtown, CT; 1990.

---

services. It can serve as an example for the dental hygienist in developing specific institutional policy. Refer to Box 21-6 ■ for the definition of an advisory role for a dental hygienist to an institution. Finally, a beneficial addition to the dental hygiene program is the use of dental hygiene students, which can bring motivation and a learning initiative to the program. See Box 21-7 ■ for a sample affiliation agreement.

BOX 21-6 Dental Advisory Role to Fones Long-Term Care Facility

A. The RDH serves on the facility's Dental Advisory Board with the Facility's Administrator, Dentist or Dental Consultant, Patient Care Coordinator, and one faculty member of UNM Division of Dental Hygiene.
B. The RDH serves as an in-house dental adviser to the staff and is responsible for guidance and instruction in the care of residents' individual oral health.

Source: Modified from Dental Advisory Role, Suzann C. Chenery, RDH, BS, Ashlar of Newtown, CT; 1990.

BOX 21-7 Coordination of Affiliation with University of New Mexico (UNM) Division of Dental Hygiene

A. The RDH in cooperation with the supervising faculty of UNM Division of Dental Hygiene plans and implements a minimum of two annual visitations of the dental hygiene students, which include

1. Orientation.
2. Tour of facility.
3. Individualized screening and counseling sessions.
4. Submission of problem-oriented data on each resident screened by the RDH.
5. In-service programs to the nursing staff concerning oral health and the dental hygiene program to be implemented.

Source: Modified from Affiliation Agreement, Suzann C. Chenery, RDH, BS, Ashlar of Newtown, CT; 1990.

SUMMARY

When deciding whether to start a dental hygiene practice in a public health setting, dental hygienists should consider their clinical skills as well as communication skills, motivation skills, knowledge of health and wellness, assessment and treatment-planning skills, and an interdisciplinary team approach to providing care. Dental hygienists can adapt these skills to working with the public in a wide variety of settings.

Author's Note

For dental hygienists interested in creating their own position, the American Dental Hygienists' Association (ADHA) document entitled *Marketing Dental Hygiene Services in Alternative Practice settings: Starting and Growing Your Own Dental Hygiene Business* can be downloaded from http://www.adha.org.

SELF-STUDY TEST ITEMS

1. Members of the public, government agencies, and other health care professionals, as well as the dental hygiene profession itself, are showing significant interest in establishing dental hygiene programs in settings other than private dental offices. Many states have expanded the dental hygienists' scope of practice.
   a. The first statement is true; the second statement is false.
   b. The first statement is false; the second statement is true.
   c. Both statements are true.
   d. Both statements are false.

2. What may be necessary to increase dental hygienists' accessibility to the underserved public?
   a. Marketing promotion
   b. Blueprint development
   c. Legislative Initiatives
   d. None of the above

3. During which phase should a target population's needs be determined?
   a. Assessment
   b. Dental hygiene diagnosis
   c. Planning
   d. Implementation

4. Continually refining the product is which part of the business plan?
   a. Service development
   b. Marketing
   c. Sales
   d. Operations

5. Which phase involves prioritizing goals and objectives?
   a. Assessment
   b. Dental hygiene diagnosis
   c. Planning
   d. Implementation

REFERENCES

1. Nathe C. *Dental Hygiene: A Career for the Future Manual.* Albuquerque: University of New Mexico; 1999.
2. *A Resource Guide for Dental Hygienists in Non-traditional Settings.* Nepean, Canada: Ontario Dental Hygienists' Association; 1998.
3. Nathe C. Dental hygienists: A needed reality [editorial]. *Contact International.* 1998;12:3.
4. Kotler P. *Marketing for Nonprofit Organizations.* Upper Saddle River, NJ: Prentice Hall; 1982.

PEARSON
myhealthprofessionskit

Multimedia Extension Activities

Use this address to access the interactive Companion Website created for this textbook. Simply select "Dental Hygiene" from the choice of disciplines. Find this book and log in using your username and password. To obtain a username and password, please register using the scratch-off access code on the inside front cover of this book.

Chapter 22

Dental Public Health Review

Meg Zayan, RDH, MPH, EdD

OBJECTIVES

After studying the chapter, the dental hygiene student should be able to:

- Describe the National Board Dental Hygiene Examination dental public health format
- Identify topics that may appear on this examination
- Identify strategies for studying for the dental public health section of boards
- Review sample test items

KEY TERMS

Joint Commission on National Dental Examinations
Licensure Requirements
   Clinical examination requirement
   Educational requirement
   Jurisprudence requirements
   Written examination requirement
National Board Dental Hygiene Examination
Testlet

COMPETENCIES

After studying the chapter and participating in accompanying course activities, the dental hygiene student should be competent to do the following:

- Adhere to state and federal laws, recommendations, and regulations in providing dental hygiene care
- Provide dental hygiene care to promote patient health and wellness using critical thinking and problem solving in an evidence-based practice
- Use evidence-based decision making to evaluate and incorporate emerging treatment modalities
- Assume responsibility for dental hygiene actions and care based on accepted scientific theories and research as well as the accepted standard of care
- Continuously perform self-assessment for lifelong learning and professional growth
- Promote the profession by engaging in service activities and having affiliations with professional organizations
- Communicate effectively both verbally and in writing with individuals and groups from diverse populations
- Provide accurate, consistent, and complete documentation for assessing, diagnosing, planning, implementing, and evaluating dental hygiene services
- Provide care to all clients using an individualized approach that is humane, empathetic, and caring
- Promote the values of oral and general health and wellness to the public and organizations in and outside the profession
- Respect the patient's goals, values, beliefs, and preferences while promoting optimal oral and general health

COMPETENCIES (continued)

- Refer patients who may have a physiologic, psychological, and/or social problem for comprehensive patient evaluation
- Identify individual and population risk factors, and develop strategies that promote health-related quality of life
- Evaluate factors that can be used to promote patient adherence to disease prevention and/or health maintenance strategies
- Evaluate and utilize methods to ensure the health and safety of patient, and the provider in delivering dental hygiene
- Identify career options in health care, industry, education, and research, and evaluate the feasibility of pursuing dental hygiene opportunities
- Develop practice management and marketing strategies to be used in delivering oral health care
- Access professional and social networks to pursue professional goals
- Assess a community's oral health needs and quality and availability of resources and services
- Provide screening, referral, and education to bring consumers into the health care delivery system
- Provide community oral health services in a variety of settings
- Facilitate client access to oral health services by influencing individuals and/or organizations to assist in providing oral health care
- Evaluate reimbursement mechanisms and their impact on a patient's access to oral health care
- Evaluate the outcomes of community-based programs and plans for future activities

Specific dental hygiene **licensure requirements,** which are the requirements dental hygienists must meet to obtain a dental hygiene license to practice in each state, vary among states, but all states have four types: (1) an **educational requirement,** which is the requirement of how much instruction and what type of degree a dental hygienist must receive, (2) a **written examination requirement,** which is the written examination a dental hygienist must pass before becoming eligible for a dental hygiene license, (3) **jurisprudence requirement,** which is the required reading and possible examination of state laws governing dental hygiene practice, and (4) a **clinical examination requirement,** which is the clinical board requirement, which is mandatory in all states. The **National Board Dental Hygiene Examination,** which is the examination given by the American Dental Association to fulfill the written examination requirement, is intended to fulfill or partially fulfill the written examination requirements, but acceptance of a national board score is completely at the discretion of the states. Alabama is the only state that does not require a dental hygiene candidate to pass the National Board Dental Hygiene Examination.

This chapter reviews the community health/ research principles section of the National Dental Hygiene Board Examination given by the American Dental Association's **Joint Commission on National**

Dental Examinations, the agency responsible for the development and administration of the National Board Dental Examinations.[1] The commission includes representatives of dental and dental hygiene schools, dental and dental hygiene practice, state dental examining boards, and the public. After completing this course and during the crucial period of studying for board, students can use this chapter as a study guide.

Did You Know?

Students can get up-to-date information regarding the content and format of the national examination for dental hygienists by contacting the American Dental Association at (312) 440-2678 or www.ada.org.

STUDY GUIDE

The board exam is comprehensive and consists of approximately 350 multiple-choice test items. It has two components. The discipline-based component includes 200 items addressing the scientific basis for dental hygiene practice (anatomic sciences, physiology, biochemistry, nutrition, microbiology, immunology, pathology, and pharmacology); provision of clinical dental hygiene clinical services (patient assessments, radiology, dental

---

BOX 22-1 Compilation of Examination Specifics

Community Health Research Principles (24)

a. Promoting Health and Preventing Disease Within Groups (5)
b. Participating in Community Programs (11)
   1) Assessing populations and defining objectives (5)
   2) Designing, implementing, and evaluating programs (6)
c. Analyzing Scientific Information, Understanding Statistical Concepts, and Applying Research Results (8)

---

hygiene care, periodontology, dental biomaterials, and professional responsibility); and community health/research principles (dental public health science).

The second component includes 150 case-based items that refer to patient cases. See Box 22-1 ■ for the composition of items in the community dental health/research principles category for the exam. This section of the exam is written using a **testlet** format that introduces a case study involving an issue pertinent to dental public health. The testlets are written in paragraph form followed by a series of multiple-choice questions. (See Table 22-1 ■.) The target populations often mentioned in these testlets may involve persons in programs such as

Head Start; preschool/elementary/middle/high school; substance abuse; geriatric (nursing homes, senior day cares, senior centers); people who are physically or mentally challenged; teen pregnancy; veterans; immigrants; ethnic groups; prisoners; migrant farmers; sport teams; caregivers; forensic; and special needs. The best preparation methods include the suggestions in Box 22-2 ■.

Test-Taking Strategies

First and foremost when taking an exam, prepare in advance and use your time wisely. Attempt to answer all questions even if you hope to go back to a question later. Look for logical clues and a word or concept repeated in both the question and the answer. Also look at the length

---

BOX 22-2 Suggestions for Exam Preparation

- Be prepared! This will undoubtedly increase your confidence!
- Organize your notes from dental hygiene school and prerequisite classes.
- Outline notes in a manner that works well for you.
- When reviewing old notes, look up in textbooks any information that is still unclear.
- Review key concepts from professors.
- Review previous board examinations.
- Study with groups and by yourself.

Table 22-1 Sample Item Format

For national board use, a multiple-choice item must have at least three and not more than five possible answers. Only one of the possible answers listed is correct.

Format	Definition
Completion	Requires correctly finishing a statement regarding a concept or idea
Question	Communicates a problem or set of circumstances
Negative	Includes a word such as *except* or *not* in capital letters and/or italics in the stem
Paired true-false	Varies only in the stem, which consists of two sentences on the same topic
Cause-and-effect	Varies only in the stem, which consists of a statement and reason written as a single sentence and connected by *because*
Testlet	Begins with one or two paragraphs that describe a case study or problem providing at least five examination items; used exclusively for the Community Health/Research Principles section

Source: American Dental Association. *National Board Dental Hygiene Examination. 2009 Candidate Guide.* Chicago, IL: American Dental Association; 2008.

of the responses; often the correct response is the longest. Eliminate potential answers involving contradictory answers.

Did You Know?

As in all areas of dental hygiene, the most important factor in taking the exam is being prepared.

Specific types of test items can be answered more effectively when you understand the test item model. Multiple-choice test items evaluate knowledge and understanding of specific concepts. These items are composed of a stem, which poses a problem and a list of possible answers to that problem. The stem may be a question, a statement, or an incomplete sentence. Only one of the possible answers is correct; the other answers are called *distractors*.

Key Concepts

The community dental activities section on the exam generally covers key concepts such as the following.

Promoting Health and Preventing Disease Within Groups

- The overall goal of dental public health programs is to reduce oral disease.
- The major aspect of dental public health programs is promotion and prevention. These are accomplished through activities to enhance positive behavior, education, and clinical services.
- *Dental health education* is defined as the teaching of oral health behaviors whereas *dental health promotion* is defined as informing and motivating individuals to adopt healthy behaviors.
- In areas where dental public health programs are indicated, the demand for dental care is low but the need is high. It is the intent of public health programs to achieve a higher demand for dental care and to decrease the need.
- Dental public health dental hygienists should concentrate on teaching those individuals who work closely with the target population including teachers, caregivers, nurse's aides, and so on.
- State dental health departments' primary purpose is to serve as a consultant regarding state dental issues for public and private health care.

- When teaching a population to adopt positive dental health behaviors, the values they may hold concerning oral health need to be changed.
- Behavior change will not be attained until value adoption is complete; providing dental health education to a population does not ensure behavior change.
- When distributing educational materials, be careful to critique them beforehand to make sure they are not blatantly promoting a dental care product, and, most importantly, that they have factual information that is not misleading.
- Water fluoridation has proven to be cost effective although opponents claim that fluoridation itself violates their human rights.
- Advocates of water fluoridation may find developing long-term strategies for adoption to be beneficial.

Participating in Community Programs

- Assessment of populations and defining objectives are important factors in such programs.
- Establishing community programs involves designing, implementing, and evaluating programs.
- Planning consists of determining consumer needs, which a dental professional can diagnose as compared with consumer demands, which can be defined as the frequency of dental visits or attempted dental visits.
- Program planning should include the dental hygiene process of care including assessment, dental hygiene diagnosis, planning, implementation, and evaluation. Many public health paradigms place the diagnosis stage in the planning stage.
- Prioritizing is a necessary component during the dental hygiene diagnosis and planning stages of program development.
- Program planning should include developing measurable objectives so that the program can be effectively evaluated and measured.
- To increase participation in a program, having personal contact with the target population is beneficial.
- Dental hygienists should include the target population or its representatives when planning a dental public health program.
- Dental hygienists working with programs that target minorities should include minority leaders during planning to obtain their support.
- When initiating a dental public health program, dental hygienists should contact the head administrator for approval and support.

- A dental sealant program should be planned to target children in the second through sixth grades to ensure they have fully erupted molars for placement of the sealants.
- Always have support from the target group. If a program involves parents, their support is crucial.

Analyzing Scientific Information, Understanding Statistical Concepts, and Applying Research Results

- *Prevalence* is the number of existing cases of a specific disease or condition in a population at a specific point in time.
- *Incidence* is the expression of the new number of cases of a disease or condition in a population at a specific point in time.
- *Mortality* is the ratio of the number of deaths from a specific disease to the total number of cases of that disease.
- *Morbidity* is the ratio of sick to well persons in a population.
- *Reliability* is the consistency or degree to which an instrument will produce the same results in the same population every time the characteristic is measured.
- *Validity* is the degree to which an instrument measures the variable that it is designed to measure.
- A *pilot study* is a trial of a research study so its variables can best be controlled during the long-term study.
- The *dependent variable* is the measure as a result of the manipulation of the independent variable.
- *Independent variable* is the manipulated measure expected to be changed under the investigator's control.
- *Measures of central tendency,* including the mean, median, and mode, measure what is typical in the sample group.
- *Measures of dispersion,* including range, variance, and standard deviation, are used to describe the variability of scores in a distribution. If a relation has a normal distribution, it is a *normal bell curve.* If a relationship has a few extreme scores, it is *skewed.*
- *Correlation* is the determination of the strength of the linear relationship between two variables. The closer the number is to 1, the stronger is the relationship.
- Research studies utilize different approaches to sample the population.

SAMPLE QUESTIONS

This section provides sample testlet questions that may be asked on the national examination. It is intended to familiarize you with necessary information about these items. Answers to the questions appear upside down at the bottom of each page.

TESTLET 1 (QUESTIONS 1–5)

The Indian Health Service approached a state department of dental public health about establishing a caries prevention program in a Native American elementary school. The school consists of grades 1–6 with twenty-five to thirty students per grade. The community is not fluoridated, and local dentists are concerned about the high incidence of dental caries recognized during the past six years. The elementary school receives state and federal funding for health care services including nursing, dental, and nutritional care. Of these children, 30 percent receive Medicaid funding to help meet medical and dental care costs. The school employs a nurse full-time as well as a dental hygienist and nutritionist two days per week A dentist volunteers his time one day per week. The Indian Health Service is asking for assistance in determining the needs of the school children and supporting the implementation of a program to reduce dental caries. It is asking for the program to include educational, therapeutic, and referral services.

1. What is the first step in developing a dental health prevention program for this school?
   a. Contacting the state's department of public health
   b. Identifying the students who will participate in the pilot study
   c. Meeting with the parents to identify the students' oral hygiene habits
   d. Developing a data collection instrument to determine caries rate
   e. Obtaining informed consent from the parents of the students

2. Possible negative reactions and conflict could be avoided by obtaining which of the following:
   a. Permission from the board of dentistry
   b. Permission from the state department of education
   c. Support of the school nurse and teachers
   d. Support from the local dental hygiene association
   e. Permission from the governor

3. If it is determined that the school vending machines contain highly sugared snacks and the removal of these machines is approved, which of the following does this action exemplify?
   a. Health prevention
   b. Disease progression
   c. Health promotion
   d. Health services

4. In this nonfluoridated community, which of the following preventive dental health programs would have the maximum cost benefit for controlling caries in these elementary school children?
   a. Pit and fissure sealant program
   b. Fluoride mouth rinse program
   c. Restorative care program
   d. Parent-teacher education program

5. The primary purpose of referring indicated children to a dentist for treatment is to
   a. Provide a follow-up activity to the program
   b. Ensure that parents are aware of their children's dental needs
   c. Increase the probability that dental disease will be reduced
   d. Create an environment in which dentists are treating more patients

TESTLET 2 (QUESTIONS 6–10)

The board of education approached a public health dental hygienist about establishing a dental health education curriculum for the students enrolled in a public school system. The board was concerned that the only dental health education students received was during Children's Dental Health Month when volunteer dental hygienists provided education to grades K, 3, 7 and 12. The classroom teachers were interested in implementing dental health education in the student's health classes but were looking for guidance with lesson plan content and activities. The school system consists of 3,500 students, grades K–12. Health care facilities, including a nurse who is available twice a week, are available at each school.

6. The primary purpose of the public health dental hygienist is to
   a. Provide dental hygiene services to the public school students
   b. Provide age-appropriate dental health knowledge and preventive techniques to improve oral health
   c. Encourage more volunteer dental hygienists to visit all classes during Children's Dental Health Month
   d. Lobby the board of education to hire a dental hygienist to work on days when the nurse is not present at the public school

7. To fully understand the oral hygiene knowledge of the public school students, the dental hygienist should
   a. Perform DMFS on all students
   b. Conduct a caries-activity test
   c. Perform clinical examinations and radiographs
   d. Conduct a discussion group with all teachers
   e. Conduct an oral hygiene questionnaire for all students and teachers

8. When the classroom teachers discuss the importance of good oral hygiene habits and the prevention of dental disease during their health classes, which of the following is(are) the *best* technique(s) for teaching this material?
   a. Lecture and question–answer session
   b. Distribution of brochures and class activities
   c. Lecture only
   d. Lecture with slides and posters
   e. Lecture with slides, posters, and class activities

9. If more funding than currently allocated is needed, which of the following strategies is the most effective in obtaining additional financial support?
   a. Partnering with other community agencies to develop a collaborative request to local foundations
   b. Approaching local businesses and industries requesting program funds
   c. Engaging community churches to conduct fund-raising efforts
   d. Sending high school students door-to-door in the affluent parts of the community to solicit funds

Answers: 2. (c) 3. (c) 4. (b) 5. (c) 6. (b) 7. (e) 8. (e) 9. (a)

10. After the program has been developed, the *most* effective role for the public health dental hygienist would be as a(an)
    a. Major provider for classroom instruction
    b. Consultant for the parents
    c. Clinical chair-side instructor
    d. Evaluator of the program's success

TESTLET 3 (QUESTIONS 11–15)

A dental hygienist employed by a dental clinic in a federal correctional institution is planning to implement a plaque control program for female prisoners. She has worked at the prison for three years and has noticed a high prevalence of gingival and periodontal disease. The prison warden has given her permission to develop a pilot program with funding for additional supplies and increased working hours. One of the first steps the dental hygienist performed was to distribute a survey to the seventy-five female prisoners involved in the pilot program. The questionnaire data indicated that 65 percent brush daily, 10 percent floss on a regular basis, and 80 percent of emergency dental cases are due to toothaches.

11. The primary purpose of implementing a pilot program is to
    a. Solicit more funding to implement the full program
    b. Encourage other federal prisons to implement similar programs into their dental clinics
    c. Perform the planned program on a small population to ascertain its success before performing it on a larger population
    d. Develop measurable objectives so that the program can be effectively evaluated

12. To further ascertain the dental needs of the prisoners, which of the following should be utilized?
    a. Preindex scores for plaque and gingival and periodontal conditions
    b. A survey regarding prisoners' dental knowledge, values, and attitudes
    c. The level of prisoners' demand for dental care
    d. Financial resources in planning treatment for the dental clinic
    e. Access to care regarding clinic hours, payment, and prisoner schedules

13. The overall goal of this plaque control program is to
    a. Reduce the amount of gingival and periodontal diseases
    b. Increase the number of prisoners seeking dental treatment
    c. Increase the amount of practicing dentists in the clinic
    d. Decrease overall expenses of dental care in the clinic

14. The statistics regarding brushing, flossing, and emergency dental care visits imply that
    a. The need for dental care is lower than the demand for dental care
    b. The need for dental care is higher than the demand for dental care
    c. The need and the demand for dental care are equal

15. If additional funding is needed, which of the following governments should be helpful?
    a. Federal government
    b. State government
    c. Local government
    d. A partnership between state and local governments

TESTLET 4 (QUESTIONS 16–20)

Several community dental hygienists conducted a five-year study on dental caries incidence rates in permanent teeth of school age children. The study compared incidence rates of dental caries in students who received sealants and routine professional fluoride treatments to those for students who received professional fluoride treatments only. The study was conducted at a public school district whose population was 5000 students in grades K–12. At the beginning of the study, no schools in the district had fluoridated water, and fewer than 20 percent of the children attending these public schools had sealants.

To decrease the number of subjects involved in the study, a sample was taken from the 5000 students; however, students who did not have their permanent first molars could not participate. When those students without permanent first molars were eliminated, the remaining students were randomly selected from each grade level and classroom. The sample size then consisted of 2000 students K–12. The sample was then further divided into two groups: Group 1 received sealants

Answers: 10. (d) 11. (c) 12. (a) 13. (a) 14. (b) 15. (a)

at the start of the study and fluoride treatments every six months for five years. Group 2 received only fluoride treatments every six months for five years.

In addition, dental caries and plaque accumulation indexes were performed on both groups. A mean plaque index score of 2.6 (based on a 3.0 scale) was recorded for both Group 1 and Group 2, and at the end of the five years, the plaque index for Group 1 was 2.0 and for Group 2 was 2.3. There was high interrater reliability among the community dental hygienists.

16. What type of research study did the dental hygienists conduct?
    a. Historical
    b. Experimental
    c. Cross-sectional
    d. Descriptive

17. The mean plaque index score for both groups at the beginning of the study revealed that the students had
    a. No plaque
    b. Slight plaque
    c. Moderate plaque
    d. Severe plaque
    e. Cannot be determined

18. The type of sampling performed for this study suggests
    a. Simple random
    b. Systematic
    c. Stratified
    d. Convenience

19. The dependent variable that is investigated in this study is
    a. Dental caries
    b. Fluoride treatments
    c. Occlusal sealants
    d. Dental plaque

20. The best way to gather information about the students' knowledge of dental health care is by
    a. Interviewing each student regarding oral hygiene habits
    b. Utilizing a plaque and calculus index
    c. Performing a DMFT survey
    d. Conducting a questionnaire

TESTLET 5 (QUESTIONS 21–25)

Three state public health dental hygienists are identifying oral health needs of persons residing in state-subsidized drug and alcohol rehabilitation centers. One study compared oral lesions in persons who smoke cigarettes to those who do not smoke. This study was performed in three state rehabilitation centers, and patient selection was done in alphabetical order by choosing every third individual from the patient list. The two dental hygienists who worked jointly for one day at each of the three sites calibrated the index.

21. The type of research utilized in this study is
    a. Historical
    b. Descriptive
    c. Experimental
    d. Ex post facto

22. The research design is an example of what type of epidemiological study?
    a. Cross-sectional
    b. Prospective cohort
    c. Case–control
    d. Longitudinal

23. Which of the following is characteristic of the type of sampling used in these data?
    a. Stratified
    b. Simple random
    c. Convenience
    d. Systematic

24. The dental hygienists established the research hypothesis as "there is no significant correlation between cigarette smoking and oral lesions." This is an example of what type of hypothesis?
    a. Positive
    b. Correlational
    c. Null

25. When the dental hygienists select the most effective index to measure oral lesions, which of the following is a necessary criterion?
    a. Predictability of outcome
    b. Ease in calibration
    c. Flexibility in measurement

TESTLET 6 (QUESTIONS 26–30)

A dental hygienist was asked to plan an in-service program to present to a group of nursing assistants in a 200-bed nursing home. Its overall purpose was to improve the residents' oral hygiene status by teaching proper toothbrushing. Using a written questionnaire, the dental hygienist first surveyed the nursing assistants concerning their understanding of dental health concepts. Following compilation and evaluation of the answers, the dental hygienist planned the program including writing goals and objectives to be met during it.

26. Which of the following private practice activities do these activities parallel?
    a. History taking and diagnosis
    b. Diagnosis and treatment planning
    c. History taking, diagnosis, and treatment planning
    d. History taking, diagnosis, and evaluation
    e. History taking, treatment planning, implementation, and evaluation

27. Before initiating the in-service training program, the dental hygienist should confer with whom?
    a. Nursing home residents
    b. Residents' family members
    c. Nursing home administrator and consulting dentist
    d. Local dental hygienist association board members

28. Utilizing the cognitive learning model, the intended outcome for this program is:
    a. Knowledge
    b. Behavioral change
    c. Attitude

29. In writing a behavioral objective, the verb should indicate what the learner is expected to do. Which of the following is the best learner performance verb?
    a. To believe
    b. To know
    c. To demonstrate
    d. To understand
    e. To feel

30. The more specific are the objectives, the more effective the intent will be communicated to the nursing assistants. In-service evaluation is more effective without objectives.
    a. The first statement is true; the second statement is false.
    b. The first statement is false; the second statement is true.

c. Both statements are true.
d. Both statements are false.

TESTLET 7 (QUESTIONS 31–35)

A high school class of twelve physically challenged students, fourteen to nineteen years of age, shows a need for improved oral hygiene. The high school nurse has asked the district dental hygienist to assess their needs and to work with the nurse to implement a dental public health program for these students. The dental hygienist plans to set up a portable dental unit to orally screen the students and to implement an evaluative tool to understand the dental health knowledge of the group. In addition, the dental hygienist plans to provide oral hygiene instruction each month during the remainder of the school year, and the nurse will follow up with the instructions once a week. The Patient Hygiene Performance (PHP) scores during the initial assessment of the class were 2.5, 2.75, 1.5, 3.0, 2.5, 2.0, 2.5, 2.75, 2.5, 2.5, 2.0, and 3.0. The mean OHI-S score of the twelve individuals was 4.8.

31. A complete dental assessment of the class should include all of the following *except* one. Which one is the *exception*?
    a. Plaque and gingival scores
    b. Dental hygiene treatment needs
    c. Individual dexterity skills
    d. Familial income and education level
    e. Level of physical disabilities

32. Based on the severity of the physical disabilities, the dental hygienist may need to make accommodations for all of the following *except* one. Which one is the *exception?*
    a. Oral hygiene instruction
    b. Transportation to area dentists if needed
    c. Utilization of the portable dental chair
    d. Selection of dental indices

33. Which of the following represents the mean PHP score?
    a. 2.45
    b. 2.0
    c. 2.75
    d. 2.25
    e. 2.95

Answers: 26. (c) 27. (c) 28. (b) 29. (c) 30. (a) 31. (d) 32. (d) 33. (a)

34. Which of the following PHP scores represents the mode?
    a. 1.5
    b. 2.0
    c. 2.5
    d. 2.75
    e. 3.0

35. When performing a correlation test between the debris and calculus scores of this class, the correlation coefficient was +.94. The relationship between gingival disease and plaque accumulation according to this test is statistically
    a. Strong
    b. Moderate
    c. Weak
    d. Not correlated

TESTLET 8 (QUESTIONS 36–40)

A dental product company became concerned with the number of dental staff personnel and patients with sensitivity to its low-cost latex gloves. Its research department investigated the need to eliminate all latex from its products. It sent a questionnaire to 250 dental offices throughout the United States that had large accounts with the company. Although most mailings were randomly selected, the department ensured that any dental office that had reported sensitivity receive the questionnaire. Its overall purpose was to determine the degree of people experiencing sensitivity, the possible causes of the latex sensitivity, and ways to prevent it. The questionnaire requested data on the dermatological signs and symptoms, medical gloves used, foods commonly eaten, other personal hygiene products used, medical care received, and health history.

36. What is the primary focus of this research questionnaire?
    a. Assessment and evaluation
    b. Service and education
    c. Therapy and promotion
    d. Referral and treatment

37. What type of research study is being conducted?
    a. Experimental
    b. Ex post facto
    c. Historical
    d. Descriptive

38. This study's overall effectiveness can be best measured by
    a. Its length
    b. Its cost
    c. The number of participants involved
    d. The degree to which the study met its objectives

39. If the research department of this dental product company concludes that a high prevalence of latex sensitivity has been reported, this should be interpreted as follows:
    a. A high number of new cases of latex sensitivity have been reported during the year.
    b. A high number of dental staff personnel and patients are sensitive to latex gloves.
    c. Many dental staff personnel are choosing alternative solutions to latex gloves.
    d. Patients are refusing to have dental office personnel wear gloves from this company.

40. What is the best action for this dental product company based on the high prevalence rate and low cost of latex gloves?
    a. Continue making only latex gloves and target sales to those not sensitive to latex
    b. Find a nonlatex product regardless of price and recall all latex gloves
    c. Continue making latex gloves and offer an alternative type of glove
    d. Change nothing at this time and have the research department continue sending out questionnaires

REFERENCE

1. http://www.ada.org/prof/ed/testing/

PEARSON
myhealthprofessionskit™

Multimedia Extension Activities

Use this address to access the interactive Companion Website created for this textbook. Simply select "Dental Hygiene" from the choice of disciplines. Find this book and log in using your username and password. To obtain a username and password, please register using the scratch-off access code on the inside front cover of this book.

Answers: 34. (c) 35. (a) 36. (a) 37. (d) 38. (d) 39. (b) 40. (c)

Appendix A
Table Clinic Presentation

A *table clinic* is a presentation on a tabletop booth setting that uses both verbal communication and visual aids to disseminate a review of the literature on a specific topic (Figure A-1 ■). The presentation may include slides, graphs, and/or pictures displayed on the poster board. The length of a typical table clinic presentation is five to seven minutes. The topic chosen may be a technique, theory, service, trend, or career opportunity in the practice of dental hygiene. See Box A-1 ■ for tips on preparing a table clinic.

RESEARCH

You can share information regarding research that you have learned about with patients, employees, and peers. It is inevitable that as health care professionals, you will be questioned about oral care products and specific techniques. The information gathered during a table clinic is a perfect way to formulate recommendations about issues that may arise.

After choosing your topic, select a theme. Brainstorm for ideas. When researching your topic, use all available resources. Your public and school libraries are great places to gather information. Don't limit yourself to books: Include journals, newspapers, and videotapes; contacting companies directly is a fantastic way to get information. Remember to keep a list of all of your resources because you will need to provide a handout that includes the main concepts of your topics and that includes a bibliography. In addition, other professionals may ask where you obtained your information.

VISUAL DISPLAY

Next, you will need to prepare your poster board. The purpose of the visual media is to inform, clarify, and/or review specific material. Begin by looking at arts and crafts stores or stores that cater to teachers. Items such as foam board, stick-on lettering, artwork, and crepe or construction paper can usually be found in these stores. You can have pictures or graphs enlarged, copied, or colored at a copy center. You can make the display board bifold or trifold by taping or gluing two or three pieces of poster/foam board together. Generally, you can purchase trifold display boards at office supply stores. The

FIGURE A-1   Table Clinic

BOX A-1 Tips on Preparing Your Table Clinic

- **Getting Started:** Choose a topic that is interesting to you.
- **Research:** Determine a theme for your presentation and work to develop it.
- **Research:** Do thorough research of your topic and have documentation of your findings available.
- **Research:** Be prepared for questions and discussion.
- **Visual Aids:** Use visual aids effectively to reinforce what you are saying.
- **Presentation:** Limit your presentation to approximately 7 minutes.
- **Presentation:** Practice your communication skills: voice projection, body language, and eye contact in front of friends and family. Ask for constructive criticism.
- **Handouts:** Prepare handouts to outline, summarize, or supplement your presentation.

---

poster/foam board should be neat, or-ganized, easy to read from a distance, and eye catching and should stimulate the audience's curiosity.

PRESENTATION

When the visual component is completed, it is time to begin the verbal section. If two speakers will make the presentation, you need to decide who will provide what information. Next, write your part of the presentation on note cards, and then practice, practice, practice. Present it to friends and family members. Be sure to practice voice projection and control, eye contact, and body language. Also practice using your visual aids, which are reinforcing what you are saying. It is best to have your speech memorized, which should not be difficult. Remember that if you are sharing the presentation, the two of you must limit it to only five to seven minutes. In addition to preparing for your speech, also be prepared for questions and controversial feedback. The best way to promote confidence about your topic is to be well versed in other areas that closely relate to it.

HANDOUTS

In addition to the display, handouts should be available. The information in a handout is used to outline, summarize, and/or supplement your presentation. It should include the table clinic's title and date of presentation, the name of the presenter(s), dental hygiene affiliation, and bibliography. The audience should be able to use your handout as a reference guide concerning your topic and, if needed, a way to contact you later.

AMERICAN DENTAL HYGIENISTS' ASSOCIATION (ADHA) GUIDELINES

Every year at the ADHA annual session, students from around the country compete in the table clinic presentations (see Box A-2 ■). More information on ADHA

BOX A-2 ADHA Rules and Regulations

- Handouts must be available and should include the clinic title, date, bibliography, and your dental hygiene affiliation.
- Only one 3 ft. × 6 ft. table is permitted for each table clinic.
- All clinics are conducted at individual tables; no more than two clinicians are permitted to be present at one time.
- Advertising matter, commercial promotion, and solicitation of sales of any type are prohibited.
- Drugs should be identified by their generic or chemical formula rather than the commercial trade name.
- Any trade name on instruments must be covered.
- You must supply all equipment, except for the table, cloth cover, identification sign, and two chairs. You may order electrical outlets, audiovisual equipment, and so on directly from the supplier. Each accepted table clinic presenter receives an order form. The charges for this equipment are your responsibility.
- You are not permitted to use patients or live models for treatment or demonstration.
- Sound devices of any kind are not permitted.
- You must have completed setup of your table clinic 30 minutes prior to commencement of judging.
- You must remain at your clinic at all times because judging times may overlap with the public viewing time.
- Charts or diagrams must be constrained to the tabletop. Easels and materials on the floor or in the aisles are not allowed.

Source: ADHA Guidelines. Chicago: ADHA; 2008.

current guidelines is available at (800) 243-ADHA or www.adha.com. The basic guidelines developed by ADHA for table clinic presentations are summarized in Box A-2. These guidelines change slightly every year, so it is a good idea to contact ADHA for current guidelines.

SUMMARY

By preparing a table clinic, you have the opportunity not only to expand you knowledge of a specific topic but also to inform others. A table clinic is also an excellent way to meet other health care professionals and possibly make new employment contacts. Often the sponsors of the table clinics present awards to the best-prepared and presented table clinic. Have fun and be creative!

Appendix B
Poster Session Preparation

A poster session presents information about an original dental hygiene research study. Basically, a poster session disseminates the study's results whereas a table clinic disseminates a literature review on a specific topic. Poster sessions actually incorporate visual media that reflect an area of dental hygiene research (please see Figure B-1 ■).

Refer to Box B-1 ■ for an outline of the format to use for the poster session. The research should have been conducted in the order the box indicates.

As with all professional endeavors, organization is the key. Faculty members should serve as mentors during research, and it is recommended that all research conducted have numerous reviews before, during, and after the process to ensure success in presenting the information. The ADHA has set criteria for preparing a poster session (Box B-2 ■).

Please see www.adha.org for the rules and regulations for research poster sessions at the American Dental Hygienists' Association annual sessions.

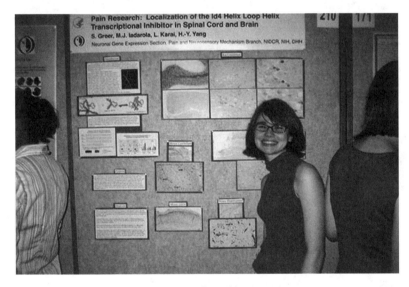

FIGURE B-1   National Institutes of Health Poster Day

BOX B-1   Poster Session Format

- Purpose of study or hypothesis tested
- Statement of the problem and significance of the study
- Brief overview of methodology
- Statistical tests employed
- Study results including statistical data analysis
- Conclusion

BOX B-2   Poster Session Criteria

- Clearly define the purpose for the research study.
- State the problem and significance of the study.
- Identify and outline the research methodology.
- Describe the results including statistical data analysis.
- Clearly state how the results support the conclusions or findings.
- Be prepared for questions and discussions.

Appendix C
Dental Terms and Phrases Translated into Spanish and Vietnamese with Spanish Pronunciation Guide

English	Spanish	Vietnamese
dentist	dentista	Nha sĩ
tooth	diente	Răng
throat	garganta	Cuống họng
neck	cuello	Cổ
mouth	boca	Miệng
head	cabeza	Đầu
face	cara	Mặt
ear	oido	Tai
nose	nariz	Muõi
tongue	lengua	Lưõ'i
tonsils	amigdalas	Hạch
denture	dentadura	Hàm răng
toothbrush	cepillar(v), cepillo(n)	Bàn chãy đánh răng
show me	enseneme	Chỉ cho tôi
relax	relajese	Bình tỉnh, thông thả
don't move	no se muera	Đừng nhúc nhích
look straight ahead	vea derecho	Nhìn thẳng phía trước
swallow	trague	Nuốc vào
open your mouth	abra la boca	Mở' miệng ra
stick out your tongue	saque la lengua	Lè lưõ'i ra
close	cerra	Đóng lại
spit	escupir	Nhổ ra
abscess	abceso	Ung, nhọt
asthma	astma	Bệnh suyễn
bleeding	sangrado	Nhảy máu
cold	frio	Lạnh
diabetes	diabetes	Bệnh tiểu đường
edema	edema	Chứng phù thủng
fracture	fractura	Chỗ nú't, chỗ gãy
headache	cefalea	Nhức đầu
high blood pressure	presion alta	Chứng cao huyết áp
hot	caliente	Nóng
infection	infeccion	Nhiễm trùng

(continued)

English	Spanish	Vietnamese
injured	herido	Bị thương
pregnant	embarazada	Mang thai
stitches	puntadas	Khâu, vá
swelling	inflamacion	Bị sưng
trauma	trauma	Chấn thương
wound	herida	Vết thương
mild	suave	Nhẹ, êm
moderate	moderado	Vừa phải
severe	severo	Nghiêm khắc
earache	dolor de oido	Bệnh đau tai
sore throat	dolor de garganta	Đau họng
difficulty swallowing	dificultad al tragar	Khó khăn khi nuốt
toothache	dolor de muela	Nhức răng
neck pain	dolor de cuello	Đau cổ
sensitive	sensible	Nhạy cảm
disease	enfermedad	Bệnh tật
medications	medicamentos	Bốc toa thuốc (dùng thuốc)
antibiotics	antibioticos	Kháng sinh
pain pills	calmantes	Thuốc đau nhức
narcotics	narcoticos	Thuốc mê
penicillin	penicilina	Thuốc trụ sinh
right	derecho (m.) derecha (f.)	Phải
left	izquierdo (m.) izquierda (f.)	Trái

English	Spanish	Pronunciation
Good day! How are you?	Buenos dias! Como esta?	Boo-eh-nus dee-ass. Kum-muh estah?
Does it hurt?	Le duele?	Leh doo-eh-leh?
When does it hurt?	Cuando le duele?	Kwan-doh leh doo-eh-leh?

All of the time?
Todo el tiempo¿
(toh-doh el tee-m-poh)

Where does it hurt?
Donde le duele¿
(dun-deh leh doo-eh-leh)

Does the cold water or air hurt you?
Le molesta el agua o el aire frio¿
(leh muh-les-tah el ah-goo-ah oh el i-reh free-oh)

Does it hurt when you bite?
Le duele cuando muerde¿
(leh doo-eh-leh kwan-doh moo-erdeh)

Open your mouth.
Abra la boca.
(ahbra lah bokah)

Close your mouth a little.
Cierre la boca un poco.
(see-ehreh lah bokah oon poh-koh)

Bite slowly.
Muerda despacio.
(moo-erdah des-pah-see-oh)

Bite again.
Muerda otra vez.
(moo-erdah oh-trah vez)

Spit out, please.
Escupa, por favor.
(ess-coo-pah por favor)

Turn your head to the right.
—to the left.
Volte la cabeza a la derecha.
—a la izquierda.
(vol-teh lah ka-beh-zah ah lah deh-reh-chah
—ah lah eez-kee-erdah)

Do not eat or drink for 30 minutes.
No coma ni beba por 30 minutos.
(noh koh-mah nee beh-bah por trentah mee-nuh-tohs)

Do not chew on this side for 24 hours.
No mastique en este lado por 24 horas.
(no mahs-teekeh en esteh lahdoh por ven-tee kwah-troh o-rahs)

Do not brush tonight.
No se cepille esta noche.
(no seh seh-peeyeh ess-tah no-cheh)

Do not rinse tonight.
No se enjuage esta noche.
(noh seh en-huah-ghe ess-tah no-cheh)

Appendix D
Standards for Dental Hygienists in Dental Public Health Education

COMMISSION ON DENTAL ACCREDITATION, DENTAL PUBLIC HEALTH STANDARDS

Dental hygiene students may attend programs that have been accredited by the Commission on Dental Accreditation, which is part of the American Dental Association. The Commission is composed of twenty members including a representative from the American Dental Hygienists' Association. The Commission has been accrediting dental hygiene educational programs since 1953.

The Accreditation Standards for Dental Hygiene Education Programs includes mandatory curriculum content. Dental hygiene students must prove competency in dental public health. Specifically, dental hygiene graduates must include and advocate for the evaluation of current literature to prepare for lifelong learning in dental hygiene practice. Faculty should integrate these principles of lifelong learning throughout the curriculum.

Moreover, content in community dental health and public health dentistry must be included in the curriculum to provide students background in the procedures of assessing, planning, implementing, and evaluating community oral health programs. Curriculum must also include experience in oral health education and preventive counseling for groups. The dental hygiene faculty must implement a mechanism for planning, supervising, and evaluating community field experiences.

Curricular requirements for community health instruction can be found in the Accreditation Standards for Dental Hygiene Education Programs, Commission on Dental Accreditation. Chicago, IL: American Dental Association; 2008. Please see http://www.ada.org/prof/ed/accred/standards/dh.pdf for these standards.

JOINT COMMISSION ON NATIONAL DENTAL EXAMINATIONS: NATIONAL BOARD DENTAL HYGIENE EXAMINATION

Prospective dental hygienists in all states except Alabama are required to take and pass the National Board Dental Hygiene Examination. The information included on this examination includes the following topics under the section entitled Community Health/Research Principles.

- Promoting Health and Preventing Disease within Groups (including media and communication resources)
- Participating in Community Programs
  1. Assessing Populations and Defining Objectives
  2. Designing, Implementing, and Evaluating Programs
- Analyzing Scientific Information, Utilizing Statistical Concepts, and Applying Research Results

Refer to Chapter 22 for a more complete discussion of the National Board Dental Hygiene Examination.

Appendix E
Guide to Scientific Writing

The following guidelines to writing can be used when writing scientifically based papers for table clinic presentations and poster presentations.[1]

TITLE PAGE

The title page should include the title of the manuscript in boldface; each author's name, credentials, rank or title, and organizational affiliation; and the primary author's mailing address and telephone, e-mail, and fax numbers. In addition, if an organization funded the investigation, its name should be noted on the bottom of the title page.

LENGTH

Manuscripts should be six to ten pages in length excluding references, tables, figures, and photographs.

PRESENTATION

All manuscripts must be written in the English language. Manuscripts must include an abstract and the following:

- Original research including an introduction, methods and materials, results, and discussion and conclusion
- Case studies including an introduction and case as described in the dental hygiene process of care; assessment, dental hygiene diagnosis, treatment planning, implementation, and evaluations; and summary
- Literature reviews containing an introduction, the significance of the topic, main body, and conclusions
- Position papers, which are written to reflect a position taken on a specific issue, including an introduction, the significance of the issue, main body, and summary

REFERENCES

All references should be numbered in the order they are cited. The following style of citation should be used:

> Periodical: Fones, AC and Newman, I: The inception of the professional dental hygienist. *J Dent Hyg* 2008;78:395–402.

> Textbook: Nathe, CN: Dental Public Health and Research. 3rd edition. Upper Saddle River, NJ: Pearson. 2010:10–12.

TABLES, FIGURES, AND PHOTOGRAPHS

All tables, figures, and photographs should be at the end of the manuscript, not inserted into it. Written permission for the use of copyrighted material must be included with the manuscript and is the author's responsibility.

ACKNOWLEDGMENTS

The authors may acknowledge one to two individuals for their assistance in manuscript preparation.

AUTHORS

Primary authors of all manuscripts must be dental hygienists or dental hygiene students; secondary authors may represent any discipline.

CONTENT

Manuscripts may be original research, case studies, literature reviews, or position papers.

REFERENCE

1. http://www.adha.org/jdh/guidelines.htm

Appendix F
Answers to Self-Study Test Items

CHAPTER 1

1. What is an example of primary public health prevention?
   a. Disease prevention
   b. Periodontal debridement
   c. Fluoride treatments
   d. Restorative materials

   ANSWER: a

2. Public health is credited with the dramatic increase in the average life span because of which of the following?
   a. Vaccinations
   b. Safety policies
   c. Family planning
   d. All of the above

   ANSWER: d

3. What is an example of secondary public health prevention?
   a. Prevention of disease
   b. Fluoride treatments
   c. Restorations
   d. Patient education

   ANSWER: b

4. What is the main health care research institution in the United States?
   a. Centers for Disease Control and Prevention
   b. Food and Drug Administration
   c. National Institutes of Health
   d. Johns Hopkins University

   ANSWER: c

5. How has malpractice directly impacted dental care delivery and quality?
   a. Enabled patients to sue
   b. Decreased the number of dental providers because of the fear of malpractice suits
   c. Decreased quality of care
   d. Increased the number of suits against dental providers

   ANSWER: a

CHAPTER 2

1. What is referred to as a constituent member in the ADHA organization?
   a. National organizations
   b. State organizations
   c. Local organizations
   d. Student organizations

   ANSWER: b

2. When is school fluoridation recommended?
   a. When an independent water source is available
   b. For children who have caries
   c. For children who have brown discolored areas on enamel
   d. None of the above

   ANSWER: a

3. Demineralization, enhancement of remineralization, and inhibition of bacterial activity are examples of what?
   a. Water fluoridation
   b. Topical fluoridation
   c. Systemic fluoridation
   d. Fluoride supplements

   ANSWER: b

4. Which type of fluoride increases children's risk of developing dental fluorosis?
   a. Supplements
   b. Systemic
   c. Topical
   d. Both a and b

   ANSWER: d

5. When are sealants most effective?
   a. When applied without etchant
   b. When an assistant is utilized
   c. In the presence of saliva
   d. When material is cured for one minute
   ANSWER: b

CHAPTER 3

1. What has been recognized as a major unmet need in the United States?
   a. Health insurance
   b. Oral Health
   c. Access to health care
   d. Geriatric awareness
   ANSWER: b

2. What branch of the federal government has a direct impact on dental care delivery?
   a. Legislative
   b. Executive
   c. Judicial
   d. All of the above
   ANSWER: b

3. Who or what directs the US Public Health Service?
   a. US Surgeon General
   b. Centers for Disease Control and Prevention
   c. Johns Hopkins University
   d. Dental Public Health Committee
   ANSWER: a

4. Which organization provides a system of health surveillance to monitor and prevent outbreak of diseases and maintain national health statistics?
   a. National Institutes of Health
   b. Centers for Disease Control and Prevention
   c. Food and Drug Administration
   d. Indian Health Service
   ANSWER: b

5. Which organization is responsible for the Head Start Program?
   a. Administration on Aging
   b. Centers for Medicare and Medicaid Services
   c. Administration for Children and Families
   d. Indian Health Services
   ANSWER: c

CHAPTER 4

1. Which European country has a history of establishing the profession of dental hygiene?
   a. England
   b. Italy
   c. Germany
   d. Portugal
   ANSWER: a

2. Which of the following is a reason for the lack of access to dental hygiene services worldwide?
   a. Insufficient funding
   b. Lack of social and cultural awareness
   c. Legal restraints
   d. All of above
   ANSWER: d

3. How many countries in the European Union report no or virtually no hygienists?
   a. 3
   b. 7
   c. 10
   d. 17
   ANSWER: b

4. In industrialized nations where do dental hygienists mainly practice?
   a. Public health clinics
   b. Educational institutions
   c. Government positions
   d. Private dental clinics
   ANSWER: d

5. What organization is a nonprofit group that unites dental hygiene associations from around the world in their common cause of promoting access to quality preventative oral services and to raise public awareness of the prevention of dental disease?
   a. American Dental Hygiene Association
   b. European Dental Hygienists' Federation
   c. International Federation of Dental Hygienists
   d. European Federation of Periodontology
   ANSWER: c

CHAPTER 5

1. Which of the following does financing of dental treatment involve?
   a. Private sector
   b. Dental practitioner
   c. Public sector
   d. Both a and c

   ANSWER: d

2. What payment is based on an office visit and is always the same regardless of the services rendered?
   a. Encounter
   b. Fee-for-service plan
   c. Capitation
   d. Barter system

   ANSWER: a

3. What term refers to a portion of the cost of each service that the patient pays—in other words, the part of the payment not covered by the third party?
   a. Insurance payment
   b. Copayment
   c. Deductible
   d. Exchange

   ANSWER: b

4. What is defined as the number given to a specific procedure as designated in the *Codes on Dental Procedures and Nomenclature* published by ADA?
   a. Premium number
   b. Procedure number
   c. Contract number
   d. Benefit number

   ANSWER: b

5. What form is sent to the patient and provider explaining the payment or denial for procedures rendered?
   a. Explanation of benefits
   b. Managed care
   c. Exclusive provider arrangement
   d. Dental claim

   ANSWER: a

CHAPTER 6

1. State agencies such as state dental boards fall within which type of law?
   a. Common
   b. Statutory
   c. Constitutional
   d. Administrative

   ANSWER: d

2. Which branch of government makes laws for the state?
   a. Legislative
   b. Executive
   c. Administrative
   d. Judicial

   ANSWER: a

3. Laws which explain what services dental hygienists can provide are found in
   a. Medicaid rules
   b. State law
   c. Federal Law
   d. Health care regulations

   ANSWER: b

4. Judges do not make laws, but they interpret them.
   a. The first statement is true, but the second statement is false.
   b. The first statement is false, but the second statement is true.
   c. Both statements are true.
   d. Both statements are false.

   ANSWER: c

5. Because federal laws regulate dental hygiene practice, federal senators are involved with state regulation.
   a. The first statement is true, but the second statement is false.
   b. The first statement is false, but the second statement is true.
   c. Both statements are true.
   d. Both statements are false.

   ANSWER: d

CHAPTER 7

1. What of the following is an individual or group who causes a social, cultural, or behavioral change, be it intentional or unintentional?
   a. Mentor
   b. Change agent
   c. Lobbying
   d. Grants writer

   ANSWER: b

2. Which of the following is *not* a way in which social advocates initiate change in dental public health?
   a. By delivering dental care
   b. By helping to sustain dental public health programs
   c. By determining the type of dental treatment rendered
   d. By determining who receives dental care

   ANSWER: c

3. What is necessary to create change?
   a. Influencing individuals who govern policy
   b. Increasing an organization's financial status
   c. Redesigning the public health facility
   d. All of the above

   ANSWER: a

4. What are the roles identified for the dental hygiene change agent?
   a. Catalyst
   b. Solution giver
   c. Resource linker
   d. All of the above

   ANSWER: d

5. Making basic changes without losing the essential components is termed?
   a. Modification
   b. Competency
   c. Application
   d. Networking

   ANSWER: a

CHAPTER 8

1. Empowerment models that focus on patient autonomy and collaborative relationships are paternalist regimens. These regimens are led by patients whose knowledge of health and disease increases the likelihood that healthy behaviors are attained.
   a. The first statement is true; the second statement is false.
   b. The first statement is false; the second statement is true.
   c. Both statements are true.
   d. Both statements are false.

   ANSWER: d

2. Which of the following aspects is part of the multi-dimensional model of health?
   a. Spirituality
   b. Knowledge
   c. Behavior
   d. Values

   ANSWER: a

3. The local dental hygiene association worked on policy change that banned sugary beverages from school vending machines. This is an example of
   a. Healthy behavior
   b. Health action
   c. Health education
   d. Health promotion

   ANSWER: d

4. For behavior change to occur, an individual must reach what milestone?
   a. Value the change
   b. Understand the healthy behavior
   c. Understand unhealthy behavior
   d. Understand why a behavior was chosen

   ANSWER: a

5. A patient who receives praise for having healthy gums during two routine dental hygiene appointments will be more likely to maintain good home care to ensure that the praise will continue at subsequent appointments. This theory is called
   a. Classical conditioning
   b. Operant conditioning
   c. Modeling
   d. Empowerment

   ANSWER: a

CHAPTER 9

1. The best way to ensure an effective presentation is to
   a. Decrease the number of participants
   b. Utilize audiovisual aids
   c. Have at least ten objectives for each presentation
   d. Be prepared

   ANSWER: d

2. "Following the presentation, the audience will be able to compare ten healthy and unhealthy snack choices" is an example of a(n)
   a. Goal
   b. Lesson plan
   c. Objective
   d. Healthy behavior

   ANSWER: c

3. Lecturing is always an effective way to teach dental health education. Lecture always includes the problem-based method of learning.
   a. The first statement is true; the second is false.
   b. The first statement is false; the second is true.
   c. Both statements are true.
   d. Both statements are false.

   ANSWER: d

4. Which verb pertains to the psychomotor domain?
   a. Demonstrating
   b. Comparing
   c. Advocating
   d. Defending

   ANSWER: a

5. When used as an objective, the verb *understand*
   a. Is easily measured
   b. Is open to misinterpretation
   c. Always requires skill
   d. Is frequently used

   ANSWER: b

CHAPTER 10

1. A group from a local church youth group could be considered a
   a. Target population
   b. Target population profile
   c. Faith-based initiative
   d. Community agency

   ANSWER: a

2. It is important not to frighten child patients. It is better not to tell the truth if a procedure could involve some discomfort.
   a. The first statement is true; the second statement is false.
   b. The first statement is false; the second statement is true.
   c. Both statements are true.
   d. Both statements are false.

   ANSWER: a

3. Faith-based initiatives funded by the federal government do not generally include health care.
   a. The first statement is true; the second statement is false.
   b. The first statement is false; the second statement is true.
   c. Both statements are true.
   d. Both statements are false.

   ANSWER: a

4. Social workers and dental hygienists can work together during programs for target populations
   a. To provide dental hygiene care
   b. To assess dental health
   c. To ensure social services for the population
   d. To implement periodontal treatment

   ANSWER: c

5. Inconvenient office hours of a dental practice can become a
   a. Target population profile technique
   b. Faith-based issue
   c. Barrier to care
   d. Long-term strategic plan

   ANSWER: c

CHAPTER 11

1. The fact that only a small number of minorities work in the oral health care professions may be considered a barrier to oral health care. A study of the racial and ethnic composition of the health care workforce reveals that the dental workforce is the least diverse of all the health professions.
   a. The first statement is true; the second statement is false.
   b. The first statement is false; the second statement is true.

c. Both statements are true.

d. Both statements are false.

ANSWER: c

2. Which of the following could prevent a patient from seeking care or reduce effectiveness of care?

a. Unhealthy behaviors

b. Severe pain

c. Language barrier

d. None of the above

ANSWER: c

3. A country in which people strive to acculturate into a new society and make valiant attempts to change their cultural patterns to those of their host society is colloquially called

a. A melting pot

b. A salad bowl

c. Jello

d. Amalgam

ANSWER: a

4. Which of the following is or are guidelines to effective communication?

a. Assess one's own cultural beliefs and values

b. Recognize those cultural influences affecting communication

c. Understand a patient's belief system

d. All of the above

ANSWER: d

5. Cross-cultural dental hygiene is the effective integration of the population's socioethnocultural background into the process of care. Recognizing how your culture influences your values, behaviors, beliefs, and decision making is part of cross-cultural dental hygiene.

a. The first statement is true; the second statement is false.

b. The first statement is false; the second statement is true.

c. Both statements are true.

d. Both statements are false.

ANSWER: c

CHAPTER 12

1. Which of the following is part of the planning phase of program planning?

a. Identify methods to measure goals

b. Assess the population's dental needs

c. Begin program operation

d. Revise program as needed

ANSWER: a

2. Dr. Fones's original paradigm for the school dental hygienist focused on

a. Restoration

b. Utilization of a case manager

c. Prevention of disease

d. All of the above

ANSWER: c

3. Which school program is particularly advantageous for middle school athletes?

a. Sealant program

b. School fluoridation

c. Case management

d. Athletic mouth guard program

ANSWER: d

4. During which stage of the program paradigm planning should the target population's needs be identified?

a. Assessment

b. Dental hygiene diagnosis

c. Planning

d. Evaluation

ANSWER: a

5. A dental hygienist employed in a nursing home could provide routine preventive care. In addition, the dental hygienists could have a collaborative relationship with a dentist, so that restorative and urgent care is provided as need.

a. The first statement is true; the second statement is false.

b. The first statement is false; the second statement is true.

c. Both statements are true.

d. Both statements are false.

ANSWER: c

CHAPTER 13

1. Program goals should be evaluated based on
   a. Measurement tools
   b. Baseline data
   c. National guidelines
   d. State surveillance records

   ANSWER: b

2. During which phase of program planning should evaluation be started?
   a. Assessment
   b. Dental hygiene diagnosis
   c. Planning
   d. Evaluation

   ANSWER: c

3. Which type of evaluation refers to the internal evaluation of a program?
   a. Formative
   b. Summative
   c. Quantitative
   d. Qualitative

   ANSWER: a

4. Which type of evaluation is a basic screening?
   a. Nonclinical
   b. Clinical
   c. Provider driven
   d. Educational

   ANSWER: b

5. An index that measures a conditioin that will not change, such as dental caries, is termed a(n)
   a. Clinical index
   b. Nonclinical index
   c. Irreversible index
   d. Reversible index

   ANSWER: c

CHAPTER 14

1. Evidence-based decisions come from research, practice, and
   a. Science
   b. Patient preferences
   c. Disciplines
   d. None of the above

   ANSWER: b

2. Informed consent is an ongoing process that is initially obtained at the first step of the research process. It should be discussed in a group setting.
   a. The first statement is true; the second statement is false.
   b. The first statement is false; the second statement is true.
   c. Both statements are true.
   d. Both statements are false.

   ANSWER: a

3. Which type of sample involves choosing every subject independently and all subjects have an equal chance of being selected?
   a. Systematic
   b. Random
   c. Convenience
   d. Judgmental

   ANSWER: b

4. "No statistically significant difference between Brand X and Brand Y toothpaste in the reduction of tooth decay" is an example of a
   a. Research question
   b. Research hypothesis
   c. Null hypothesis
   d. Positive hypothesis

   ANSWER: c

5. Data analysis involves
   a. Assessing the research question
   b. Developing the hypothesis
   c. Analyzing the data
   d. Performing statistical regression techniques

   ANSWER: c

CHAPTER 15

1. Which of the following is a descriptive approach to research?
   a. Case study approach
   b. Experimental approach
   c. Retrospective approach
   d. Prospective approach

   ANSWER: a

2. Which studies combine descriptive and historical research to establish patterns from the past and present to predict future occurrences?
   a. Document analysis studies
   b. Correlational studies

c. Trend studies

d. Prospective studies

ANSWER: c

3. In a split mouth study, one side of the mouth is used for the test treatment. The other side of the mouth is used for the control treatment.
   a. The first statement is true; the second statement is false.
   b. The first statement is false; the second statement is true.
   c. Both statements are true.
   d. Both statements are false.

ANSWER: c

4. A quasi-experimental study is designed as an experimental study but lacks inherent control. However, results from a quasi-experimental study may be used when planning further studies.
   a. The first statement is true; the second statement is false.
   b. The first statement is false; the second statement is true.
   c. Both statements are true.
   d. Both statements are false.

ANSWER: c

5. Studying the relationship between obesity and oral health is an example of which type of study?
   a. Experimental
   b. Quasi-experimental
   c. Correlational
   d. Analytic

ANSWER: c

CHAPTER 16

1. *Epidemiology* has been defined as the study of the nature, cause, control, and determinants of the frequency and distribution of
   a. Disease
   b. Disability
   c. Death
   d. All of the above

ANSWER: d

2. The agent of disease is the biologic or mechanical cause of the disease or condition. Examples of agents are the specific bacteria in relation to dental caries or brushing with a hard toothbrush in relation to abrasion.

   a. The first statement is true; the second statement is false.
   b. The first statement is false; the second statement is true.
   c. Both statements are true.
   d. Both statements are false.

ANSWER: c

3. The occurrence of an illness in excess of normal expectancy in a community or region, usually occurring suddenly and spreading rapidly, is termed a(n)
   a. Endemic
   b. Epidemic
   c. Pandemic
   d. All of the above

ANSWER: b

4. Which study attempts to relate outcome with exposure to a suspected risk factor using data that are available for the population?
   a. Case–control
   b. Case study
   c. Ecological
   d. Time Series

ANSWER: c

5. What is a modifiable attribute or exposure that is known to be associated with a health condition?
   a. Risk ratio
   b. Risk factor
   c. Risk attribute
   d. Risk indicator

ANSWER: b

CHAPTER 17

1. Tobacco use, excessive alcohol use, and inappropriate dietary practices contribute to a number of diseases and disorders. In particular, tobacco use is a risk factor for oral cavity and pharyngeal cancers, periodontal diseases, candidiasis, and dental caries, among other diseases.
   a. The first statement is true; the second statement is false.
   b. The first statement is false; the second statement is true.
   c. Both statements are true.
   d. Both statements are false.

ANSWER: c

2. Which gender does periodontal diseases affect the most?
   a. Males
   b. Females
   c. Both are effected the same
   d. Teen and elderly females

   ANSWER: a

3. In which teeth are early childhood caries most evident?
   a. Permanent molars
   b. Permanent anteriors
   c. Primary anteriors
   d. Primary molars

   ANSWER: c

4. Early detection frequently affects the outcome of
   a. Oral cancer treatment
   b. Cleft lip rates
   c. Cleft lip and palate rates
   d. None of the above

   ANSWER: a

5. When toothaches are not prevented, which services might individuals seek?
   a. Medical
   b. Dental hygiene
   c. General dentistry
   d. Cosmetic Dentistry

   ANSWER: a

CHAPTER 18

1. Which variable is made up of distinct and separate units or categories but is counted only in whole numbers?
   a. Quantitative
   b. Qualitative
   c. Continuous
   d. Discrete

   ANSWER: d

2. Which scale of measurement contains all of the characteristics of the preceding scales and has an absolute zero point determined by nature?
   a. Interval
   b. Ordinal
   c. Ratio
   d. Numerical

   ANSWER: c

3. Which type of correlational relationship would the following statement indicate: as the consumption of fluoridated water increases, the caries rate decreases.
   a. Positive
   b. Inverse
   c. Strong
   d. Weak

   ANSWER: b

4. The research hypothesis, also called the *alternative* or *positive hypothesis,* is the logical opposite of the null hypothesis. The research hypothesis can indicate a direction of difference.
   a. The first statement is true; the second statement is false.
   b. The first statement is false; the second statement is true.
   c. Both statements are true.
   d. Both statements are false.

   ANSWER: c

5. The chi-square test (χ^2) is the most commonly used nonparametric statistic. It is used to determine whether a significant difference exists between frequency counts of nominal (categorical or dichotomous) data by comparing the observed frequencies to expected frequencies.
   a. The first statement is true; the second statement is false.
   b. The first statement is false; the second statement is true.
   c. Both statements are true.
   d. Both statements are false.

   ANSWER: c

CHAPTER 19

1. The ADA Seal of Approval program is regulated by the FDA. It is mandatory for all over-the-counter dental care products.
   a. The first statement is true; the second statement is false.
   b. The first statement is false; the second statement is true.
   c. Both the statements are true.
   d. Both the statements are false.

   ANSWER: d

2. PubMed is a service of the US National Library of Medicine (NLM). It includes more than 17 million citations from MEDLINE and other life science journals for biomedical articles back to the 1950s.
   a. The first statement is true; the second statement is false.
   b. The first statement is false; the second statement is true.
   c. Both the statements are true.
   d. Both the statements are false.

   ANSWER: c

3. Which of the following is/are part of a research report's methods and materials section?
   a. Research design
   b. Ethical considerations
   c. Sample size
   d. All of the above

   ANSWER: d

4. Which of the following terms defines the review of manuscripts for content and accuracy before they can be included in refereed journals?
   a. Critique
   b. Double Blind
   c. Primary evaluation
   d. Peer reviewed

   ANSWER: d

5. *Statistical significance* means that the result was not caused by
   a. Control
   b. Chance
   c. Placebo effect
   d. Sugar pill

   ANSWER: b

CHAPTER 20

1. Dental hygienists initially are eligible to be a US PHS Commissioned Officer with which of the following credentials?
   a. Certificate in dental hygiene
   b. Associate's degree in dental hygiene
   c. Bachelor's degree in dental hygiene
   d. Master's degree in dental hygiene

   ANSWER: c

2. Civil service employment falls under the state department. Many times hygienists are employed at a VA Hospital as a civil service employee.
   a. First statement is true; the second statement is false.
   b. First statement is false; the second statement is true.
   c. Both statements are true.
   d. Both statements are false.

   ANSWER: c

3. Students are eligible for the COSTEP program during their dental hygiene education. The COSTEP program is part of the US Department of Defense health care system.
   a. The first statement is true; the second statement is false.
   b. The first statement is false; the second statement is true.
   c. Both statements are true.
   d. Both statements are false.

   ANSWER: a

4. Dental hygienists can work on military bases in the United States as
   a. Military officers
   b. PHS officers
   c. Contract employees
   d. None of the above

   ANSWER: c

5. Which of the following are goals of the US Public Health Services?
   a. Prevent and control disease
   b. Identify health hazards in the environment
   c. Help provide health care to Native Americans
   d. All of the above

   ANSWER: d

CHAPTER 21

1. Members of the public, government agencies, and other health care professionals, as well as the dental hygiene profession itself, is showing significant interest in establishing dental hygiene programs in settings other than private dental offices. Many states have expanded the dental hygienists' scope of practice.
   a. The first statement is true; the second statement is false.
   b. The first statement is false; the second statement is true.
   c. Both statements are true.
   d. Both statements are false.

   ANSWER: c

2. What may be necessary to increase dental hygienists' accessibility to the underserved public?
   a. Marketing promotion
   b. Blueprint development
   c. Legislative initiatives
   d. None of the above

   ANSWER: c

3. During which phase should a target population's needs be determined?
   a. Assessment
   b. Dental hygiene diagnosis
   c. Planning
   d. Implementation

   ANSWER: a

4. Continually refining the product is which part of the business plan?
   a. Service development
   b. Marketing
   c. Sales
   d. Operations

   ANSWER: a

5. Which phase involves prioritizing goals and objectives?
   a. Assessment
   b. Dental hygiene diagnosis
   c. Planning
   d. Implementation

   ANSWER: c

GLOSSARY

A

Abstract Section of a study report that outlines its content by concisely stating its purpose, significance, previous findings, methodology, results, and suggestions for future studies in no more than 250 words.

Acculturate To assimilate or adapt to another culture by assuming its practices and beliefs.

Administrative law Body of rules, regulations, orders, and decisions created by a government's administrative agencies.

Affective domain Name of a category that includes feelings, attitudes, and values and is not easily measured.

Agent factor Biological or mechanical means for causing diseases or conditions.

Alternative restorative treatment (ART) Technique by which the provider removes carious lesions with hand instruments and restores the resultant cavity and adjoining fissures with a dental sealant.

American Association of Public Health Dentistry (AAPHD) Organization that represents American public health dentists, dental hygienists, and the science of dental public health.

American Association of State and Territorial Dental Directors Organization that represents state dental departments.

American Dental Association (ADA) Organization that represents American dentists and the science of dentistry.

American Dental Hygienists' Association (ADHA) Organization that represents American dental hygienists and the science of dental hygiene.

Assessment Process of care that analyzes the program's target group and resources.

Assimilate *See* acculturate.

Athletic mouth guard Removable oral appliance that protects the hard and soft tissues of the oral cavity and brain during contact sports.

B

Barrier to care Limitation on an individual's ability to receive dental services.

Barter system Method used only in the private sector by which the dental provider and patient negotiate payment that involves exchanging goods and services without using money.

Behavior change Act of changing behavior such as daily flossing.

Benefit Amount that an insurance entity will pay for covered dental services described in its policy.

Bioethics Established norms of conduct in performing research that distinguish between morally acceptable and unacceptable behavior.

Biostatistics Data analysis and interpretation in health care research.

Blueprint Skeletal framework developed before implementing a program.

Bodies of law Rules of conduct or action prescribed or formally recognized as binding or enforced by a controlling authority; in the United States: common, statutory, constitutional, and administrative.

Branches of government Sections of federal and state governments: legislative, executive, and judicial.

C

Calibration Process of ensuring consistency within and among examiner(s).

Capitation plan Plan in which a dental provider contracts with a third party to provide all or most of the services to a specified group of people in return for a fixed monthly payment, which is determined according to the number of individuals or families in the group.

Causality Concept that certain exposure will result in a particular outcome.

Change agent Individual who intentionally or unintentionally causes social, cultural, or behavioral change.

Children's Health Insurance Program (CHIP) Federal program created to cover medical care for children whose families have incomes too high to qualify for state medical assistance but cannot obtain private insurance; all states participate, but some do not cover dental care.

Civil service employment Employment category that refers to all people holding appointed positions in the executive, judicial, and legislative branches of the federal government other than military positions or individuals contracting with a governmental or private placement agency.

Claims processing Entering procedures rendered and determining whether payment will be approved or denied.

Clinical evaluation Study or appraisal supported by clinical data such as basic screenings and epidemiological examinations that utilize dental indices.

Clinical examination requirement The clinical board requirement, which is mandatory in all states.

Clinician Person who provides dental hygiene clinical care to a population.

Coalition Alliance among individuals or groups in which they cooperate in collaboration, each in its own self-interest.

Cognitive domain Category that consists of intellectual skills.

Collaboration Process of working together toward a common goal.

Collaborative practice Science of the prevention and treatment of oral disease by providing education, assessment, preventive, clinical, and other therapeutic services in a cooperative working relationship with a consulting dentist.

Commercial insurance plan Plan that operates for a profit.

Commissioned Officer Student Training and Extern Program (COSTEP) Program that enables students to enhance their educational background and provides hands-on experience to those committed to future employment.

Common law Legislation created by courts through judicial decisions that in many cases other courts can change; contains ideas of common sense and precedent.

Community dental health *See* dental public health.

Community water fluoridation Addition of fluoride to community water supplies.

Complementary alternative medicine (CAM) Use of herbs, natural products, and practices such as massage or yoga in health care.

Component organization Local member of the American Dental Hygienists' Association.

Congressman *See* representative.

Constituent organization State or regional component of the American Dental Hygienists' Association.

Constitutional law Interpretation and implementation of a government's codified constitution.

Consumer advocate Person who provides dental health consultation to various target populations.

Continuous variable Variable that can be expressed by a large and infinite number of measures along a continuum and in a fraction, and considered quantitative.

Contract Legal agreement between an entity such as a insurance company and a group or individual.

Control Group in a study that does not receive treatment or therapy, receives a placebo, or receives the standard treatment or drug.

Copayment Portion of the cost of each service a patient pays.

Correlation Relationship or association between variables that can be measured mathematically.

Cultural competency Awareness and understanding of cultural difference.

Cultural diversity Integration of an individual's or population's socioethnocultural background into dental hygiene care.

Cultural sensitivity Awareness and understanding of cultures different from one's own.

Culture and cycle of poverty Exploration of the culture of poverty and the cyclical change of poverty.

D

Data Information collected by a researcher using various methods from questionnaires to clinical testing.

Data analysis Application of statistical tests to data to organize, describe, summarize, and analyze them to answer a research question or test a hypothesis.

Deductible Amount an individual enrolled in an insurance plan must pay for covered services before the insurance entity begins paying.

Defluoridation Process of removing excessive natural fluorine from water supplies.

Degrees of freedom Number of values or observations that are free to vary when computing a statistic.

Demand Particular or desired frequency of dental care by a population.

Dental assistant Professional who assists the dental hygienist and/or dentist.

Dental care delivery Way that dental care is provided to the public.

Dental claim Patient's formal request for insurance payment for a dental procedure that was rendered.

Dental claim form Standard dental document used to file a claim or request authorization for a procedure.

Dental hygiene Art and science of preventive oral health.

Dental hygiene diagnosis Formal diagnosis of a population's current dental hygiene status.

Dental hygiene movement Inception and evolution of the use of the dental hygienist to provide dental care.

Dental hygiene process of care Assessment, dental hygiene diagnosis, planning, implementation, and evaluation of dental hygiene care of a target population.

Dental hygiene treatment Comprehensive dental hygiene treatment including assessment, dental hygiene diagnosis, planning, implementation with a focus on periodontal debridement and oral hygiene instruction, and evaluation provided by a dental hygienist.

Dental hygienist Professional who provides clinical and educational dental hygiene services to the public.

Dental index Standardized quantitative method for measuring, scoring, and analyzing oral conditions in individuals and groups.

Dental necessity Service provided by a dental provider that has been determined as a generally acceptable dental practice for a specific diagnosis and treatment.

Dental nurse Term used in New Zealand for a school dental staff member; *see also* dental therapist.

Dental public health Oral health care and education with an emphasis on the utilization of the dental hygiene sciences to deliver care to a target population.

Dental sealants Plastic resins placed on tooth surfaces to prevent dental decay; sometimes called *pit and fissure sealants.*

Dental therapist Provider of restorative care under the general supervision of dentists, found mostly in the United Kingdom and in former countries of the British Commonwealth, such as Australia, Canada, and Nigeria.

Dentist Professional who provides clinical and educational dental services to the public.

Dentistry Art and science of restorative oral health.

Dependent variable In clinical study, variable that is being tested.

Descriptive approach Variety of methods, including surveys, case studies, developmental studies, document or content analysis, trend studies, and correlational studies used in research.

Descriptive statistics Procedures that are used to summarize, organize, and describe quantitative data.

Determinants of health Factors that interact to create specific health conditions, including physical, biological, behavioral, social, cultural, and spiritual.

Developmental disability Disability that occurs during uterine development.

Discrete (categorical) variable Variable made up of distinct and separate units or categories and counted only in whole numbers; also referred to as *mutually exclusive.*

Disease rate Number of disease cases or deaths among a population or target group during a given time period expressed as a ratio.

Double-blind study Type of most experimental research in which neither the subjects nor the investigators know who is in the control (or placebo) group and who is in the other (independent variable) group that receives the experimental treatment.

E

Early and periodic screening, diagnosis and treatment (EPSDT) Service for persons under twenty-one years of age for medical, dental, and vision care paid for by Medicaid.

Early childhood caries Dental caries that affect children, sometimes referred to as *nursing bottle decay* or *baby bottle decay.*

Early Head Start Federal program that promotes the economic and social well-being of pregnant women and their children up to age three.

Educational requirement The requirement of how much instruction and what type of degree a dental hygienist must receive.

Educator Person who teaches about and promotes dental health issues to various target populations.

Empower To coordinate change or cause others to take action or make a change.

Encounter fee plan Plan that basically pays for each care encounter regardless of the service provider.

Endemic Relatively low but constant level of occurrence of a disease or health condition in a population.

Epidemic Disease or condition occurring among many individuals in a community or region at the same time and usually spreading rapidly.

Epidemiology Study of the nature, cause, control, and determinants of the frequency and distribution of disease, disability, and death in human populations.

Epidemiology triangle Factors—host, agent, environment—organized by epidemiologists to demonstrate the interaction and interrelatedness of these factors over time in bringing about a disease or condition.

Ethics Guiding principles for individuals or groups based on what is right and what is wrong.

Ethnocentrism Belief that one's own culture or traditions are better than other cultures.

Etiology Theory of causation for a disease or condition.

Eurocentric Reflecting a tendency to interpret the world in terms of western and especially European or Anglo-American values and experiences.

Evaluation Part of the dental hygiene process of care that encompasses evaluation of a dental public health program.

Evidence-based practice Inclusion of experience, research, clinical practice, and patient preference when providing dental hygiene care.

Exclusive provider arrangement (EPA) Contract between dental care providers and an employer (which eliminates the third party) stating the negotiated fees for services offered to the employer's employees.

Executive branch Government entity that executes, or carries out, the laws passed by the legislature.

Experimental approach Research study also known as a *clinical trial* that studies an experimental treatment or intervention.

Explanation of benefits Form sent to the patient and provider explaining the approval or denial of payment for procedures rendered.

F

Facilitator Person who conducts meetings, brings diverse ideas together, and helps a group work to reach goals.

Faith-based initiative Community-based actions that are valued and essential partners to assist Americans in need.

Federal National; of or pertaining to the United States of America.

Fédération Dentaire Internationale (FDI) Organization that represents the international community of dentists.

Fee-for-service plan Charge based on a fee scale for all covered services; bills the patient for services rendered by a dental hygienist, dentist, or denturist; most common payment method used in the United States.

Fee slip Form a dental practice uses to detail the services rendered a patient.

Fluoridation *See* community water fluoridation.

Fluoride Salt of hydrofluoric acid.

Fluoride varnish Varnish of fluoride applied to teeth to prevent dental caries; particularly effective in the prevention of early childhood caries.

Fluorosis Form of enamel hypomineralization due to excessive ingestion of fluoride during the development of the teeth.

Formative evaluation Internal examination of a program's process usually conducted while planning the program.

Frontier Geographic area even more sparsely populated than a rural area.

G

Government Method or system of controlling people.

Government branches Three sections of the US government: legislative, executive, and judicial.

Grantmanship Art of obtaining grants for funding projects.

Graph Diagram showing the variation of a variable in comparison with one or more other variables; also called a *chart*.

Grass roots Local efforts to affect change and help guide policy-making decisions.

Group *See* target population.

H

Habit Act of behavior change that becomes automatic, such as daily flossing.

Head Start Federal program that promotes the economic and social well-being of families and children from three to five years of age.

Health education Instruction regarding health behaviors that bring an individual to a state of health awareness.

Health Maintenance Organizations (HMOs) Organizations that provide comprehensive health care to enrolled individuals and families in a specified region by participating physicians and financed by fixed periodic payments.

Health promotion Process that informs and motivates people to adopt healthy behavior to enhance their health and prevent disease.

Healthy behavior Action that helps prevent illness and promote health.

Healthy People 2010 Report released by federal government stating the goals and objectives necessary to improve the health and quality of life for individuals and communities.

Historical approach Research designed to determine the meaning of past events by reviewing records and literature and conducting interviews.

Hypothesis Question that is developed to be answered by a study.

I

Implementation Part of the dental hygiene process of care that includes the actual operation of a program.

Incidence Number of new cases of a disease in a population over a given period of time.

Independent contractor Person who works for himself or herself and can perform contracted work for a governmental agency or another business.

Independent practice Practice of dental hygiene without the supervision of a dentist, although the dental hygienist refers all dental needs to a dentist; sometimes called *unsupervised practice* or *collaborative practice.*

Independent variable In a clinical study, the variable that is being manipulated.

Index *See* dental index.

Inferential statistics Data generally presented by describing and summarizing them to make inferences or generalizations about a population based on data taken from a sample of that population.

Informed consent Ethical consideration that requires educating a subject in a research study to be educated about the study's purpose, duration, experimental procedures, alternatives, risks, and benefits.

Institutional review board (IRB) Entity charged with reviewing the ethical implications of every research study.

International Federation of Dental Hygienists (IFDH) Organization representing the international community of dental hygienists.

Interpretation Explanation of results that is used in a research report.

Interval scale of measurement Device with equal distance between any two adjacent units of measurement but without a meaningful zero point.

J

Joint Commission on National Dental Examinations Organization whose purpose is to assist state boards in determining qualification of the dental hygienist who seeks licensure to practice dental hygiene by being in charge of the community health/research principles section of the National Dental Hygiene Board Examination.

Judicial branch Government section composed of courts that interpret the laws the legislature passes but do not make them.

Jurisprudence requirement The required reading and possible examination of state laws governing dental hygiene practice.

L

Learning domain Category that includes a way to differentiate the individual types of learning.

Legislative branch *See* legislature.

Legislative initiative Proposal to change or enact laws.

Legislators Collective term used to describe senators and representatives/congressmen.

Legislature Section of a government that makes the laws.

Lesson plan   Written document used in planning a presentation.

Licensure requirement   The requirements dental hygienists must meet to obtain a dental hygiene license to practice in each state.

Literature review   Examination of all pertinent reports and studies to determine what is currently known about a specific topic or issue.

Lobbying   Attempting to influence or sway others to take or support a desired position or action; the "art of the sell."

Long-term care facility   Facility that provides live-in care for patients with medical complications.

M

Malpractice   Dental hygiene professional's negligence by act or omission when the care provided is not within the accepted standards of practice and negatively affects the patient's well-being.

Managed care   Integration of health care delivery and financing.

Manager   Developer and coordinator of dental public health programs; sometimes referred to as *administrator.*

Manpower   Available personnel to do a job; referred to as *labor force.*

Manpower shortage   Inadequate availability of personnel to perform a job.

Marketing   Organized approach to selecting and servicing markets and informing the public of a service as distinct from an impromptu approach to selling a service.

Mean   Average of scores.

Measurement   Act or process of using a particular method to gauge or evaluate something.

Measures of central tendency   Measures used to describe the central tendency of data within a research study.

Measures of dispersion   Identification of how much variation is present in a group of data and description of the distribution of data within a research study.

Median   Midpoint of scores.

Medicaid (Title XIX)   Federal program that traditionally distributes funds to states for health care services provided to certain groups including aged, blind, and disabled people; those with low incomes; and certain members of families with dependent children.

Medicare (Title XVIII)   Federal program that distributes funds to states for health care services provided to certain groups including aged, blind, and disabled people; those with low incomes; and certain members of families with dependent children.

Mentor   Role model who actively works with an individual to enhance that person's professional knowledge and abilities.

Metropolitan   Large population nucleus consisting of a city and surrounding suburban areas.

Modality   Clinical or educational dental hygiene treatment.

Mode   Score that occurs most often.

Morbidity   Ratio of "sick" (affected) individuals to well individuals in a community.

Mortality   Ratio of the number of deaths from a given disease or health problem to the total number of cases reported.

Motivation   Will of the individual to act.

Multifactorial   Approach that assumes that a disease or condition has multiple causes.

N

National Board Dental Hygiene Examination   The examination given by the American Dental Association to fulfill the written examination requirement.

National Health Service Corps (NHSC)   Part of the Health Resources and Services Administration, a PHS agency "committed to improving the health of the nation's underserved by uniting communities in need with caring health professionals and supporting communities' efforts to build better systems of care."

Need   Normative, professional judgment as to the amount and kind of health care services required to attain or maintain health.

Networking   Sharing resources or services to cultivate productive relationships.

Nominal scale of measurement   Organizes data into mutually exclusive categories that have no rank order or value.

Nonclinical evaluation   Study or appraisal employing questionnaires, individual or group interviews, telephone interviews, focus groups, direct observations, document analysis, and survey rather than being based on, relating to, or conducted in a clinic.

Nonparametric statistics Quantification that should be used for hypothesis testing when variables are discrete, sample size is small, population distributions are not normal, or group variances are not equal.

Normal distribution Curve in which the majority of subjects will fall under the large part of the middle with a few low and high outliers; a bell curve, representing the mean, median, and mode.

Null hypothesis Initial negative statement of belief about the value of a population parameter, for example, that two groups do not differ on as to a variable.

Nursing home *See* long-term care facility.

O

Oral epidemiology Study of the amount, distribution, determinant, and control of oral disease and oral health conditions among given populations.

Ordinal scale of measurement Scale that organizes data into mutually exclusive categories that are rank ordered based on some criterion but the difference between ranks is not necessarily equal.

Outreach workers Dental hygienists working "outside" the dental practice to bring patients in need of restorative dental care to private dental practices while providing preventive services outside the dental practice, such as in a school setting.

P

P.A.N.D.A. Acronym for Prevent Abuse and Neglect through Dental Awareness; educational program aimed at helping dental providers recognize and report child abuse.

Paradigm Outstandingly clear or typical example or framework that explains or illustrates a concept or theory.

Parameter Numerical characteristic of the population.

Parametric statistics Quantity of a sample computed from a sample to test a hypothesis when the data meet certain assumptions.

Partnership Intense form of collaboration, state, or condition of associating or participating with others regularly in pursuit of a joint interest.

Peer reviewed Published articles that have been reviewed for content and accuracy by peers.

Pilot study Version of a proposed study that is carried out on a small, sometimes intentionally chosen sample.

Placebo Independent variable used with a research control group that is not the factor being studied but a nontreatment, sometimes referred to as a "sugar pill" but more likely to be either a standard drug of choice for a disease or a standard treatment procedure against which the experimental one is being compared.

Planning Part of the dental hygiene process of care that includes the development of a program.

Policy Written description of rules, regulations, and stipulations to govern individual actions and procedures.

Poster session Method utilized to disseminate original research findings.

Practice Act Statute that defines the practice of dental hygiene or dentistry.

Practice management Process of planning, organizing, and managing resources to bring about the successful completion of specific project goals and objectives.

Preceptorship The on-the-job training of dental hygienists, sometimes referred to as alternative education.

Preexisting condition Medical condition that exists prior to a person's coverage by an insurance entity.

Preferred Provider Organizations (PPOs) Organizations practitioners contract with to provide dental care services for lower than average fees in order to attract patient subscribers who are seeking lower costs.

Premium Amount a group or an individual pays to the insurance entity for coverage.

Prepaid group practice Large group of dental providers contracted to provide services to groups of patients.

Prevalence Number of all existing cases of a disease in a population measured at a given point.

Prevention program Program designed to prevent disease in a target population.

Primary prevention Employment of strategies and agents to forestall the onset of disease, reverse its progress, or arrest its process before treatment becomes necessary.

Procedure number Identification given to a specific procedure as designated in the *Codes on Dental Procedures and Nomenclature* published by the ADA.

Program planning Process of developing a dental public health program that includes the stages of assessment, diagnosis, implementation, and evaluation.

Promulgate To put a law into practice as done by state dental boards.

Proposal Written description of a planned program or project intended to motivate an entity to adopt it.

Provider Legally licensed dental hygienist or dentist operating within a scope of practice.

Psychomotor domain Name of a category that describes actions.

Public health *See* dental public health.

Public health goals Goals that guide all public health activities.

Public health officer *See* US Public Health Service Officer.

Public health services Services that help attain goals of public health.

Public relations Practice of managing the dispersion of information between an organization and its public.

PubMed Web site that includes more than 17 million citations from MEDLINE and life science journals for biomedical articles back to the 50s.

p-**value** Probability that the findings of a study are due to chance.

Q

Qualitative evaluation Answering the why and how of a dental public health program or research project.

Quantitative evaluation A numerical evaluation of a dental public health program or research project.

Quasi-experimental approach Research design that lacks inherent control.

R

Range Number determined by subtracting the highest score from the lowest score.

Ratio scale of measurement Scale containing all characteristics of the preceding scales and an absolute zero point determined by nature.

Refereed Description of publications that include peer-reviewed articles.

Regulation Rules of order imposed by an executive authority or government agency governing practice.

Reliability Consistency or degree to which an instrument will produce the same results on repeated trials within the same population every time the characteristic is measured.

Representative Elected member of the US or individual state house of representatives.

Request for proposal Request for proposal (RFP) by groups or agencies; also called *request for applications, notice of funding availability,* or *program announcement.*

Research approach Type of research used to obtain information; all types involve observation, description, measurement, analysis, and interpretation of occurring phenomena.

Research design Overall plan for conducting a study.

Researcher Person who conducts research germane to the study of health and disease.

Research proposal Protocol or detailed plan for a study.

Retrospective (ex post facto) approach Research that looks backward (ex post facto, or after the fact) to investigate a group of people with a particular disease, usually via medical records.

Risk factor Characteristic of an individual or population that may increase the likelihood of experiencing a given health problem.

Rural Geographic area that is sparsely populated.

S

Sample Subgroup of a target population.

Sample size Referring to an adequate number of subjects within a research study.

Sampling technique Technique used when selecting a sample from a population to study.

Scales of measurement Classification of data as (1) nominal (or categorical), (2) ordinal, (3) interval, and (4) ratio.

Scientific method Body of techniques using observation, reason, and experimentation to gather evidence that is empirical and measurable.

Secondary Prevention Routine treatment methods to terminate a disease process and/or restore tissues to as near normal as possible and can be termed restorative care.

Self-regulation Governing of dental hygiene practice by dental hygienists.

Senator Elected member of the US or individual state senate.

Single procedure Specific process designated by a specific code.

Skew Tail of a distribution formed by a few extreme scores.

Skewed distribution Description of distribution of asymmetrical scores causing the curve to be distorted, or skewed.

Social worker Professional who works to help individuals or the community enhance their capacity for social functioning.

Sociocultural theory Theory proposed by Lev Vygotsky that an individual's social interaction as a child leads to continuous changes in thought and behavior that can vary greatly from culture to culture.

Socioeconomic status (SES) Individual's comparative social and economic standing within a community.

Sound natural teeth Either primary or permanent teeth that have adequate hard and soft tissue support.

Stakeholder Individual in an organization who has a vested interest in a specific topic, issue, or initiative.

Standard deviation Measure of dispersion.

Statistical decision Determination made about the null hypothesis based on the results of the inferential statistics.

Statistical significance Research study whose results show the quality of being statistically important.

Statute Law enacted by a government's legislature.

Statutory law Legislature-enacted, written law, which serves to promote justice.

Subculture Group of people with a culture that differentiates them from the larger culture to which they belong.

Summative evaluation Examination of a program's merit after it has been implemented.

Supply Amount of dental care services available.

Surgeon general Appointed administrator of the US Public Health Service.

Surveillance Ongoing observation, persistent watching over, scrutiny, constant monitoring, and assessment of changes in populations related to disease, conditions, injuries, disabilities, or death trends.

T

Table clinic Method utilized to disseminate past research studies and literature reviews of a specific topic.

Target population Clearly identified segment of the population.

Target population profile Comprehensive overview of the target population that includes specific descriptions.

Teaching strategy Plan or method used in instruction.

Tertiary prevention Strategy to replace lost tissues through rehabilitation.

Testlet Format that introduces a case study involving an issue pertinent to dental public health in the community dental health/research principles category for the Board Examination.

Therapeutic services Services the dental hygienist provides that benefit the patient; can include periodontal debridement, polishing, fluoride application, local anesthesia, dental sealants, education, and behavior modification interventions.

Three-party system Program in which a dental provider renders the service for which the patient's sponsor (insurance company or employer) pays.

Tobacco cessation program Program to encourage patients to quit using tobacco.

Transcultural communication skill Ability to interpret and transmit information to someone from a different culture.

TRICARE Health care program serving active-duty service members, National Guard and Reserve members, retirees, their families, survivors, and certain former spouses worldwide; formerly known as Civilian Health and Medical Program of the Uniformed Services (CHAMPUS).

Two-party system Program in which a dental provider renders the service for which the patient pays.

Type I error Error that occurs when the null hypothesis is rejected but is actually true; also called an alpha error.

Type II error Error that occurs when the null hypothesis is accepted but is actually false and should have been rejected; also called a beta error.

U

US Public Health Service Commissioned Corps Unit of highly trained and mobile health professionals who conduct programs to promote the health of the nation, understand and prevent disease and injury, ensure safe and effective drugs and medical devices, deliver health services to federal beneficiaries, and provide health expertise in time of war or other national or international emergency.

Urban Concentrated human settlement, usually consisting of at least 2500 people.

Usual, customary, and reasonable (UCR) fee Average dentist fee per service in the immediate local region.

Utilization Number of dental care services actually consumed, not just desired.

V

Validity Degree to which a research study measured what it was supposed to measure (internal) and that can be generalized to the entire population (external).

Values Ideas and beliefs a person possesses that influence behavior, giving meaning to life.

Variables Quantity whose value may change over the course of a research study.

Variance Squared deviation of each score from the mean's sum.

W

Washout period Period of time in research with no treatment; in drug trials, period allowed for all of any administered drug to be eliminated from the body.

Water fluoridation *See* community water fluoridation.

Workforce Workers whose members deliver health care to the public.

World Health Organization (WHO) Body that addresses unmet oral health needs of global populations in its commitment to improve oral health as an integral part of general health.

Written examination requirement The written examination a dental hygienist must pass before becoming eligible for a dental hygiene license.

X

Xylitol Sugar substitute found in berries, fruit, vegetables, mushrooms, and birch wood that has shown promising results in reducing dental decay and ear infections.

Z

Zone of proximal development Difference between a child's actual level of development displayed by unassisted performance and the child's potential level as indicated by assisted performance.

INDEX